Ophthalmology: Investigation and Examination Techniques

We dedicate this book to our families:
Jane, Richard, Edward;
Alison, Stephen, Sarah, Charlotte, Kathryn.

Commissioning Editor: Belinda Kuhn
Development Editor: Louise Allsop
Project Manager: Kathryn Mason
Design Manager: Jayne Jones
Illustration Manager: Bruce Hogarth
Illustrator: Ian Ramsden
Marketing Manager UK: Jeremy Bowes
Marketing Manager US: Lisa Damico

Ophthalmology

Investigation and Examination Techniques

Edited by

Bruce James MA DM FRCS (Ed) FRCOphth
Consultant Ophthalmologist
Eye Unit, Stoke Mandeville Hospital, Aylesbury, Buckinghamshire, UK

Larry Benjamin DO FRCS (Ed) FRCOphth
Consultant Ophthalmologist
Eye Unit, Stoke Mandeville Hospital, Aylesbury, Buckinghamshire, UK

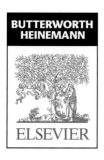

BUTTERWORTH
HEINEMANN

ELSEVIER

BUTTERWORTH HEINEMANN

An imprint of Elsevier Limited

First published 2007

EAN: 978-0-7506-7586-4
ISBN: 0-7506-7586-1

British Library Cataloguing in Publication Data
A catalogue record for this book is available from the British Library

Library of Congress Cataloging in Publication Data
A catalog record for this book is available from the Library of Congress

Notice
Medical knowledge is constantly changing. Standard safety precautions must be followed, but as new research and clinical experience broaden our knowledge, changes in treatment and drug therapy may become necessary or appropriate. Readers are advised to check the most current product information provided by the manufacturer of each drug to be administered to verify the recommended dose, the method and duration of administration, and contraindications. It is the responsibility of the practitioner, relying on experience and knowledge of the patient, to determine dosages and the best treatment for each individual patient. Neither the Publisher nor the author assume any liability for any injury and/or damage to persons or property arising from this publication.
The Publisher

Printed in China
Last digit is the print number: 9   8   7   6   5   4   3   2   1

Contents

Contributors

Larry Benjamin DO FRCS FRCOphth
Consultant Ophthalmologist
Eye Unit
Stoke Mandeville Hospital
Aylesbury, Buckinghamshire, UK

Bruce James MA DM FRCS FRCSOphth
Consultant Ophthalmologist
Eye Unit
Stoke Mandeville Hospital
Aylesbury, Buckinghamshire, UK

Ramona Khooshabeh MD FRCS FRCOphth
Consultant Ophthalmic and Oculoplastic Surgeon
Department of Ophthalmology
Wycombe General Hospital
High Wycombe, Buckinghamshire, UK

Andrew McNaught MD FRCOphth
Consultant Ophthalmologist
Eye Unit
Cheltenham General Hospital
Cheltenham, Gloucestershire, UK

Manoj V. Parulekar MS FRCS DNB
Specialist Registrar
Oxford Eye Hospital
Oxford, Oxfordshire, UK

Gerardine Quaghebeur MBBCh FRCS FRCR
Consultant Neuroradiologist
Department of Neuroradiology
Radcliffe Infirmary
Oxford, Oxfordshire, UK

David Sculfor BSc
Head of Optometry
Eye Unit
Stoke Mandeville Hospital
Aylesbury, Buckinghamshire, UK

Asifa Shaikh FRCS FRCOphth
Glaucoma Fellow
Oxford Eye Hospital
Oxford, Oxfordshire, UK

Richard Smith MBChB FRCS FRCOphth
Consultant Ophthalmologist
Eye Unit
Stoke Mandeville Hospital
Aylesbury, Buckinghamshire, UK

Carlos Eduardo Solarte MD
Medical Director
Flying Eye Hospital
ORBIS International
Toronto, Ontario, Canada

Preface

Ophthalmology is an exciting and rapidly advancing field. Our understanding of ocular anatomy, physiology and pathology has increased considerably over the last few decades. The treatment of eye disease has developed enormously with significant innovations in microsurgery, pharmacology and laser treatment. With these developments have come advances in the techniques we use to examine the eye, the orbit and the structural and functional integrity of the visual pathway.

Despite this rapid progress it remains as important as ever to understand how to use both old and new examination techniques to arrive at an accurate diagnosis with the minimum of inconvenience to the patient and the greatest degree of accuracy. It is also important to learn how to communicate with other specialists who may be involved in the investigation of ophthalmic disease, to appreciate what information they require to tailor their work. A complete understanding of the shortcomings of the equipment or test procedures is also vital if the results are to be interpreted correctly and given the correct weight in arriving at a diagnosis or developing a treatment plan.

Some of the newer diagnostic instruments described in this book rely on complex technology, produce a vast array of data and often beautiful and sometimes beguiling pictures. Although these may add greatly to our ability to detect, diagnose and treat ophthalmic disease, we must be sure that we understand something of the basis on which these machines work. Their limitations and sometimes the inevitable uncertainty as to where they currently lie in the diagnostic armoury must also be considered. Those working in the field of ophthalmology are fortunate in being able to visualise most of the eye directly. A detailed anatomical and functional examination of the eye, its movements and surrounding structures, can be made with relatively little complex equipment. We still remain dependent on the skilful use of the slit lamp and other simple techniques for arriving at most of our diagnoses. This book describes both old and new examination and investigative techniques that those involved in eye care will use or may encounter in their work. The authors of each chapter not only describe how to undertake each test or examination but also outline the problems and pitfalls that will be encountered in their performance and interpretation.

No book can hope to replace a skilled teacher well versed in the examination of the eye. Practical teaching must remain the cornerstone of learning how to examine the ophthalmic patient. Similarly, time spent discussing the most appropriate test to perform with colleagues working in associated areas, for example optometrists, orthoptists, ophthalmologists, neurophysiologists, neurologists or radiologists, is never wasted. We hope that this book will provide a sound framework for this practical teaching and discussion.

Bruce James
Larry Benjamin

Acknowledgements

We are enormously grateful to the contributors to
this book who have worked so hard to produce
their chapters. Many others have also helped with
advice, reading manuscripts, the provision of
pictures and, above all, encouragement. We would
like to acknowledge their help.

Tom Meagher
Tony Bron
Imran Akram
Paul Foster
Janet Sear
Edward James
Moorfields Electrodiagnostic Department
Palvi Bhardwaj
Consuela Moorman
Cate Ames
Hazel Nyack

The assessment of vision

DAVID SCULFOR and BRUCE JAMES

Introduction

The ophthalmic examination requires detection of abnormal structure and function. Vision, the ability to see, the fundamental function of the eyes, can be assessed in various ways:

- *Visual acuity* is a measure of the visual system's ability to discriminate two high-contrast points in space.
- *Contrast sensitivity* is a measure of the minimum contrast required for the visual system to discriminate these points from the background.
- *Colour vision* is the ability of the visual system to differentiate light of different wavelengths.
- *Dark adaptation* is the ability of the visual system to adapt to reduced luminance.
- *Motion detection* is the ability to detect movement (see Ch. 7).
- *Visual field* is the area over which the visual system is able to detect light (see Ch. 7).

Distance visual acuity

The Snellen chart

Measurement of visual acuity is commonly performed in adults with the Snellen chart (Fig. 1.1). The chart uses standard letters of different size with approximately equal legibility, and measures high-contrast visual acuity. The letters are constructed on a 5×5 or 5×4 grid such that, when viewed at the intended distance, each limb subtends 1 min arc at the eye, and the whole letter 5 min arc (Fig. 1.2a). Snellen acuity is written as a fraction:

$$\frac{\text{Distance at which the chart is viewed}}{\text{Distance at which the letter subtends 5 min arc}}$$

Normal vision is taken to be 6/6 (although 6/4 is not unusual), so a letter on the 6/6 line subtends 5 min arc at the eye at 6 m. Vision of 6/60 means that, at 6 m from the chart, the subject can just read a letter which someone with normal vision would be able to see from 60 m away.

Practically, care must be taken to ensure that the chart is well illuminated and that the patient is at the correct distance from the chart. Distance glasses should be worn for the test. A pinhole will overcome moderate degrees of refractive error but will also compensate for some media opacities such as cataract. Each eye is tested separately. If only some of the letters on a line are seen, the acuity is recorded as the completed line minus the number of letters missed, or plus the number of letters seen on the next line, whichever is smaller.

The Landolt C test is similar in principle to the Snellen test and attempted to overcome the problem that some of Snellen's optotypes were more recognisable than others (Box 1.1). It used a broken ring or C in different orientations (Fig. 1.2b). It has been used more in research than in clinical practice.

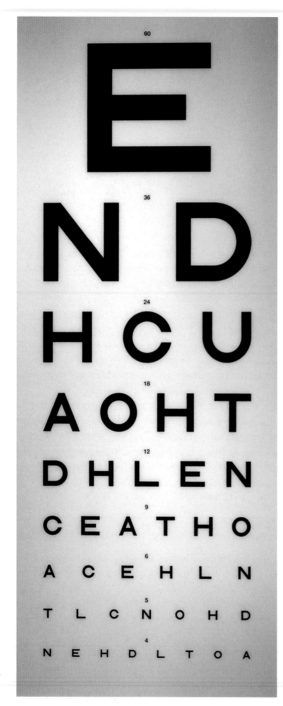

Fig. 1.1 A Snellen acuity chart.

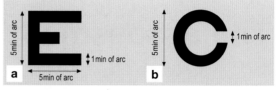

Fig. 1.2 (a) A 6/6 Snellen's letter; **(b)** a Landolt C 6/6 symbol.

For illiterate patients a Tumbling E chart is available with the letter E rotated in various positions. The examiner points to a letter and the patient uses a cut-out E to match its position. The conventional Snellen chart can also be used with patients matching the indicated letter to one on a sheet in front of them, similar to the Sheridan–Gardiner test for children, described below.

logMAR charts

To overcome some of the problems with the Snellen chart, a number of alternatives have been proposed. Those based on the logMAR scale have clear advantages and are increasingly used in clinical work, while being mandatory for research.

Bailey–Lovie chart

Two Australian optometrists, Ian Bailey and Jan Lovie-Kitchen, developed the first commercially available logMAR chart. Designed for use at 6 m, it has five letters per line, each letter based on a 5×4 grid.

logMAR is short for $\log_{10}$ minimum angle of resolution. If normal vision is the ability to see a letter 5 min high where each limb is one-fifth of the height, then the minimum angle of resolution is 1 min. The $\log_{10}$ of 1 is zero, so the logMAR equivalent of 6/6 is 0.00. Similarly, the logMAR equivalent of 6/60 is 1.00. For acuities less than this, the testing distance can be halved, and the score simply doubled, with 3/60 being logMAR 2.00. One slight disadvantage is that acuity better than 6/6 has a negative logMAR score, with 6/3 being logMAR −0.30.

This minor disadvantage is outweighed by several key advantages: a 0.1 logMAR progression in letter size, an equal number of letters on each line, the spacing between the letters is equal to the letter width, and the spacing between lines is equal to the

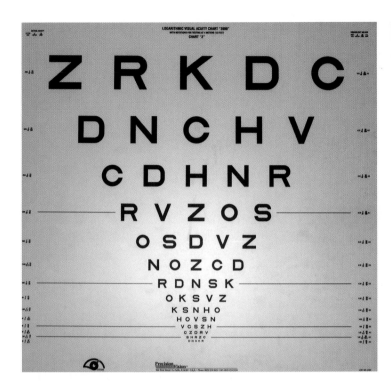

Fig. 1.3 An Early Treatment in Diabetic Retinopathy Study (ETDRS) chart.

height of the line below. Thus each line presents a task of equal difficulty with letter size being the only variable. This has the further advantage of allowing accurate scoring of incompletely seen lines. Since each line represents a 0.1 step, and there are five letters per line, each letter seen scores 0.02. Thus, if all the 6/6 equivalent line is seen, the score is logMAR 0.00, but three letters more would be –0.06, and three letters less would be 0.06. Similarly, if the 0.2 line is seen, but only two letters on the next line, the score is 0.2 – 0.04, giving a logMAR of 0.16.

Early Treatment in Diabetic Retinopathy Study (ETDRS) chart

The ETDRS chart was developed from the Bailey–Lovie chart (Fig. 1.3). It uses letters based on a 5×5 grid, chosen from the Sloan character set where each letter has similar legibility. A further revision ensured that the letters were mixed in such a way as to ensure equal legibility for each line. Three charts were used in the ETDRS study to reduce the learning effect: one each for right and left eyes, and one for refraction. It is scored in a similar way to the Bailey–Lovie chart. Alternatively the number of letters read can be recorded and this is particularly useful in patients with poor vision where acuity can be measured with greater accuracy than is possible with a Snellen chart. Increasingly used clinically, this test is the gold standard for acuity testing in vision research. Front- and back-lit versions of the chart are available. They are designed to be used at 4 m; versions designed for use at shorter distances are also available.

Near vision

This is assessed with a reading test-type book (Fig. 1.4). The patient should wear reading glasses if necessary and position the book a comfortable distance from the eyes. Various test-type books are available, including the Faculty of Ophthalmologists' near-acuity book. This is the commonest chart used in the UK. It is based on a printer's block where N72 comprises a lower-case letter 13.5 mm high. The Jaeger near-acuity book is rarely used now.

It is important to ensure that the book is adequately illuminated. The size of the test type seen with either eye, and then both eyes simultaneously, is recorded, together with the distance at which it is held.

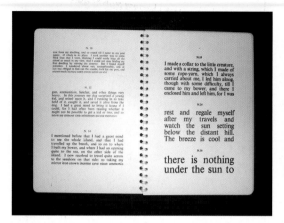

Fig. 1.4 Near-vision test type.

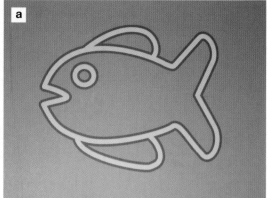

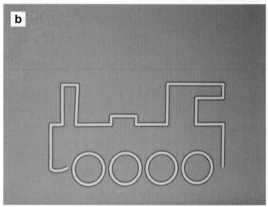

Fig. 1.5 (a, b) Cardiff cards. Note the difference in the width of the outline between the two cards.

Children's vision

The assessment of visual acuity in children requires special methods until they are at least able to match pictures or letters on a chart. Until a child is 6 months old, vision is assessed by the ability to fixate and follow an object. As the child reaches 6 months the ability to detect hundreds and thousands cake decoration shapes is a traditional test. Similarly the size of fixation objects can be varied and the ability of the child to maintain fixation assessed.

The first formal test between 6 months and 3 years is performed with a preferential looking test, for example, Cardiff cards (Fig. 1.5) or Keeler acuity cards. These are based on the premise that children prefer to look at a picture or pattern rather than a plain card. Cardiff cards use a variety of targets consisting of a simple picture drawn by a white band bordered by two black bands, on a grey background. The mean brightness of the picture is equal to that of the background so that as the width of the bands decreases, the object becomes harder to see because it merges into the background. The card is presented either with an object on the top or on the bottom. The direction of the child's gaze is noted. When the examiner is unable to detect the position of the object from the direction of the child's gaze the child is assumed not to have seen the object.

From the age of 2 years matching tests can be performed with children matching a picture at 6 m to one in a book held close to them by the examiner.

This provides a more repeatable measure of visual acuity. Initially charts with single pictures of differing sizes are used. Kay pictures and the Sheridan–Gardiner letter tests are examples of this type of test (Fig. 1.6). Kay pictures can be presented in a crowded form to reproduce the crowding phenomenon mentioned in the description of Snellen visual acuity.

The Keeler logMAR crowded test, also known as the Glasgow acuity test (Fig. 1.7), is a letter-matching test that can also test single letters or reproduce the crowding phenomenon. The progression of letter size is similar to the Bailey–Lovie chart. It is usually measured at a distance of 3 m. If both tests are performed the crowding ratio can be calculated as the uncrowded acuity divided by the crowded acuity.

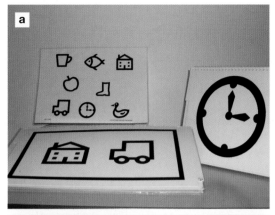

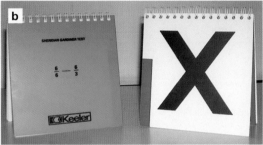

Fig. 1.6 (a) Kay pictures: both crowded and single test plates are shown. **(b)** Sheridan–Gardiner letter test.

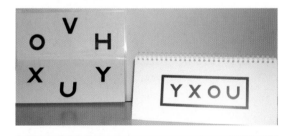

Fig. 1.7 The Glasgow acuity test.

The distance Snellen chart can be used from about 4 years of age onwards.

It is important that all these tests are conducted patiently and quietly in an environment with few distractions. The test chart must be well illuminated and correctly positioned. The child should be alert and not acutely unwell.

Colour vision

Colour is a visual experience, not a physical property of light. As might be expected for a psychophysical experience, even for a normal observer the ability to detect a difference in wavelength is not perfect, and varies across the spectrum. The human retina is able to detect a difference of 1 nm in wavelength between blue-green (490 nm) and yellow (585 nm). At the violet (430 nm) and red (650 nm) ends of the visible spectrum a greater difference exceeding 4 nm is required for a difference to be appreciated. Discrimination is even worse with dark or pale colours, and for those with colour vision deficiencies (the term 'colour-blind' should usually be avoided). Three types of cone with different but overlapping spectral sensitivities, L, M, and S (approximating to red, green and blue), are responsible for colour detection (Fig. 1.8). Shorter wavelengths tend to stimulate all three cone classes.

Colour can be specified using three properties: (1) hue, which is closely related to wavelength, and which is used to name a colour; (2) saturation, which describes the intensity of a colour; and (3) brightness, which indicates the intensity of light emitted or reflected by the surface.

Colour vision may be affected by both congenital and acquired defects. Congenital colour deficiencies are characterised by abnormal colour-matching, colour-naming confusion where different colours

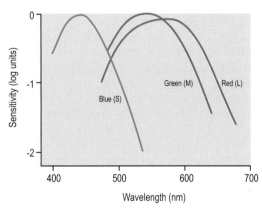

Fig. 1.8 Sensitivity of L, M and S cones at different frequencies. (Adapted from Wald G. The receptors of human colour vision. Science 1964; 145: 1007.)

Table 1.1	Congenital deficiencies in colour vision		
Number of functioning cone pigments	**Defect type**	**Category and cone type affected**	**Hue discrimination**
None	Monochromat	Typical or rod monochromat	None
One	Monochromat	Cone monochromat	None
Two	Dichromat	Protanope (L cones) Deuteranope (M cones) Tritanope (S cones)	Severely impaired
Three (one abnormal)	Anomalous trichromat	Protanomalous (L cones) Deuteranomolous (M cones) Tritanomalous (S cones)	Severe to mild impairment
Three	None	Normal trichromat	'Normal'

appear the same, and, in one case, a reduction in apparent brightness. They are caused by missing or abnormal cone pigments.

Table 1.1 summarises these deficiencies. Note that only monochromats with only one class of pigment are completely 'colour-blind'. Dichromats with two functioning pigments have severely impaired colour vision, while trichromats who have three pigments, of which one is abnormal, show mild to severe impairment.

In order to simplify the specification of colour, in 1931 the International Commission on Illumination (CIE) published the CIE chromaticity diagram (Fig. 1.9). It is an invaluable aid to describing colour vision defects and colour vision tests.

The elliptical area contains all the colours that appear in the spectrum, plus, along the lower straight edge, purple, which is not a spectral colour. The centre is neutral (white), and any line drawn from the centre to the edge will have constant hue, but increasing saturation.

As stated earlier, the normal observer does not have perfect colour discrimination, and if asked to match one colour with another, will make small errors. If one standard deviation of the scatter of those errors is plotted on the CIE diagram, they form small ellipses known as isochromatic (i.e. identical in hue) zones. These were first plotted in 1942 by David McAdam. For anomalous trichromats those ellipses

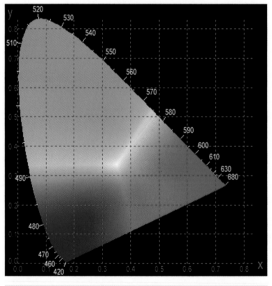

Fig. 1.9 The 1931 International Commission on Illumination (CIE) chromaticity diagram. Any colour can be specified in terms of its hue and saturation using x and y coordinates. z is used for brightness. Note that it is not possible to reproduce the colours accurately, either by printing or on a computer screen.

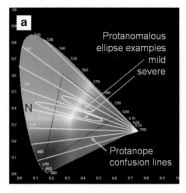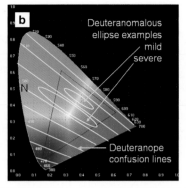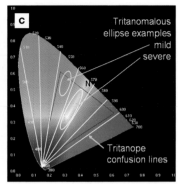

Fig. 1.10 International Commission on Illumination (CIE) chromaticity diagram showing confusion lines and examples of: isochromatic ellipses for **(a)** protan defects; **(b)** deutan defects; and **(c)** tritan defects.

become very much larger, while for dichromats the isochromatic zones become isochromatic lines.

Figure 1.10 shows the confusion lines and examples of isochromatic ellipses for the three classes of congenital deficiencies.

Note that for each of the three colour deficiencies the major axes of the ellipses and the origin of the isochromatic lines lie in characteristic directions, which means that they make colour confusions specific to that defect. This is the basis of all colour vision tests for congenital defects. The confusion lines for protan and deutan lie very close together, and hence they are classified as a red/green defect. It can be very difficult to determine whether a subject is protanomalous or deuteranomalous.

Screening tests utilise colours that lie close together on the CIE diagram, and along the confusion lines for the defect that is being detected. Grading tests use colours that are further apart, and which lie on a circle centred on the white area.

Pseudoisochromatic plates

The best known pseudoisochromatic (PIC) plate test is the Ishihara (Fig. 1.11). It uses the principle of colour camouflage where the dot matrix breaks up the shape of the figure or shape on the plate. The dots are isochromatic: there is no difference in contrast between them. For example, the 'disappearing digit' comprises a number made up of green dots of various shades, surrounded by dots of yellow and orange. To a colour-normal person, the green dots are clearly different from the yellow/orange, and the

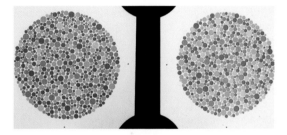

Fig. 1.11 Ishihara plate.

number is seen. A subject with a red/green defect will perceive the figure and the surrounding dots as being similar, and the figure will not stand out from the background. The colours are chosen to lie along confusion lines specifically to test for red/green colour deficiencies. The Ishihara test is not designed to pick up tritan defects.

The plates must be read in daylight or artificial light resembling daylight. The book should be held 75 cm from the patient at right angles to the line of vision. The patient should be given a maximum of 3 s to identify each plate. The maze plates are use for illiterate patients. All patients, unless vision is particularly poor, should be able to see the control plate. A full explanation of the interpretation of the results accompanies the book.

Variants on the test, including Hardy–Rand–Rittler plates, are also available. Here geometric shapes have to be identified. This test series includes plates to test for yellow/blue colour deficiencies.

Table 1.2	Differences between inherited and acquired colour defects	
Congenital	**Acquired**	
Constant through life	Type and severity vary	
Readily classified	Classification difficult	
Binocular	Monocular differences	
Visual acuity etc. unaffected (except monochromats)	Visual acuity and visual field loss also	
Red/green commonest	Tritan common	
Males most affected	Male/female equal	

PIC plates can be used with caution in detecting acquired colour deficiency. Table 1.2 outlines the differences between inherited and acquired defects.

Two limitations apply: (1) around 8% of males have an inherited defect; and (2) the confusion lines in acquired defects do not correspond with those of inherited defects. However, the plates can give an indication of impaired colour discrimination. The examiner assesses whether or not a number is seen, recording the number of plates correctly identified. A difference between the two eyes is particularly helpful in identifying ocular disease. In acquired conditions macular disease tends to cause abnormalities in the blue/yellow region, whereas optic nerve disease causes red/green defects, but this is not invariable. In severe disease of either tissue there is a global reduction in colour perception.

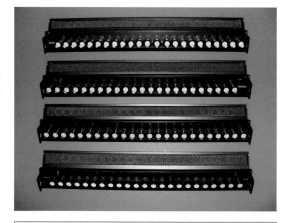

Fig. 1.12 Farnsworth–Munsell 100-hue test.

Hue discrimination and arrangement tests

The two arrangement tests in common use are the D15 and the Farnsworth–Munsell 100-hue test. Each comprises an array of chips of different colour which have to be sequenced (Fig. 1.12). The colours are approximately evenly spaced around the colour circle, and colour-deficient patients make specific errors in the sequencing of the chips. In the D15 test, using 15 tiles, more severely affected subjects can make colour confusions that cross the colour circle, while those who are mildly affected confuse adjacent colours. As might be expected, the confused colours lie along the confusion lines for the defect concerned. Figure 1.13 shows a typical D15 result for a tritan defect.

A more sensitive version, the Lantony desaturated D15, is also available.

The 85 chips in the 100-hue test are divided into four boxes to prevent confusions being made across the circle. Instead, errors tend to be clustered around the points where confusion lines form a tangent with the colour circle, and are again characteristic for the defect concerned.

Arrangement tests can be useful for detecting acquired tritan defects, and will give an indication of the severity of the defect.

While it is not a strictly accurate description, the City University test (Fig. 1.14) can be thought of as the D15 test in book form. It comprises four screening plates and six classification plates. It is designed

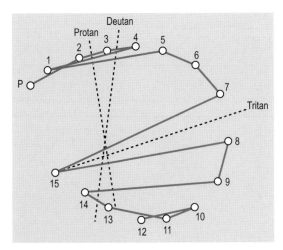

Fig. 1.13 Typical D15 result for a tritan defect. P represents the reference point. A person with no colour deficiency would lay out the colours from 1 to 15 in order. This is represented by a circle. A patient with a tritan defect will, for example, put colour 15 after colour 7 and make other mistakes along the tritan line. Note that the axes for protan and deutan defects lie close together, making differentiation difficult.

to be less sensitive than the Ishihara test, but will detect 'significant' defects, including tritan. Comprehensive instructions are included, together with a scoring sheet. It is suitable for use in the clinic as the illumination used is less critical than with some other tests.

Anomaloscopes

In these tests the subject is asked to use a mixture of two colours to match a standard sample, commonly red and green being matched with yellow. The brightness of the sample can also be adjusted. The proportion of red and green required indicates the presence of a deficit, together with its severity, while the brightness required will help classify the defect.

The Nagel anomaloscope (type I) firstly requires the subject to match the yellow sample by adjusting the mixture of red and green together with the brightness of the yellow. Protanomalous subjects require excessive amounts of red to obtain a match, and deuteranomalous subjects require more green than normal. Next, the examiner chooses a red/green mixture, and the subject is asked to make a match

altering only the brightness of the yellow. Dichromats will accept any match, simply by adjusting the brightness of the yellow, and protans in particular lower the brightness of the yellow when a red-dominated mixture is offered for matching. The type II Nagel anomaloscope can be used to test those with short-wavelength deficiencies. An aqua test light is matched to a violet and blue/green mix.

The Neitz anomaloscope is similar to the Nagel, and computerised anomaloscopes are also available.

Red desaturation

This can be particularly helpful in identifying uniocular optic nerve disease. The patient is asked to look at a red object with both eyes and report which eye sees the object as most red. Patients with optic nerve disease in one eye will report that the object is less red in that eye than the normal eye (see Ch. 5).

Contrast sensitivity

These tests provide a more detailed understanding of the working of the visual system. For a target to be visible, it must not only be of sufficient size, but also have sufficient contrast with the background so that it stands out. If the object is too pale, it will not be seen, however large it is. Contrast threshold is the minimum contrast required for a given target to be visible. Contrast sensitivity is defined as 1/contrast threshold.

Commonly, contrast sensitivity is tested using a sinusoidal grating of light and dark lines which blend gradually into each other. The interval between the contrasting lines, known as spatial frequency, can be varied, with coarse gratings having low spatial frequency. The ratio between light and dark (contrast) can also be varied. For a particular spatial frequency contrast is increased until the bars can just be seen (contrast threshold). The contrast sensitivity at a number of different spatial frequencies is measured to construct a contrast sensitivity curve. This can be compared to a normal range. Note that greater contrast is required to see gratings of high and low spatial frequency.

Alternatively, uniformly sized letters of varying contrast are viewed. While a grating has only one spatial frequency, letters are composed of a mixture of high, medium and low spatial frequencies, as are real-life objects. It is reasonable to think of Snellen visual acuity as a measure of the greatest spatial

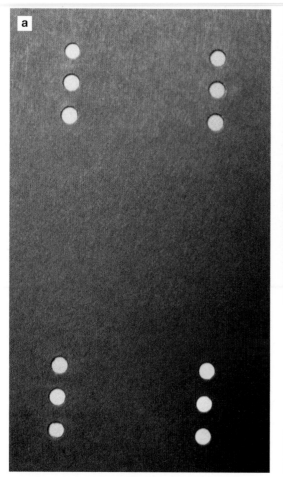

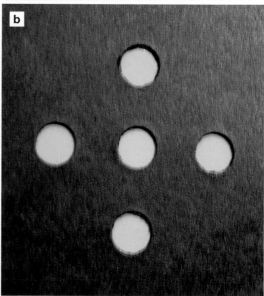

Fig. 1.14 City University test. **(a)** Screening plates; **(b)** differentiation plates.

frequency that is detected at near maximum contrast, for here the size of the letters varies but not the contrast.

Measurement of contrast sensitivity

Testing formats use either gratings or low-contrast letters.

Grating methods

The Vis Tech chart and, more recently, the functional acuity contrast test (FACT) chart are formed from photographs of sinusoidal gratings at different spatial frequencies and contrasts (Fig. 1.15). The Vis Tech chart is arranged in five rows with gratings of 1.5, 3, 6, 12 and 18 cycles per degree and nine contrast levels with an average step size of 0.25 log units. The gratings are oriented vertically or at 15° to

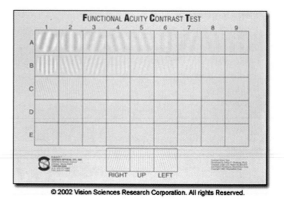

Fig. 1.15 A functional acuity contrast test (FACT) chart.

the left and right. The FACT chart is similar to the Vis Tech chart but has smaller contrast steps (0.15 log units). The size of the gratings is also larger, thus presenting more cycles at low spatial frequency, which is a problem with the Vis Tech chart.

The chart is uniformly lit at normal room lighting levels with no glare. To ensure repeatable illumination a light meter can be used. The viewing distance is about 3 m (10 ft). If the patient is new to the test the demonstration patches at the bottom of the chart can be used to explain the orientation of the gratings. The patient indicates the last patch where lines can be seen and describes the orientation of the lines. If incorrect the patient is asked to describe the next patch to the left. If correct, even if no lines can be seen, the patient is asked to describe the orientation of lines in the next patch to the right. The patch with the lowest contrast that is correctly identified is recorded on a chart which indicates the normal range (Fig. 1.16).

The Cambridge low-contrast gratings are arranged in an A4 booklet: on one side is a low-contrast square-wave grating, on the other a uniform grey square. The patient has to identify the side with the

grating. Spatial frequency is constant (4 cycles per degree at 6 m) but the contrast varies. The highest contrast plates are presented first and the tests proceed until the patient makes a mistake. The test is repeated four times in total to obtain a score of the contrast sensitivity. Normative data are available.

Letter methods

The Pelli–Robson chart uses a letter chart viewed at 1 m to measure contrast sensitivity (Fig. 1.17). The spatial frequency is constant at about one cycle per degree, dictated by the size of the letters. The letters are arranged into groups of three, with two groups per line. The contrast between the letter and the background is reduced between one group and the next. The patient identifies the letters on each line, starting at the top left corner until the contrast is insufficient to allow recognition. It is important to ensure uniform illumination of the chart. The group of letters with the lowest percentage contrast that the patient can see is recorded.

Alternatively visual acuity can be assessed using low-contrast charts (the Regan low-contrast letter

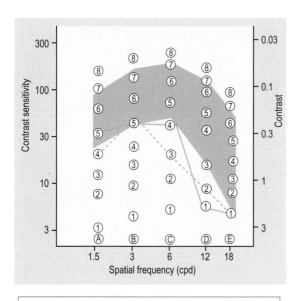

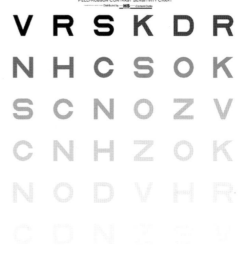

Fig. 1.16 Example of a Vis Tech contrast sensitivity result. The continuous and interrupted lines represent results from the right and left eyes. The shaded area indicates the normal range. Note the loss of sensitivity at high spatial frequencies.

Fig. 1.17 The Pelli–Robson chart.

charts have a contrast of 96%, 7% and 4%) and a contrast sensitivity curve plotted.

Clinical use

Eye conditions that reduce contrast sensitivity may cause visual problems despite relatively good Snellen acuity. It is important to realise that loss of contrast sensitivity can be just as much a handicap as loss of acuity. Cataracts may affect both higher and lower spatial frequencies, in part depending on the nature of the opacity. The reduction in vision may be more readily measured with contrast sensitivity than Snellen acuity. Optic neuropathies affect the middle range of spatial frequencies. Contrast sensitivity may also demonstrate that the vision in an amblyopic eye is worse than suggested by Snellen acuity. In practice, however, the tests have not been as useful as initially thought.

The charts may also be used in low-vision-aid prescribing.

Dark adaptation

The eye is sensitive to light over a 6 log range (1:1 000 000). During dark adaptation the normal eye takes about 20 min to change in sensitivity by 3 log units (Fig. 1.18). The first part of the curve corresponds to cone adaptation and the second part to rod adaptation. Retinal disease may affect dark adaptation, usually by reducing the threshold. In some diseases the time course of dark adaptation is also changed.

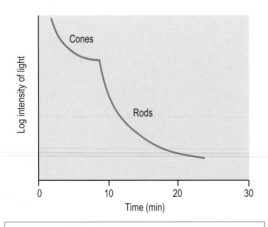

Fig. 1.18 A dark adaptation curve.

Measurement

The Goldmann–Weekers dark adaptometer and the LKC SST-1 whole-field scotopic sensitivity tester have been designed to measure dark adaptation.

The subject is dark-adapted for at least 30 min. A dimly lit target is then presented to the eye to be tested. The weakest light stimulus a patient is able to see, starting at a low level and working upwards, is recorded, giving the dark-adapted threshold.

A dark adaptation curve can be recorded by measuring the time taken during dark adaptation for the subject to see a stimulus of a particular intensity. When this is seen the intensity is reduced and the time at which this dimmer light is seen is then noted.

Summary

Different aspects of vision may be measured in a number of ways. The examiner must choose the method that is both best suited to the patient and most likely to answer the clinical problem posed. No one method will have universal applicability.

> Assessment of vision involves a large number of parameters, including:
> - Acuity
> - Contrast
> - Colour
> - Visual field
>
> Each of these can be assessed in a variety of ways
> Special techniques are needed for children

Further reading

Bailey IL, Lovie JE. New design principles for visual acuity letter charts. Am J Optom Physiol Opt 1976; 53: 740–745.

Birch J. Diagnosis of defective colour vision, 2nd edn. Edinburgh: Butterworth Heinemann; 2001.

Green J. On a new series of test-letters for determining the acuteness of vision. Trans Am Ophthalmol Soc 4th Meet 1868; 4: 68–71.

McGraw PV, Winn B. Glasgow acuity cards; a new test for the measurement of letter acuity in children. Ophthalmol Physiol Opt 1993; 13: 400–404.

Wald G. The receptors of human colour vision. Science 1964; 145: 1007.

The slit lamp

BRUCE JAMES

Introduction

One of the basic tools of the ophthalmologist is the slit lamp, designed to give a magnified, three-dimensional view of the eye. It relies on the observation of light reflected from the structures of the eye to produce an optical section.

Gullstrand developed the first slit-lamp illuminator in the early twentieth century. Initially a slit of light was viewed with an independent binocular loupe. Subsequently, a compound binocular microscope was placed on the same stand as the slit lamp. In the modern slit lamp, devised by Goldmann, the slit lamp and microscope are arranged on a common column, although each may be adjusted independently. Both are focused at the same point (coincident) and independently of the angle between the two.

Additional equipment allows the optical measurement of corneal thickness (*pachymetry*) and anterior chamber depth. The use of special contact and non-contact lenses permits a three-dimensional view of the retina (*fundoscopy*) and the iridocorneal angle (*gonioscopy*). Attaching the Goldmann tonometer allows measurement of intraocular pressure (*tonometry*).

Effective use of the slit lamp requires an understanding of its structure and controls. It must be appropriately set up by the examiner prior to use. Both patient and examiner must be comfortably positioned and a full explanation of the procedure given to the patient.

The instrument

This description is based on the Haag–Streit type of slit lamp; the position of controls may differ on other machines but the general principles still apply (Fig. 2.1).

Table

The slit lamp is mounted on a stand or table (Box 2.1). The height of the table or the height of the examination chair is adjustable so that the patient can be comfortably positioned. Ideally the table should have wheels or a movable stand to obtain the most comfortable distance between the patient and the instrument. This applies particularly when examining disabled patients.

Stage

Both the microscope and the slit lamp illuminator are mounted on a stage in a single column. A joystick allows the stage to be moved to the left and right, forwards and backwards over a low-friction plate screwed to the table. Additionally, rotation of the joystick moves the central column up and down. The microscope can be focused roughly by moving the stage manually, using the joystick to achieve fine focus within the eye. If the stage moves roughly or sticks on the plate, it should be thoroughly cleaned with an oily cloth. A locking screw can be used to prevent movement of the base plate when moving the slit lamp from one place to another.

Microscope

The binocular microscope (Fig. 2.3) has two eyepieces that can be adjusted independently to correct for the examiner's refractive error.

The magnification of the microscope itself can also be adjusted. In the Haag–Streit type slit lamp this is accomplished by a lever below the eyepieces, while in the Zeiss slit lamp it is achieved by rotating a knob at the side. These manoeuvres change the power of the objective lens. Additional magnification is achieved by changing the power of the eyepiece lenses: 10× and 16× oculars are usually provided with each slit lamp. Multiplication of the power

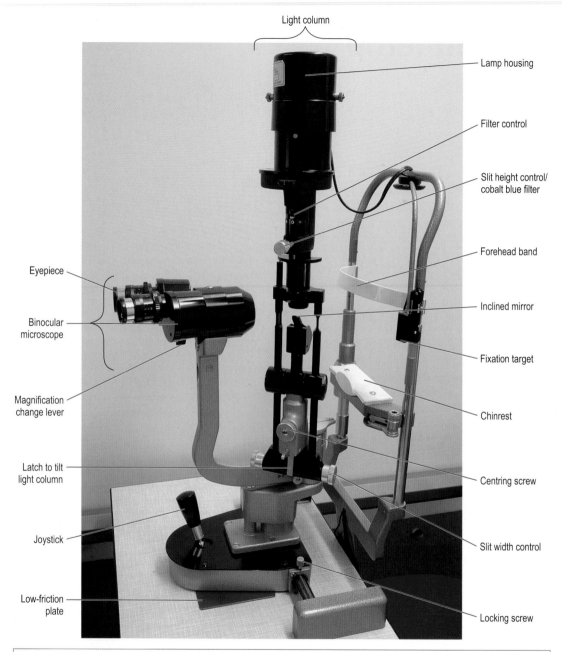

Fig. 2.1 An overall view of the slit lamp.

of the ocular and objective lens gives the total magnification. In the Haag–Streit this is 10× and 16× for the low-powered (10×) eyepiece and 16× and 25× for the high-powered eyepiece. The greater the magnification, the less the depth of focus.

The eyepieces may also have rubber guards, which are generally extended for non-spectacle wearers and folded in if glasses are worn when looking through the eyepieces. This maintains the correct distance between the observer's eyes and the objective lenses.

Setting up the slit lamp

- Switch on power supply
- Adjust eyepieces to correct for examiner's refractive error and interpupillary distance. Younger users can set a small minus correction so that accommodation can be used to increase the depth of focus
- Check focus and centration of slit lamp by viewing the slit on the matt black surface of the centring (or focusing) rod placed in the central fixation hole with the flat surface perpendicular to the microscope. The microscope and illumination columns should coincide exactly, that is, the angle between the microscope and the illumination column should be

set at zero. This should be repeated with the high-power oculars if they are to be used. Each eye should be checked separately (Fig. 2.2). It is important to check the focus, even if emmetropic, because using a microscope stimulates accommodation (instrument myopia) by some −1.5 to −2 D
- A thin beam should appear sharp and in the centre of the rod, with the grainy nature of the surface apparent. If it appears to one side, check that the decentration screw is tightened
- Check that the correct mirror is in place and that all controls are functioning

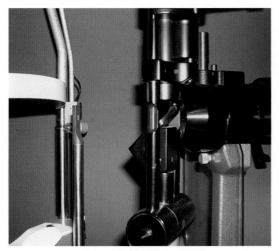

Fig. 2.2 Checking the centration and focus of the slit lamp.

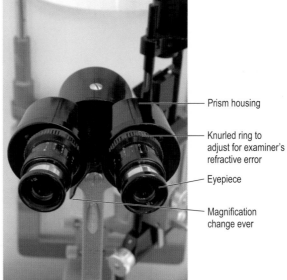

Prism housing

Knurled ring to adjust for examiner's refractive error

Eyepiece

Magnification change ever

Fig. 2.3 The slit-lamp microscope.

The distance between the eyepieces can also be adjusted for different interpupillary distances by turning the prism housing of the microscope. The microscope can be swung on the central pillar through an arc of 180°. A locking screw fixes its position if required.

The slit illuminator

The projection of a uniformly sharp slit of light to the plane of focus is essential for clear observation of ocular structures.

The intensity, height, width, angle (both horizontal and vertical) and colour of the slit beam can

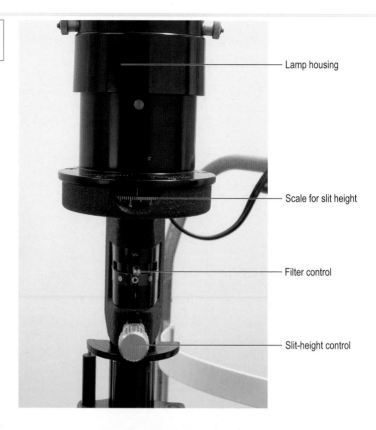

Fig. 2.4 The contols on the light column.

Lamp housing

Scale for slit height

Filter control

Slit-height control

all be adjusted. The slit illumination can also be displaced away from the centre of the field of vision (decentred or decoupled) by loosening the centring screw (see Decentration, below). In the Haag–Streit machine light is projected vertically from an incandescent lamp, passes through a condenser lens and is then reflected into the eye by an inclined mirror. The voltage to the lamp can be adjusted to vary its brightness, with either a three-position switch or a continuously variable rheostat.

Adjustment of slit size

The width of the slit is adjusted by a knurled knob on the lower part of the slit lamp housing. The scale provided does not indicate the actual width of the slit but allows a previous setting to be re-established. A knurled knob at the top of the slit lamp adjusts the vertical height of the slit beam. This either changes the height by fixed amounts or provides a continuously variable adjustment (between 1 and 8 mm), which can be used to measure the size of ocular structures. On some machines this control

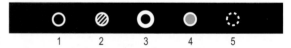

1 = **Open** 2 = **Heat absorption screen** 3 = **10% filter**
4 = **Red-free filter** 5 = **Open** (on some slit lamps, a cobalt blue filter)

Fig. 2.5 The filters on the light column.

also allows a cobalt blue exciter to be inserted into the beam at maximal slit height to view the eye after application of fluorescein (Fig. 2.4).

Filters

The filter control lever can be used to place additional filters in the slit beam (Fig. 2.5). With the lever straight ahead a grey, neutral-density filter is inserted in the beam which reduces the intensity of the light. Moving the lever one click to the left places a heat absorption screen in the path of the light. This should be used when the lamp is powered with the maximum voltage and the slit is fully open. The next click to the left places no filter in the path of the light. Moving to the right of the central position, the lever provides a green (red-free) filter, which causes red objects such as blood vessels and haemorrhages to appear black, with increased contrast. A further click allows for the provision of additional, specialised filters. In some machines this may be the location of the cobalt blue filter.

Illuminator movement

The slit illumination can be moved around the vertical axis and from left to right. A latch on the bottom of the column allows movement on the horizontal axis between 0 and 20°, permitting a horizontal optical section to be produced; this is useful in examining the iridocorneal angle, vitreous and fundus. At the base of the column scales are embossed on both the illuminator arm and the microscope arm. The long central mark on the microscope arm indicates the angle between the microscope axis and the illumination unit. The short marks on the microscope on either side of the long mark indicate a 6.5° angle to the left and right between the microscope and the illumination unit. This position is used with the short mirror in place (see below). A support roller clicks in position when the illumination and microscope columns are directly aligned and when at 10° to the left or right of one another.

Mirrors

The slit lamp is provided with a long and a short inclined mirror (Fig. 2.6). The long mirror is generally used for anterior-segment examination when the angle between the illuminating column and the microscope is generally more than 10°. If the angle between the microscope and the illuminating column is between 0 and 10°, for example when examining the vitreous, part of the long mirror obstructs the microscope and the short mirror is used instead. To maximise illumination, the column should be tilted vertically by 10° when the short mirror is used.

Decentration

The centring screw is found on the lower part of the column. When tightened, the illumination is at the centre of the microscope field as the slit beam and microscope focus are coincident. Loosening the screw allows the illumination column to be rotated

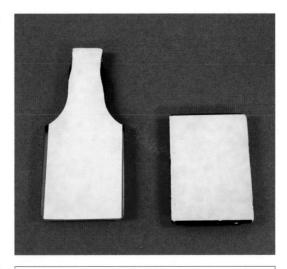

Fig. 2.6 The long and short mirrors. They are front silvered and therefore have delicate optical surfaces.

manually on its vertical axis so that it is offset from the centre of the field. This is necessary when specialised examination techniques, described below, are used (Fig. 2.7).

Headrest

The headrest is securely fastened to the front of the instrument. The chinrest can be moved by turning the knob on the side of the rest to allow the position of the subject's head to be adjusted. The patient's eyes should be aligned with the marker on the side of the frame (Fig. 2.8). Tissue-paper pads can be attached to the chinrest with two small rivets. The subject's forehead should press into the forehead band (Box 2.2).

Fixation target

Attached to the headrest is a fixation target, which rotates across the top of the headrest and can be positioned in front of the right or left eye. Additional movement of the fixation target can be obtained by turning the knurled knob on the top of the headrest. The correct position of the fixation light is indicated when the reflection of its disc is seen in the cornea. Movement of the fixation light will then always be within the subject's visual field. A small lever on the fixation light sleeve allows the focus of the light to be adjusted for the subject's distance spectacle correction by bringing an illuminated target into

Fig. 2.7 Coupled and uncoupled illumination.

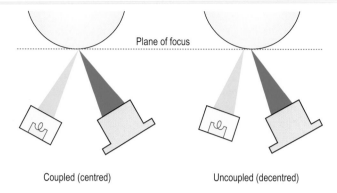

Plane of focus

Coupled (centred)   Uncoupled (decentred)

Fig. 2.8 Correct positioning at the slit lamp.

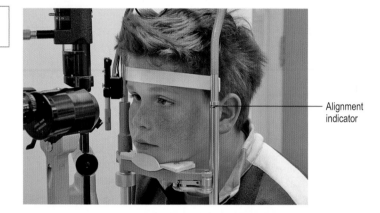

Alignment indicator

Box 2.2

Patient positioning

- Ensure that the patient is comfortably seated. Adjust the patient chair height, slit-lamp table height and examiner's chair height for maximum comfort
- Position the patient's head on the chinrest and adjust the position of the chinrest to align the eyes with the eye-level marker
- Ensure that the patient's forehead is touching the forehead-restraining band
- At this stage the patient should have a straight back, the neck aligned with the back and be leaning forwards slightly. The shape of some patients may not allow for this ideal positioning! A small drawer underneath the slit table may also prevent the correct positioning of some patients' knees unless it is opened
- Children may need to stand, or alternatively they can sit on a parent's lap or kneel on a stable chair. Beware of the position of the tonometer plate, which may poke into a child
- It is helpful in a clinic to have at least one slit-lamp table without a central bar so that wheelchair-bound patients can be examined more easily
- Indicate the position of the hand grips to patients in case they wish to use them
- Inform patients of each step in the examination process *before* it is carried out. Reassure patients and warn them that the light may appear bright
- Make sure that you too are correctly and comfortably positioned

focus. This limits accommodation and associated convergence of the eyes.

Guide plates, slides and pegs

Ancillary equipment can be attached to the slit lamp. On the bottom of the column a plate can be slotted into a central fixation hole so that a Goldmann tonometer can be attached. The central fixation hole also allows for the insertion of the centring (or focusing) rod required during the setting-up of the instrument.

Although largely replaced by modern indirect lenses, slit lamps are also equipped with an attachment for a Hruby indirect fundoscopy lens. This fits into a slide underneath the chinrest and then into the central fixation slot on the base plate (see Ch. 5).

A peg in the centre of the microscope enables a pachymeter to be attached for the assessment of corneal thickness and anterior-chamber depth.

Illumination techniques

Both direct and indirect illumination is used in slit-lamp examination of the eye. Use the lowest level of illumination that provides a good view of the eye and keep examination time to a minimum.

Direct examination

Direct diffuse illumination is commonly used in photography; it is also useful in the initial quick assessment of the eye. A wide slit beam is used. The light can be further diffused with the placement of an additional diffusing screen. High-contrast structure such as the lids can be viewed in this way but more transparent structures require different techniques. Remember that the higher the magnification, the less the depth of focus: it is better to start the examination with a low magnification.

Narrowing the slit allows the creation of the classical optical section (Fig. 2.9). The varying refractive indices of the transparent structures of the eye scatter light differently to produce the qualitative features of this section. A thin bright beam gives the greatest clarity to the section. The cornea, iris and lens are swept by moving the light column from side to side with a narrow full-length beam looking for abnormalities in structure and shape. The position of the microscope is adjusted to obtain a clear view of the structure being examined. A very narrow and short slit is used to examine the anterior chamber,

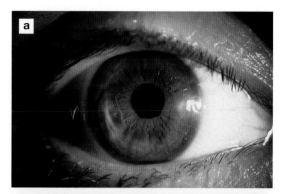
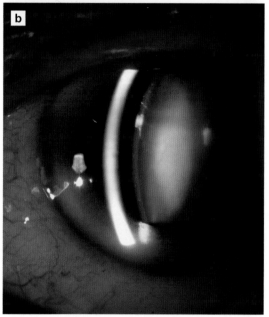

Fig. 2.9 Low-power view of the anterior segment under **(a)** diffuse illumination and **(b)** the classical slit view. Note the appearance of a nuclear cataract.

particularly when looking for cells and flare. The ambient light level needs to be low. The cobalt blue filter is useful for detecting iron lines in the cornea and to examine the eye following instillation of fluorescein (Box 2.3). The characteristics of the tear film and meniscus can be assessed and any staining of the conjunctiva and cornea noted. Staining of the conjunctiva is seen better if a yellow absorption filter is placed in the optical pathway to filter out blue light reflected back from the sclera (Bron et al. 2003).

Abnormalities may be more apparent in the shadow of an obliquely placed slit beam, thus avoiding the bright reflection from the tear film. A beam placed at the edge of a corneal abnormality will be scattered into the surrounding tissue, thus emphasising the perimeter of the abnormality. The latter two techniques are really indirect methods of illumination.

Specular reflection

This is most commonly used to examine the corneal endothelium. It can also be used to examine the lens of the eye.

To examine the cornea the illuminator is placed at 30° to the midline and the microscope at 30° on the opposite side. Initially, with a low magnification, set the illumination (narrow slit, short height) so that it produces a dazzling reflex from the corneal epithelium, and a duller reflex from the endothelium (the first and second Purkinje images formed because each refracting interface acts as a spherical mirror). Slightly adjust the angle of the illuminating beam and the focus of the microscope to obtain a clear view of the second image. Switch to high magnification, widen and dim the illumination and look at the side of the slit beam towards the microscope. A low-contrast view of the endothelial surface should be apparent. It is the irregularity of the surface causing reflection of light at different angles that provides the specular image. It is only seen monocularly, for only one eyepiece will subtend the correct angle with the illuminating beam. The position of the slit lamp or direction of gaze will have to be adjusted to view different parts of the curved surface of the cornea (Fig. 2.10).

Indirect illumination

Sclerotic scatter

The examination room should be as dark as possible, as the reflection of light from the iris and pupil reduces the contrast of the image produced by this technique. The slit lamp is initially focused on the corneal apex. The slit beam is then decentred to project a slit of light 1–2 mm width and 4–5 mm high on to the temporal limbus. If the beam comes from the right then the offset is also to the right. The light enters the cornea and is reflected by total internal reflection to leave the cornea at the opposite limbus, where it produces a halo around the cornea. Opacities or altered structures within the cornea scatter the light and allow the corneal changes to be viewed (Fig. 2.11). The cornea is viewed with the microscope perpendicular to the cornea at low magnification to maximise the depth of focus.

Retroillumination

Incident light is both absorbed by the illuminated structure and reflected. Retroillumination makes use of the reflected light to illuminate a structure diffusely from behind.

Iris retroillumination

The slit is offset by 45°. To view corneal pathology the slit is aimed on the iris either immediately behind (direct) or to the side (indirect) of the corneal pathology. The microscope is focused on the corneal pathology, which will appear relatively dark. The illuminated patch of iris retroilluminates the features of interest. If the apex of the cornea or high magnification is to be used, the slit beam is decentred. For lesions at the limbus, for example

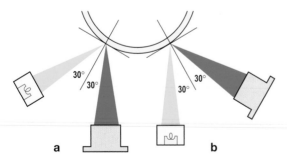

Fig. 2.10 Specular reflection. Note how the slit lamp must move (a to b) to view different parts of the cornea.

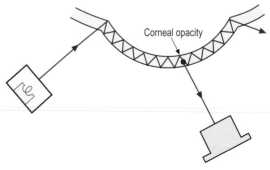

Fig. 2.11 Scleral scatter.

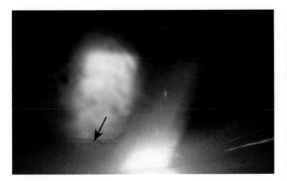

Fig. 2.12 Iris retroillumination demonstrating pigmentation on the endothelium.

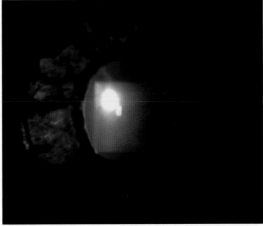

Fig. 2.14 Iris transillumination defects.

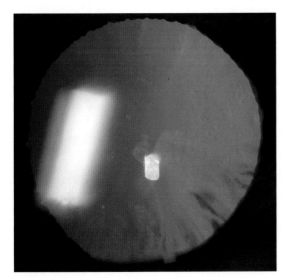

Fig. 2.13 Fundus retroillumination highlighting the appearance of a cataract.

corneal vascularisation, decentration is not necessary (Fig. 2.12).

Fundus retroillumination

This is particularly useful in examination of the cornea or lens, particularly in identifying vacuoles, fluid clefts and abnormalities in the region of the posterior capsule (Fig. 2.13). The patient should be dilated, the illuminator and microscope almost coaxial and the beam height just smaller than the pupil diameter. Offsetting the beam may facilitate

retroillumination. The lens is viewed against an orange glow of light reflected from the choroid. The technique can also be used to highlight opacities in the anterior vitreous. Transillumination is a modification used to detect defects in iris pigmentation. Here the illuminator and microscope are coaxial, all the light must pass through the pupil and the microscope is focused on the iris; the defects found in the iris are transillumination defects (Fig. 2.14).

Scleral retroillumination

This is useful in examining the conjunctiva, particularly in looking for microcystic changes following a trabeculectomy. A narrow slit beam, slightly offset, illuminates the sclera and the microscope is focused on the conjunctiva just to the side of the illuminating beam (Fig. 2.15).

Assessment of anterior-chamber depth

Accurate measurement of anterior-chamber depth requires a pachymeter (see below) attached to the slit lamp. An approximate assessment can be made with the slit lamp. Peripheral anterior-chamber depth, important in determining the possibility of angle-closure glaucoma occurring, can be estimated as follows.

Van Herrick's method

The patient looks straight ahead. To measure the temporal peripheral depth the microscope is

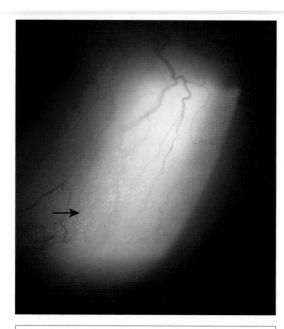

Fig. 2.15 Scleral retroillumination demonstrating the presence of microcysts in a functioning trabeculectomy bleb.

perpendicular to the eye and the light source is at 60°. The space between the most peripheral corneal endothelium and the iris is measured in terms of the peripheral corneal thickness (Fig. 2.16). A depth of less than 0.25% corneal thickness suggests the possibility of angle closure.

Central anterior-chamber depth
This can be measured as described by Smith (1979). A horizontal slit initially 1–2 mm in height is used

and viewed uniocularly through the microscope (right eye for patient's right eye, left eye for patient's left eye). The illuminating column and microscope are separated by 60°. A reflex from the cornea and iris/lens will be seen. Adjusting the height of the beam will cause the two reflexes just to overlap. The slit height (providing it is less than 2.8 mm) multiplied by 1.31 gives the anterior chamber depth at the apex of the cornea.

With practice, however, the examiner learns to estimate anterior-chamber depth without recourse to this method.

Additional lenses

The use of additional contact and non-contact lenses with the slit lamp allows a stereoscopic view to be obtained of the angle, vitreous gel and the fundus. These are fully described in Chapters 4 and 5.

Measurement of corneal and anterior-chamber depth (pachymetry)

Ultrasound techniques are commonly used to assess corneal thickness and anterior-chamber depth. Optical depth measurement can also be performed using a pachymeter attachment for the slit lamp, which fits on to the peg on the microscope housing (Fig. 2.17). This enables a narrow slit of light to be projected on to the cornea or anterior chamber. The microscope and illumination column are each set at 30° to the normal and the brightest, thinnest visible slit is used to illuminate the cornea. An eyepiece with a horizontal slit and a doubling prism is used to view the eye. This produces two images of the slit section. A lever on the pachymeter moves the position of one image relative to the other. To

Fig. 2.16 Van Herrick's method of peripheral anterior-chamber depth estimation.

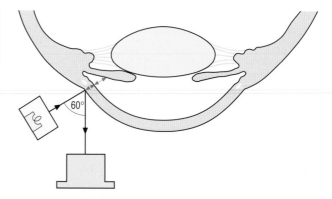

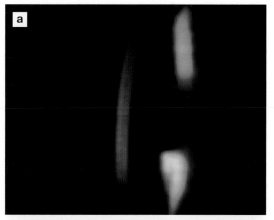

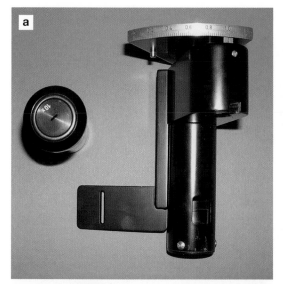

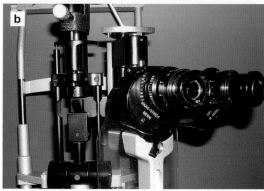

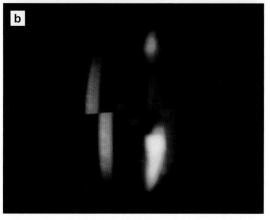

Fig. 2.17 Measurement of corneal and anterior-chamber depth. **(a)** The optical pachymeter; **(b)** the pachymeter attached to the slit lamp.

Fig. 2.18 The view through the pachymeter eyepiece when the images are aligned in the measurement of corneal thickness. **(a)** The corneal image appears complete. **(b)** The slit section of the cornea has been separated so that the endothelial layer of the top image is aligned with the epithelial layer of the bottom image. The corneal thickness is simply read from the scale on the pachymeter.

measure corneal thickness the lever is adjusted until the epithelium of the lower image just touches the endothelium of the upper image (Fig. 2.18a, b). The thickness of the cornea is then read from the scale. Similarly, but using a differently scaled attachment, the anterior lens surface is aligned with the corneal endothelium to assess anterior-chamber depth. A more accurate measure of anterior chamber depth is made by measuring the distance from the corneal epithelium to the lens surface and subtracting the corneal thickness. The measurements should be repeated two or three times and an average taken.

The slit-lamp examination

It is important to record the findings of the examination clearly. To do this it must be performed in a logical sequence using appropriate methods of illumination.

The appearance of the lids is first noted. Abnormalities of the lashes, lid margin, meibomian glands and puncta are noted.

The tarsal and bulbar conjunctiva are next examined. If necessary, the appearance of the tarsus

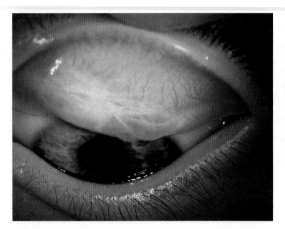

Fig. 2.19 The lid has been everted to reveal fibrosis of the tarsal conjunctiva.

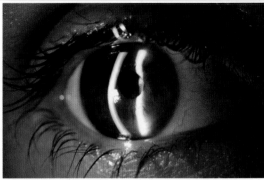

Fig. 2.20 The shape of the cornea is observed. Keratoconus can be seen with a steep central curvature.

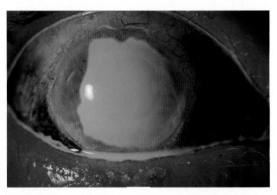

Fig. 2.21 A corneal ulcer stained with fluorescein.

under the upper lid is examined by everting the lid over a blunt-ended object (Fig. 2.19). The presence, site and depth of inflammation, haemorrhage or masses arising from the conjunctiva is noted.

Focusing through the bulbar conjunctiva, the sclera can be observed. Is there thinning (as in scleromalacia) or inflammation? Is the inflammation localised (perilimbal in uveitis, associated with a muscle insertion as in myositis or dysthyroid eye disease)?

The tear film is examined (see Ch. 8).

The cornea is examined and any abnormalities of shape or thickness noted (Fig. 2.20). The layers are then examined from epithelium to endothelium with appropriate illumination techniques, and abnormalities recorded. Dyes may be applied to highlight corneal epithelial abnormalities (Figs 2.21 and 2.22) (and abnormalities of the conjunctiva and tear film: Fig. 2.23 and Box 2.3).

The anterior chamber is next examined, noting its central and peripheral depth and the presence of any cells (red or white) or flare (indicating the presence of protein in the aqueous). Use a small-diameter circular light beam with the highest light intensity and the highest magnification when looking for cells. A more accurate determination requires a laser cell flaremeter, principally used in research. The inferior sector of the anterior chamber should be examined for the presence of a hyphaema or hypopyon (Fig. 2.24).

Abnormalities of the iris are next recorded, looking for frank defects (e.g. coloboma or structural abnormalities associated with mesodermal dysgenesis); in anterior penetrating eye injuries the iris may become plugged in the wound, causing pupillary distortion. Look for abnormalities of pigmentation (heterochromia or pigmented lesions), rubeotic blood vessels, masses growing on or distorting the iris and abnormalities of the pupillary margin (e.g. ectropion uveae or pseudoexfoliation material). Choroidal retroillumination will reveal transillumination defects found in pigment dispersion syndrome. Note how the iris responds to the light (e.g. the vermiform movements seen in patients with an Adie's pupil; see Ch. 10). Look for areas where the iris has become stuck to the lens (posterior synechiae (PS); Fig. 2.25) and gross peripheral anterior synechiae (PAS) where the iris has become attached to the peripheral cornea.

Box 2.3

Corneal and conjunctival dyes

- First make sure that patients are not wearing contact lenses. These dyes will stain soft lenses!
- Warn patients that the drop will cause the vision to change, appearing yellow (fluorescein) or crimson (rose Bengal)
- Warn the patient that the drops will sting, particularly rose Bengal
- A complete assessment requires that the upper lid is gently raised

Fluorescein

This is readily available as a strip which requires wetting with normal saline or a 2% sterile unit dose solution. It absorbs light in the blue wavelength and emits a green fluorescence. At 0.1% it is highly fluorescent but at 2% it is non-fluorescent

Precorneal tear film

Following application of a dilute solution of fluorescein (e.g. by applying a drop from a wetted strip to the lower tarsal conjunctival surface), patients are asked to blink and then keep the eye open. The fluorescein-stained tear film, illuminated with a cobalt blue filter, initially forms a uniform coating over the eye which gradually breaks down. The time it takes for the film to start to degrade is recorded. It should normally be more than 10 s.

Topical fluorescein is also used in the assessment of epiphora (see Ch. 8)

Epithelial defects

A dilute solution is again applied to the eye and the cobalt blue filter used for illumination. Conjunctival and corneal epithelial lesions are highlighted (Fig. 2.21). Fluorescein stains cellular defects and intercellular spaces, not cells themselves. It will thus show corneal abrasions. It is also used to assess patients with dry eyes. It is important to observe the staining pattern as quickly as possible following application because the dye rapidly diffuses and punctate staining will become poorly delineated. This observation is usually performed immediately after the tear break-up time has been measured. To maximise the visibility of any staining, a yellow-orange barrier filter should be used over the slit-lamp objective to remove the scattered blue light from the sclera, which degrades the image

Aqueous leaks

A more concentrated 2% solution is used to detect aqueous fluid leaking from the eye. The leaking aqueous dilutes the fluorescein, which starts to fluoresce as the concentration falls, becoming bright green (Fig. 2.22)

Rose Bengal

This iodine derivative of fluorescein stains dead and dying epithelial cells of the cornea and conjunctiva which have lost their mucin coating. It will not stain cells that are covered by mucin. It will also stain the mucus of the precorneal tear film. A 1% solution is applied to the upper bulbar conjunctiva of the eye following the application of a topical local anaesthetic (the drop is more painful than fluorescein). Staining of the skin can be avoided by pulling the lower lid down at the time of instillation; a tissue is used to mop up excess dye before the lid is released. Any further spillage of dye should also be rapidly mopped up. The staining pattern can be viewed using red-free light; if a white light is used, contrast is improved by placing a green filter over the microscope objective lens. To avoid prolonged discomfort for the patient it is better to wash the dye out of the eye at the end of the examination with normal saline solution. The dye is particularly useful in examining patients with keratoconjunctivitis sicca (Fig. 2.23). An alternative dye is lissamine green, which is less irritant. It can be obtained in strips or solution. The staining pattern of both these dyes persists longer than fluorescein

---

The lens is best viewed through a dilated pupil. This is particularly important if looking for pseudo-exfolliative material on the anterior lens surface (Fig. 2.26). Look for abnormalities in the shape of the lens (e.g. posterior lenticonus). The type and position of any lens opacity are next observed using both direct and retinal retroillumination (Fig. 2.13). Determine the type of cataract present. This can be

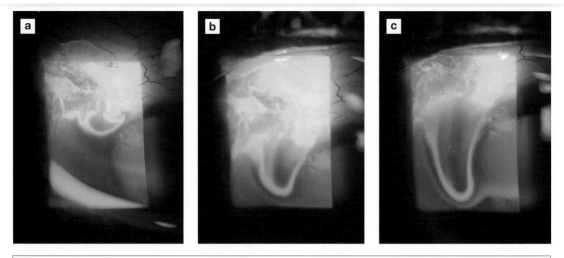

Fig. 2.22 (a–c) Aqueous leaking from a trabeculectomy bleb highlighted with fluorescein. Note how the 'teardrop' extends with time.

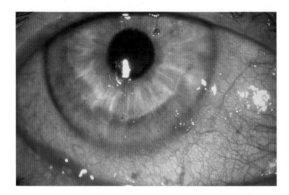

Fig. 2.23 Rose Bengal staining of a dry eye.

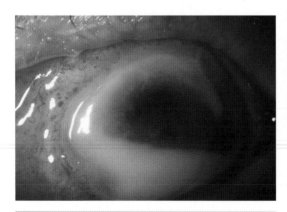

Fig. 2.24 An hypopyon.

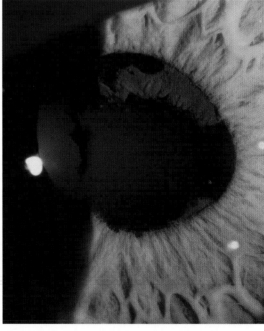

Fig. 2.25 Iris pigment on the lens superiorly; inferiorly, posterior synechiae.

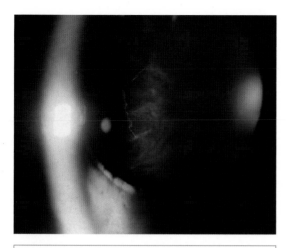

Fig. 2.26 Pseudoexfoliation.

graded according to the lens opacities classification system (LOCS III). This uses a system of coloured direct and retroillumination pictures to grade degrees of nuclear, cortical and subcapsular cataract.

If the patient has an implant lens following cataract surgery, determine the clarity of the posterior capsule. This may again be made easier if it is viewed by retinal retroillumination.

Abnormal movements of the lens (phakodonesis) and iris (iridodenesis) should also be recorded. The observer focuses on the pupil and the patient is asked to look to the side and then straight ahead again. The observer notes any iris or lens shake as the eye comes to a sudden stop in the primary position.

The anterior vitreous is the last part of the eye that is readily visible without the aid of special lenses. Look for the presence of cells or pigment granules and condensations of the vitreous gel. The angle between the microscope and the illumination will have to be small, particularly if the deeper vitreous is to be visualised. The illumination column should also be tilted. Lenses used to examine the retina (for example, the 90 D; see Ch. 5) can be used to examine the posterior vitreous.

The examination continues with tonometry if appropriate. The retina and iridocorneal angle are then viewed through special lenses (gonioscopy, see Ch. 4).

The experienced slit-lamp user will be able to perform an accurate assessment of an eye quickly: it requires much practice, however.

Summary

It is important to spend time learning the basic controls of the slit-lamp methods of illumination and use of attachments and special lenses. Correct examination technique and an orderly progression through the structures of the eye will enable what might otherwise be subtle abnormalities to be readily seen.

- The slit lamp is essential for a detailed examination, in three dimensions, of the anterior segment
- It utilises reflections from various optical interfaces to visualise different structures
- Illumination may be varied in height, intensity, angle, colour and concentricity
- Magnification to a cellular level (endothelium) is available
- Various pieces of adjunctive equipment allow examination of the posterior segment, the drainage angle, corneal thickness, anterior-chamber depth and intraocular pressure

Further reading

Bron AJ, Evans VE, Smith JA. Grading of corneal and conjunctival staining in the context of other dry eye tests. Cornea 2003; 22: 640–650.

Smith RJH. A new method of estimating the depth of the anterior chamber. Br J Ophthalmol 1979; 63: 215–220.

van Herick W, Shaffer RN, Schwartz A. Estimation of width of anterior chamber. Incidence and significance of the narrow angle. Am J Ophthalmol 1969; 68: 626–629.

Tonometry

BRUCE JAMES

Introduction

Measurement of intraocular pressure is key to the diagnosis and treatment of glaucoma. Manometric measurement, whilst being the most accurate method, requires the insertion of a cannula into the eye and is not clinically possible. Indirect methods (tonometers) for assessing intraocular pressure have thus been developed. There are two major types of tonometer: indentation and applanation.

Indentation tonometry

The Shiotz indentation tonometer measures the extent to which a plunger of known weight indents the globe in a supine patient (Fig. 3.1). The higher the intraocular pressure, the less the plunger is able to indent the cornea. Intraocular pressure is measured by converting the scale reading with a nomogram. Errors in measurement occur because not all eyes will respond to indentation in the same way. Variation in ocular rigidity and corneal shape will necessarily lead to errors in measurement. The weight of the tonometer on the eye is also responsible for a gradual reduction in pressure. This

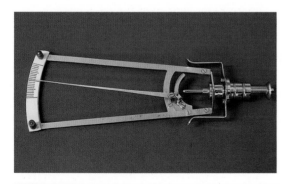

Fig. 3.1 The Shiotz tonometer.

method of intraocular pressure measurement has largely been replaced by applanation tonometers.

Applanation tonometry

The Goldmann applanation tonometer remains the gold standard against which other tonometric methods are assessed (Fig. 3.2). It is used in conjunction with the slit lamp. Its principle is based on the Imbert–Fick law, which states that:

An external force (W) against a sphere equals the pressure in the sphere (Pt) times the area of flattening (A) (assuming the sphere to be perfectly spherical, dry, so no other forces such as surface tension effects are involved, infinitely thin and flexible).

$$W = Pt \times A$$

The eye does not fulfil any of these criteria, however! The technique relies on an assumption that for a particular area of flattening of the inner aspect of the cornea, surface tension pulling the head of the tonometer towards the eye is balanced by the lack of flexibility of the cornea. An external diameter of corneal flattening of approximately 3 mm (no greater than 3.5 mm) allows this assumption to be made. Additionally, allowance must be made for the effect of the thickness of the cornea, which is obviously not infinitely thin, thus the area flattened on the outside of the cornea is not the same as the area flattened on the inside. It is further assumed that if the displaced volume resulting from corneal flattening is small, then ocular rigidity will not significantly affect the result.

The Goldmann tonometer

The Goldmann tonometer allows the application of a variable force to a transparent head or prism which

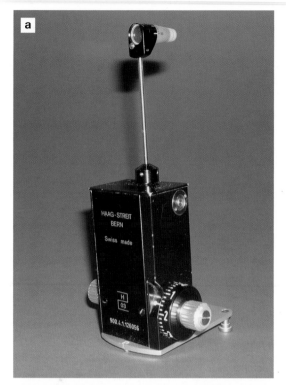

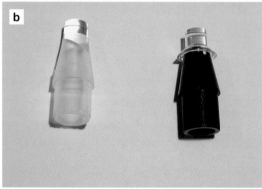

Fig. 3.2 (a) The Goldmann tonometer;
(b) disposable prisms for the tonometer.

force must be applied to the head to flatten this uniform area of cornea; if the pressure is lower, less force must be applied.

When the head touches the eye a meniscus forms. The applied force is increased to enlarge the area of contact and size of meniscus until the endpoint is reached, when both have a diameter of 3.06 mm. Observing the meniscus through a split prism contained within the head reveals it displayed as two separate semicircles (Fig. 3.3a). These gradually increase in size until they just overlap. This is the point at which the correct area of the cornea has been applanated (Fig. 3.3b). The force required to achieve this uniform area of corneal flattening, and thus the corresponding intraocular pressure, can then be read from the tonometer scale. The semicircles must be equal; if not, the cornea has not been properly applanated (Fig. 3.3c).

Measurement of intraocular pressure with the Goldmann tonometer

- The patient is seated at the slit lamp; any tight neckwear should be loosened. The technique is explained and the patient asked to breathe normally. The patient is warned that the anaesthetic drops will sting but that the procedure itself does not hurt; the fluorescein will make things appear yellow for a short time. The slit lamp is set as usual on low magnification. The cobalt blue filter is inserted in the illumination path and the slit diaphragm opened completely, with the lamp switch turned to maximum illumination. Reduced illumination may cause intraocular pressure to be underestimated.
- A drop of local anaesthetic is instilled in both eyes with the addition of a weak fluorescein solution (proxymetacaine 0.5% + fluorescein is probably the least painful and is convenient, ensuring a repeatable concentration of fluorescein every time). Applanation without fluorescein significantly underestimates intraocular pressure.
- The tonometer head is cleaned. Solutions of 70% isopropylalcohol and 3% hydrogen peroxide can be used to sterilise the tip, but it is also vital to ensure that there is no organic matter on the surface of the tonometer and that any disinfectant is removed prior to applanation. Concern about the spread of slow viruses and

contacts or applanates the cornea. The diameter of the head is set at 3.06 mm. This meets the theoretical requirements laid out above and simplifies the conversion of the applied force into an intraocular pressure measurement. An external force of 1 g flattening an area of cornea with a diameter of 3.06 mm corresponds exactly to an intraocular pressure of 10 mmHg. If the pressure is higher, more

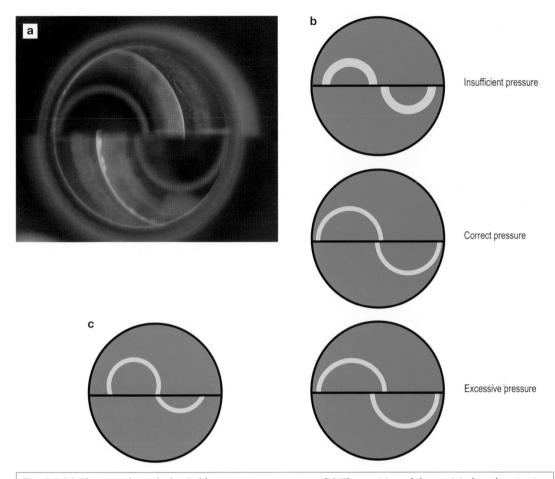

Fig. 3.3 (a) The view through the Goldmann tonometer prism. **(b)** The position of the semicircles when (top) insufficient, (middle) correct and (bottom) excessive pressure has been applied by the tonometer arm to the cornea. **(c)** The tonometer is not central; the semicircles are unequal.

possible transmission by tears has led to the production of disposable tonometer heads and disposable caps (Fig. 3.2b). It is likely that these will become increasingly used.

- The tonometer is located on the slit lamp base plate. It is viewed uniocularly, set either for the observer's right or left eye by placing the pin on its base into either the right or left hole of the horizontal guide plate on the slit lamp. The microscope is perpendicular to the eye. This may require the microscope to be turned nasally to allow for convergence by the patient. The correct positioning of the tonometer arm is indicated when it clicks into position. The illuminating column is placed at 60° to illuminate the end of

the head. On some heads a coloured band indicates where the illumination should be focused. In some cases the tonometer is attached to the accessory peg and is swung into position. The measuring drum is set to about 10 mmHg (Fig. 3.4).

- The tonometer head is slowly advanced until it just contacts the eye; observing from the side, the limbus will suddenly glow with a blue light. The examiner may have to hold the lids apart gently. If this is done it is important not to use force or apply pressure to the globe, as this may cause an artificial elevation of intraocular pressure. It is usually possible to rest the fingers holding the lids on the orbital rim. The observer

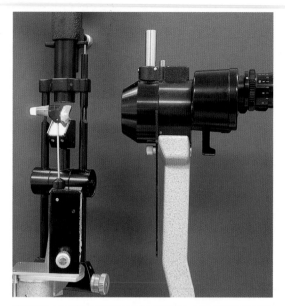

Fig. 3.4 Setting up the tonometer for use.

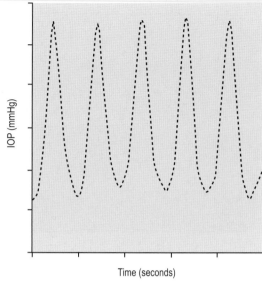

Fig. 3.5 The pulsatile variation in intraocular pressure.

now looks through the eyepieces, gently manipulating the microscope until the two semicircles are viewed. They should be equal in size and shape, about 0.3 mm thick and in the middle of the field of view.

- By rotating the measuring drum the semicircles are made to overlap on their inner edge (Fig. 3.3). It is usual to see a pulsatile movement of the semicircles. This corresponds to the inflow and outflow of blood from the eye during each heart beat (Fig. 3.5). If there is significant pulsatile movement the semicircles are adjusted so that the inner-edge overlap represents the midpoint of their excursion.
- The pressure is read from the rotating drum, multiplying the figure by 10 to find the intraocular pressure in mmHg.

Problems encountered in using the Goldmann tonometer

- The fluorescent band is too wide. This usually occurs if there is a deep tear meniscus or if the lids are in contact with the tonometer head. Dry the tonometer head and start again, otherwise the pressure will be overestimated.
- The fluorescent band is too narrow. The tear film is insufficient. Withdraw the prism and ask

the patient to blink several times. A narrow band underestimates the pressure.
- There is a large overlap of the semicircles unresponsive to rotation of the measuring drum. In this case, the tonometer head has been pressed too firmly against the eye. Withdraw the microscope and start again.
- Repeated measurement of intraocular may result in lesions of the corneal epithelium, which will stain with the fluorescein dye. These are rarely severe and cause the patient no distress, although they may cause a little temporary blurring of vision.
- Multiple measurements of intraocular pressure may lead to a gradual reduction in pressure readings due to massaging of the eye (tonographic effect). The first reading in a patient is often higher than repeated second readings, particularly if the patient is anxious and squeezing the eye. If this is the case, the first reading should be discarded.
- The pressure unexpectedly becomes very low. Beware: the patient is probably about to faint!

Measurement in patients with significant astigmatism

The tonometer head is marked in degrees between 0 and 180 (Fig. 3.6). If there is less than 3 D of

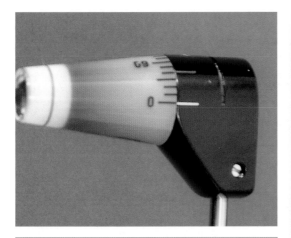

Fig. 3.6 Adjusting the tonometer prism in patients with significant astigmatism. Note the white and red lines on the tonometer housing.

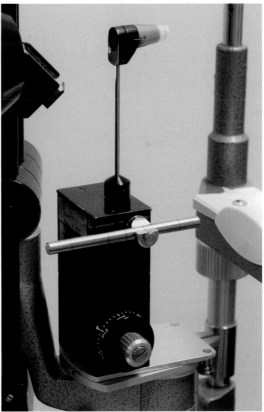

Fig. 3.7 Calibrating the Goldmann tonometer. Ensure correct alignment of the calibrations on the rod and the holder by viewing them perpendicularly.

astigmatism, the head is aligned horizontally. That is, the 0° mark is aligned with the *white* line on the head-holder. If more than 3 D of astigmatism is present the semicircles will be elliptical and the pressure not correctly estimated unless the tonometer head is rotated such that it is positioned at 43° to the *meridian* of the lowest power. The 43° position is indicated with a red line on the prism housing (Fig. 3.6).

Example
Corneal astigmatism 44 D 50°, 40 D 140°: the tonometer head is rotated until the 140° mark is aligned with the *red* line on the holder. If focimetry is used to determine astigmatism from the patient's glasses, the head is set to the *axis* of the minus cylinder.

An alternative technique proposed by Holladay et al. (1983) for regular astigmatism suggests measuring the intraocular pressure with the head in the horizontal position and then at 90° in the vertical position. The two intraocular pressure readings are then averaged.

Patients with irregular astigmatism or abnormal corneas may have unreliable intraocular pressure measurements made with the Goldmann tonometer.

Calibration
The Goldmann tonometer should be regularly calibrated. The calibration arm fits into a slot on the side of the tonometer (Fig. 3.7). The rod is positioned so that the central mark is aligned with the mark on its holder. The measuring drum is placed at 0; the pressure arm should gently rock forwards and backwards with slight pressure. Moving the measuring drum between −0.5 and +0.5 mmHg should likewise cause the pressure arm to rock. The rod is advanced to the next mark and the process repeated at 20 mmHg and then 60 mmHg. The tonometer arm should rock between 19.5 mmHg and 20.5 mmHg and 59 mmHg and 61 mmHg respectively. In practice, a slightly greater tolerance may have to be accepted. If the calibration is incorrect, the tonometer must be returned to the manufacturer.

A simple way to test calibration, which should be used at the start of each clinic, is to check that the arm rocks around zero by moving the dial

0.5 mmHg (the width of the calibration mark on the scale) either side of zero with the prism in place. Once again, a unit may decide on a slightly higher tolerance. If the tonometer is calibrated at 0 mmHg it is unlikely to be significantly out at 20 and 60 mmHg, although these levels should be checked periodically, as described above.

The effect of corneal thickness

Recent research has suggested that in patients with thin corneas the intraocular pressure may be underestimated whilst in those with a thick cornea the pressure will be overestimated.

The Ocular Hypertension Treatment Study has graphically demonstrated the importance of corneal thickness in tonometry. Patients with a thick cornea were much less likely to convert to glaucoma than those with a thin cornea and thus a thicker sclera. Although structural protective effects of a thick cornea cannot be ruled out, it is likely that the finding is most readily explained by an overestimation of intraocular pressure in patients with thick corneas. Similarly, the cornea has been shown to be thinner in patients with normal-tension glaucoma, suggesting that in these patients the intraocular pressure may be underestimated.

There is also concern that corneal laser refractive surgery may alter the accuracy of applanation pressure measurement as the corneal thickness is reduced by laser refractive surgery.

No algorithm enabling an accurate allowance for corneal thickness on intraocular pressure yet exists. Nonetheless, pachymetry (see Ch. 6) is increasingly important in the glaucoma clinic, particularly in ocular hypertension, to allow an approximate correction of intraocular pressure to be made. The automated conversion programs that some ultrasound pachymeters have for adjusting intraocular pressure to the measured corneal thickness should be used with caution.

Additional tonometers

Perkins tonometer

In some patients positioning at a slit lamp may be impossible because of immobility or because they are under an anaesthetic. In these cases a hand-held version of the Goldmann tonometer can be used (Fig. 3.8). The principle of operation is the same.

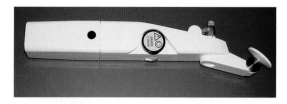

Fig. 3.8 The Perkins tonometer.

Anaesthetic and fluorescein are applied to the eye. The instrument is switched on by rotating the knurled measuring wheel; again this should be set at 10 mmHg. The light with a prefitted cobalt blue filter illuminates the end of the prism. The forehead rest is fitted to the top of the tonometer.

With the patient comfortably positioned the rest is applied to the forehead and the tonometer head gently moved towards the eye. When the limbal blue flush is seen the observer views the tonometer head through the fitted magnifying lens. The endpoint is exactly the same as with the Goldmann tonometer. Care must be taken to ensure that the light is as strong as possible; even at maximal brightness it is considerably dimmer than that available on the slit lamp.

The Pascal tonometer

This new tonometer (Fig. 3.9) has an electronic pressure sensor embedded within a contour-matched (concave) tonometer tip. This tip has a shape similar to that of the cornea. The cornea takes up the shape of the tip and then the pressure sensor measures intraocular pressure. It is thought that by measuring pressure in this way the effects of corneal thickness and other biomechanical properties of the cornea are removed. The tip is also covered with a disposable rubber membrane, improving the sterility of the procedure.

The rapid acquisition of pressure measurements (100 per second) allows the pulsatile change in intraocular pressure to be measured. A mean pressure, together with a measurement of the difference between systolic and diastolic pressure (pulse amplitude), is displayed on the screen. The tonometer also assesses the quality of the pressure recording. The exact role that this device will have remains to be ascertained.

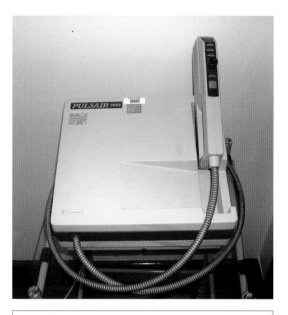

Fig. 3.10 Non-contact tonometer.

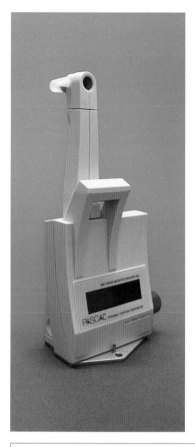

Fig. 3.9 The Pascal tonometer.

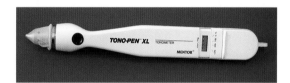

Fig. 3.11 The tonopen.

Non-contact tonometers

These are primarily for screening use. A number of different types are available (Fig. 3.10). They also work on the applanation principle but use a jet of air to flatten a uniform area of the cornea. The intraocular pressure is calculated from the time taken to flatten the cornea or the force of air needed to flatten the cornea. As the reading is instantaneous, the average of three or four readings should be taken. This machine is most commonly used to screen patients for raised intraocular pressure.

Tonopen XL

This is a small, extremely portable machine (Fig. 3.11). The area of contact with the cornea is only 1.5 mm^2. It uses a strain gauge working on the Mackay–Marg principle. The pressure exerted by the applanating plunger on the cornea is recorded electronically from the strain gauge. A liquid crystal display (LCD) screen displays the average result of four readings. A disposable rubber tip makes it particularly useful in patients with possible ocular infection. The small area of contact may also make it suitable for use in patients with corneal abnormalities, although significant measurement errors may still occur in these patients.

The eye is anaesthetised and, once the calibration procedure has been undertaken, the tonopen is gently placed on the cornea. A beep will be heard when the reading is taken and the individual reading will appear on the screen. An average will appear with 4–6 readings together with a percentage indicating the confidence level of the reading.

Summary

It is important to select the appropriate tonometer for the proposed purpose. The machine used will differ if it is used for screening, accurate clinic measurement or assessing pressure in a disabled patient. All instruments require frequent accurate calibration and a detailed knowledge of the factors that cause measurement errors.

Tonometry is by applanation (flattening) or indentation of the corneal surface

    Factors affecting accuracy include:

- Corneal thickness (thicker cornea = higher reading)
- Astigmatism
- Increased tear film
- Pressure on the globe from holding the eyelids open
- Poor calibration of tonometer

References and further reading

Brusini P, Miani F, Tosoni C et al. Corneal thickness in glaucoma: an important parameter? Acta Ophthalmol Scand 2000; 232: 41–42.

Doughty MJ, Zaman ML. Corneal thickness and intraocular pressure. Surv Ophthalmol 2000; 44: 367–408.

Holladay JT, Allison ME, Prager TC. Goldmann applanation tonometry in patients with regular corneal astigmatism. Am J Ophthalmol 1983: 96: 90.

Kass MA, Heur DK, Higginbotham EJ et al. The OHTS study. Arch Ophthalmol 2002; 120: 701–713.

Kaufmann C, Bachmann LM, Thiel MA. Comparison of dynamic contour tonometry with Goldmann applanation tonometry. Invest Ophthalmol Vis Sci 2004; 45: 3118–3121.

Whitacre MM, Stein R. Sources of error with the Golmann-type tonometers. Surv Ophthalmol 1993; 38: 1–30.

Gonioscopy

BRUCE JAMES

Introduction

Gonioscopy allows a biomicroscopic view of the iridocorneal angle, which is vital for both classification of glaucoma and for correct management of the patient.

Many mistakes in glaucoma management occur because gonioscopy was not performed. The technique requires knowledge of the structure of the iridocorneal angle.

Principle of gonioscopy

It is usually not possible to see the iridocorneal angle directly. Light from the angle is reflected back into the eye because the critical angle of the cornea–air interface is exceeded. Applying a contact lens to the eye can overcome this problem by removing the cornea–air interface. A new contact lens–air interface can then be created. In direct gonioscopy the lens is very convex, thus the critical angle is not reached and light reflected from the iridocorneal angle passes to the observer's eye. In indirect gonioscopy a mirror reflects the light through a plano anterior contact lens surface, again ensuring that the critical angle is not reached (Fig. 4.1).

Indirect lenses are the most commonly used type of lens in ophthalmic clinics.

Indirect gonioscopy

The Goldmann single-mirror gonioscopy lens, the Magna view goniolens (and the gonioscopic lens in the Goldmann three-mirror lens)

This technique provides a beautifully clear picture of the iridocorneal angle. It is particularly useful in assessing detailed angle anatomy.

- The lens, illustrated in Figure 4.2, is used with the slit lamp. The patient must be fully informed of the procedure prior to lens placement.

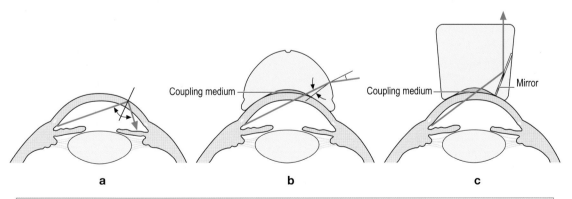

Fig. 4.1 The principles of the gonioscopy lens. **(a)** The normal eye: light from the iridocorneal angle is reflected back into the eye and thus cannot be seen. **(b)** The direct goniolens. As the index of refraction of the lens is similar to that of the cornea, the light enters the lens and is then refracted by the lens to enable the observer to view the angle. **(c)** The indirect goniolens. The principle is similar to the direct lens but, once light has entered the lens, it is reflected by a mirror.

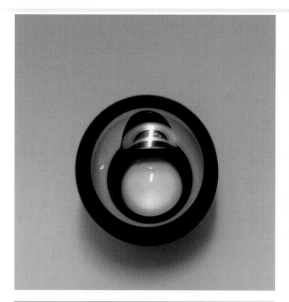

Fig. 4.2 The Goldmann single-mirror gonioscopy lens.

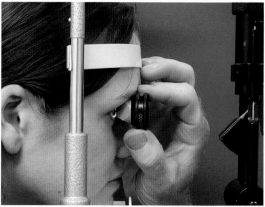

Fig. 4.3 The gonioscopy lens applied to the eye.

- The cornea is anaesthetised (with proxymetacaine 0.5%). Some patients may need tetracaine.
- The lens is cleaned (70% isopropyl alcohol or 3% hydrogen peroxide solutions can be used): it is also vital to ensure that there is no organic matter on the surface of the lens and that any disinfectant is removed prior to placement. Concern about the spread of slow viruses and possible transmission by tears has been expressed but disposable diagnostic lenses are not available.
- A coupling agent, saline or a more viscous artificial tear preparation is placed in the central well of the lens that will contact the eye. Viscotears (carbomer 90) or hydroxypropyl methylcellulose (HPMC) 0.5% are ideal; 2% HPMC is too viscous.
- Gently holding the lids apart and asking the patient to look upwards, the lens is carefully and gently placed on the eye. The inferior edge is placed first to avoid losing the coupling agent. If saline is used this manoeuvre must be accomplished quickly and is probably best avoided by the novice! The patient is asked to try and avoid squeezing the lids on the lens. Only gentle pressure should be required to keep

the lens in place. If excessive pressure is used this will not only be uncomfortable for the patient but will distort the true appearance of the angle.
- The angle is viewed through 360° by rotating the lens (Fig. 4.3). Remember that when the mirror is at the top of the eye, the inferior angle is being viewed. If the angle is narrow it may be necessary to ask the patient to move the eye in the direction of the mirror, but beware: this may distort the appearance of the angle.
- Corneal oedema, for example in acute angle-closure glaucoma, can be cleared with a 50% glycerol drop to allow a view of the angle.

Four-mirror goniolenses (Zeiss, Posner)

These lenses are particularly useful in identifying anatomical features that will allow the examiner to decide if the angle is closed due to reversible apposition or permanent synechiae.

Applying the lens to the patient requires no coupling agent: the posterior radius of curvature of the lens is closer to the anterior radius of curvature of the cornea (Fig. 4.4). Some are provided with a handle. They are otherwise applied in the same way as the Goldmann lens. This, together with the four mirrors, means that the entire angle can be viewed with only slight movement of the lens around the eye, thus speeding up examination time slightly. An additional advantage of the lens comes from the reduced area of contact with the eye. By applying gentle backward pressure on the lens an angle

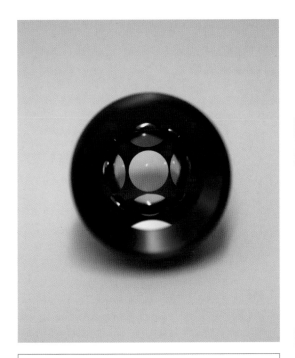

Fig. 4.4 Four-mirror goniolenses.

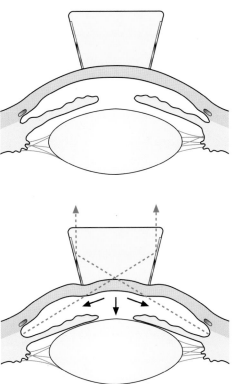

Fig. 4.5 Compressive gonioscopy. The gonioscopy lens indents the cornea, compressing the aqueous and thus pushing the iris backwards and artificially opening the iridocorneal angle.

suspected of being narrow can be opened and the structures of the angle can be viewed (*compressive or indentation gonioscopy*; Fig. 4.5). This helps confirm a diagnosis of narrow-angle glaucoma and ascertain whether there is adherence between the iris and the angle structures (posterior anterior synechiae). The view obtained is less stable, however, and may also be less clear.

Indentation will not be effective if the patient has a surgical iridectomy but will work if a small iridotomy is present. Care must be taken, however, not to apply backward pressure during the initial examination or a narrow or closed angle may be opened. If folds are seen in the cornea during the initial examination, too much pressure is being applied.

Direct gonioscopy

The use of direct gonioscopy lenses is principally re-stricted to surgical treatment of congenital glaucoma because of the practical problems associated with its routine diagnostic use. The advantage of the lens is that it allows the viewing angle to be varied so that structures that may otherwise be hidden by a convex iris can be viewed. Indentation indirect gonioscopy will overcome this to some extent. Bilateral simul-taneous gonioscopy is also possible with a lens placed on each eye, and is useful to compare the angle in both eyes. The Koeppe lens is made in different sizes (Fig. 4.6), and with different posterior radii of curvature. The patient must be horizontal (this in itself may cause the angle to appear more open than it really is). The lens is placed on the anaesthetised eye with a bridging fluid. A hand-held biomicroscope is used to view the angle directly through the lens. The examiner moves until all 360° have been examined. A separate source is used to illuminate the angle (this can be attached to the biomicroscope).

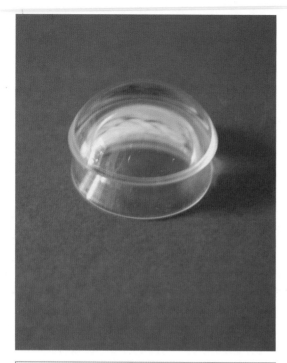

Fig. 4.6 The Koeppe lens.

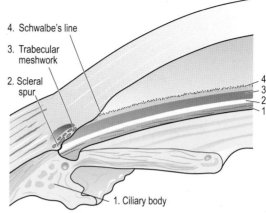

Fig. 4.7 The angle structures.

Gonioscopy in patients with epithelial oedema

It may be important to assess the iridocorneal angle in a patient with an acute elevation of intraocular pressure and epithelial oedema. The application of a drop of 50% glycerol will help to clear the cornea and allow angle structures to be viewed.

Identification of angle structures

In most eyes the angle structures are readily identified (Fig. 4.7). The examination is best started with the mirror at 12 o'clock, thus looking at the 6 o'clock angle.

It may be easier to try and find the scleral spur first as this is usually present as a prominent white band, although in some eyes it may be obscured by uveal tissue, particularly nasally. It may not be seen if the angle is very narrow. It is often most easily seen at 12 o'clock (mirror at 6 o'clock). The other structures lying anterior and posterior to this band can then be identified.

Schwalbe's line, the termination of Descemet's membrane and the most anterior structure of the iridocorneal angle may have pigment scattered around and on it (in pseudoexfoliation syndrome this is termed Sampaolesi's line), particularly inferiorly at 6 o'clock (mirror at 12 o'clock). This helps with its identification. If there is difficulty in finding Schwalbe's line and other structures are not easily visible to work back from (usually due to the absence of pigmentation), the following method of identification may help. Use a high-magnification, good gonioscopy lens (for example, the Magnaview lens). Narrow a bright, short slit beam which should be at 10–15° to the microscope. Look for the apex formed by the reflection of light from the anterior and posterior surfaces of the cornea as they approach the angle. The apex marks the position of Schwalbe's line; in practice it may be difficult to determine accurately until one is familiar with the differing shapes that the corneal wedge takes (Fig. 4.8).

The trabecular meshwork lies between Schwalbe's line and the scleral spur. It is divided into the posterior, usually pigmented (and presumed most functional) meshwork and the anterior non-pigmented meshwork. If the posterior meshwork has little pigmentation it appears as a grayish, slightly granular band. Blood in Schlemm's canal is sometimes visible beneath the posterior meshwork.

The ciliary body band is the most posterior structure. It lies between the insertion of the iris into the ciliary body and the scleral spur. It is usually dark brown in colour.

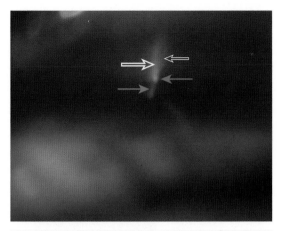

Fig. 4.8 Finding Schwalbe's line using the corneal wedge. The reflection from the corneoscleral junction (fat horizontal arrow) and the corneal endothelium (thin horizontal arrow) meet at Schwalbe's line, visible as a brighter, white area at the apex (red arrow). A heavily pigmented trabecular meshwork is visible posterior to this (blue arrow). (Courtesy of Paul Foster.)

Recording gonioscopic findings

The appearance of the angle is usually described with reference to four quadrants but variation within the quadrants must also be recorded. It is better to note the most posterior structure that is actually seen in each of the quadrants rather than to rely on a numeral when recording findings. This structural assessment forms the basis of the Scheie classification (Fig. 4.9).

Additional points should also be recorded:

- Amount and quality of pigmentation of the various structures. Assess whether the pigment is dark and granular (from the iris pigment epithelium) or the same colour as the stroma. The latter suggests that contact between the iris and iridocorneal angle has occurred.
- The level of insertion of the iris (this may require indentation gonioscopy to be performed).
- The presence of bands of uveal tissue between the iris and the angle (iris processes). These are more noticeable in younger patients and do not extend anterior to the trabecular meshwork.
- The presence of peripheral anterior synechiae.
- The presence of abnormal blood vessels. Blood vessels are not normally visible in the angle, although sometimes loops from the major arterial circle may be visible. Circumferential and radial vessels may also be seen in the ciliary body band if there is little pigment. Abnormal vessels do not normally follow a circumferential or radial course; they continue on to the surface of the iris and may pass anteriorly across the trabecular meshwork and have frequent branches.
- Any other abnormality in the angle. In trauma the ciliary body band may be focally enlarged (recessed), iris processes may be ruptured and damage to the trabecular meshwork may be present. The ciliary body may become detached from the scleral spur, allowing the white underlying sclera to be seen (cyclodialysis cleft). In uveitis there may be inflammatory deposits in the angle.

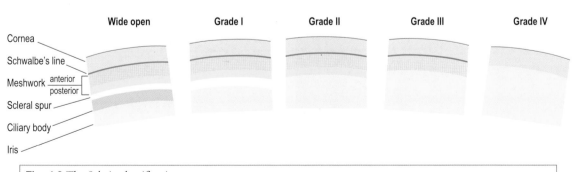

Fig. 4.9 The Scheie classification

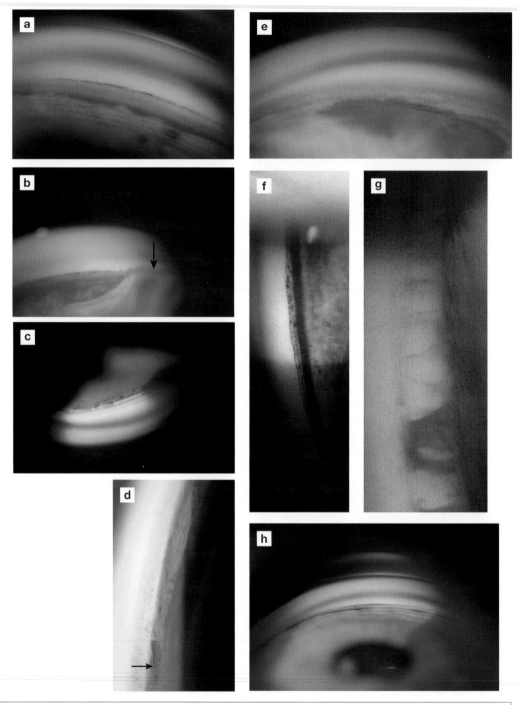

Fig. 4.10 The iridocorneal angle. **(a)** In open-angle glaucoma. **(b)** Peripheral anterior synechiae formation (arrowed). **(c)** Angle recession; note that the ciliary body band appears extended. (Courtesy of Paul Foster.) **(d)** Cyclodialysis cleft inferiorly (arrowed) with angle recession superiorly. **(e)** Iris naevus approaching angle. **(f)** In pigment dispersion syndrome, note the pigment in the trabecular meshwork. **(g)** Iris processes. **(h)** The angle appearance in plateau iris.

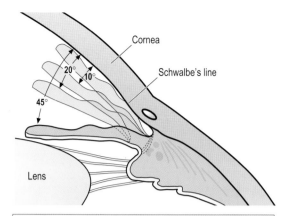

Fig. 4.11 Estimating the iridocorneal angle.

Table 4.1	The Shaffer grading system
Grade	Angle
Grade 4	40°
Grade 3	30°
Grade 2	20°
Grade 1	10°
Grade 0	Closed

Examples of some of these changes are shown in Figure 4.10.

In addition, comment should be made on the angle formed between the iris, taking a point perpendicularly from just anterior to Schwalbe's line and the trabecular meshwork (Fig. 4.11). The slit beam should be at 30° to the microscope. Shaffer based his grading system on this (Table 4.1). The narrowest angle is often seen superiorly.

Iris contour

It is also important to describe the contour of the peripheral iris. This may be flat (normal), bowed backwards (myopia, pigment dispersion syndrome) or bowed forwards (as in angle closure).

Spaeth classification system

Determination of these three elements (the level at which the iris inserts or appears to insert into the cornea or angle, the Shaffer angle and the iris profile) forms the foundation of the Spaeth system for recording angle structure, which gives the most complete picture on which to base diagnosis and therapy.

Summary

Accurate gonioscopy is the key to glaucoma diagnosis and management. It should be performed on all new cases of glaucoma and repeated periodically during follow-up.

- Warn the patient what to expect
- Select the gonioscopy lens
- Gently apply the lens to the cornea without compressing the cornea
- Identify the scleral spur if visible, or Schwalbe's line if not
- Assess which angle structures are visible in each quadrant
- Assess the level of iris insertion
- Estimate the angle the iris forms with a line connecting Schwalbe's line and the posterior trabecular meshwork
- Assess the contour of the iris
- Look for additional anomalies of the angle

Further reading

Allington RR, Damji KF, Freedman S et al. (eds) Shields textbook of glaucoma. Philadelphia: Lippincott, Williams and Wilkins; 2004.

Schie HG. The width and pigmentation of the angle of the anterior chamber. A system of grading by gonioscopy. Arch Ophthalmol 1957; 58: 510.

Shaffer RN. Symposium primary glaucomas. III. Gonioscopy, ophthalmoscopy and perimetry. Trans Am Acad Ophthal Otol 62; 112: 1960.

Spaeth GL. The normal development of the human anterior chamber angle: a new system of descriptive grading. Trans Ophthalmol Soc UK 1971; 91: 709–739.

Examination of the retina and optic disc

LARRY BENJAMIN and BRUCE JAMES

Introduction

The retina and optic disc (optic nerve head) may be examined both anatomically and functionally. Anatomical examination involves the use of direct observation via an illuminated system. It is best done through a dilated pupil. Fundus fluorescein angiography provides further information about retinal anatomy and pathological changes (see Ch. 16). New techniques for imaging the optic nerve head, nerve fibre layer and retina itself (see Ch. 17) provide additional anatomical details. Tests of retinal function include various forms of visual acuity measurement and visual field measurement. Electrophysiological testing gives information about the electrochemistry of the retina as well as retinal pigment epithelial function and nerve conduction between the eye and the brain. This chapter deals with observational techniques for studying retinal anatomy.

The decision as to which diagnostic lens to use depends on the clinical situation. For example, retinal screening in diabetic retinopathy requires a reasonably wide angle of view but still demands the ability to resolve detail to the level of a micro-aneurysm. On the other hand treating a maculopathy discovered at screening may require higher magnification, and a control of eye movements. In the first instance a 90 D lens is satisfactory and, although it can be used for treatment, a macular contact lens gives better visualization of the details at the posterior pole and some control over eye movements.

The direct ophthalmoscope

This instrument consists of a single aperture through which light is projected into the subject's eye and the examiner views the eye. It provides a magnified image (×15) and a field of view of some 6.5–10

degrees. A set of corrective lenses can be dialled into the aperture. These enables the focal point of the instrument to be adjusted (Fig. 5.1). The rack of lenses usually contains equal numbers of positive and negative spheres which can be dialled up to take account of the patient and/or examiner's refractive status. If examiners wish to wear their glasses, they can do so, and effectively they will need a zero lens in the eyepiece. The patient's refraction must also be taken into account and the relevant lens dialled into place. With highly myopic or hypermetropic patients, their glasses can be left on and used to nullify the effect of the refractive variation. Alternatively plus and minus 10 or 20 D lenses can be positioned in the sight aperture to take account of very high hypermetropia or myopia.

The size and brightness of the illumination spot can be varied with the appropriate controls.

Additional features vary among the different models but include a slit filter, producing a vertical slit of light which can be used to examine contours or elevations on the fundus, a grid for assessing the size of a fundus lesion, and a green filter for red-free viewing. This latter filter will make red features, such as haemorrhages, stand out due to increasing contrast between the various shades of red and orange which reflect from the fundus. Some ophthalmoscopes also include a cobalt blue filter for use with fluorescein dye.

The view obtained with this instrument has a narrow angle of view and a high magnification. The more myopic the patient, the more effective the magnifying effect. This is useful for examining the optic nerve head; however the view is monocular and two-dimensional. The various features of the optic disc and its vasculature, as well as the optic cup, can be examined in some detail. The macular region can also be observed. Although a view of the more peripheral retina is possible, because of the

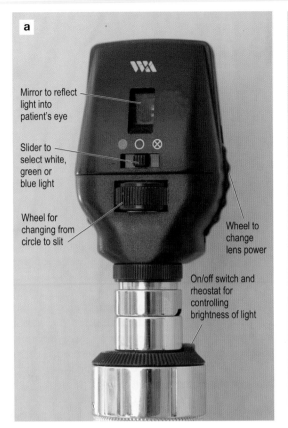
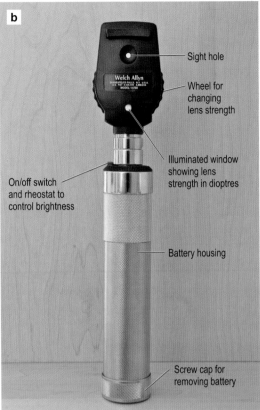

a

Mirror to reflect light into patient's eye

Slider to select white, green or blue light

Wheel for changing from circle to slit

Wheel to change lens power

On/off switch and rheostat for controlling brightness of light

b

Sight hole

Wheel for changing lens strength

Illuminated window showing lens strength in dioptres

On/off switch and rheostat to control brightness

Battery housing

Screw cap for removing battery

Fig. 5.1 The direct ophthalmoscope. **(a)** Patient's view; **(b)** examiner's view.

narrow angle of view and high magnification, it is not possible to ensure that the whole retina has been covered systematically with this instrument.

Method of use

Inform patients that you are going to look at their eye with a bright light and that you will have to get very close to their face. Instruct them to breathe normally.

The instrument is held to the examiner's eye with the illumination system switched on and for steadiness and ease of use a hand can be placed on the patient's shoulder (Fig. 5.2). The examiner's right eye is used for the patient's right eye and the examiner's left for the patient's left eye. If the examiner finds it difficult to close one eye, or the other, then it can be left open – with practice the brain manages to ignore the image from the non-examining eye. The correct lens, as described above, is dialled into the aperture. The

patient is asked to fix on a distant object and is told to maintain that fixation, regardless of whether the examiner gets in the way. The examiner thus knows roughly where the patient's macula is situated and the optic disc will be just nasal to this. The examiner then points the instrument's illumination beam into the patient's pupil and obtains a red reflex from a distance of about half a metre and slowly moves towards the patient. At this point media opacities such as cataract can be seen as black features against the red reflex. The rheostat is used to adjust the brightness of the light for the patient's comfort. If required, the front of the eye, cornea, iris and lens can be examined with a +10 lens dialled into the instruments lens bank. Following this part of the examination the lens dial is progressively turned towards zero to focus further back into the patient's eye and eventually reach the retina. It must be stressed that the head of the ophthalmoscope

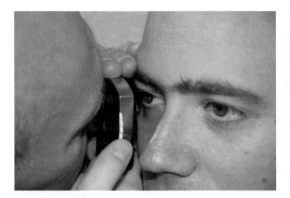

Fig. 5.2 Using the direct ophthalmoscope. Note the proximity of the examiner and the patient. The right eye is used to examine the patient's right and the left to examine the patient's left.

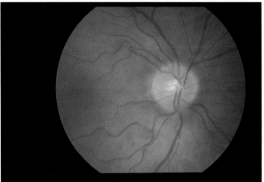

Fig. 5.3 Normal fundus appearance.

must be held very close to the patient's eye in order to gain the maximum field of view.

System for fundus examination

It is important to develop a system for optic disc and fundus examination to ensure that no features are forgotten. The following system is appropriate for all methods of retinal examination. The normal fundus appearance is shown in Figure 5.3.

The optic disc

A retinal arteriole is found and traced back towards the optic disc from which all the retinal vessels emanate. Once the disc is found, it should be examined for colour, shape and definition of its margin (is this easy to see or ill-defined, suggesting disc swelling?). The size of the optic cup compared to the overall size of the entire disc should be estimated to derive a measure of the cup-to-disc (CD) ratio. The neuroretinal rim is examined. This is normally broadest inferiorly, then superiorly then nasally and thinnest temporally (the ISNT rule) (Fig. 5.4, Fig. 5.5a). This is a useful observation to make. If the optic disc is large it may have a big cup but the area of the neuroretinal rim will be the same as a smaller disc with a smaller cup (Fig. 5.6). Although an estimate of optic disc size can be made by comparing the size of the disc to the size of the spot, this is probably more accurately performed with a 90 D indirect lens (see later).

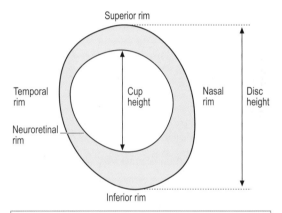

Fig. 5.4 Features to note when examining the optic disc.

Other associated features of the disc, such as splinter haemorrhages on the neuroretinal rim margin, abnormal blood vessels arising from the disc and spontaneous pulsation in the retinal veins as they course over the disc, should also be looked for (Fig. 5.5). All patients should exhibit spontaneous venous pulsation if the intracranial pressure is normal, but some have a pulsation that is in the anteroposterior direction and this can be difficult to see. Loss of the pulsation should alert the examiner to the possibility of raised intracranial pressure.

Retina

Start at the disc and then follow each of the main retinal vessels out towards its extremity. Look at the vessel size and any abnormality within its wall;

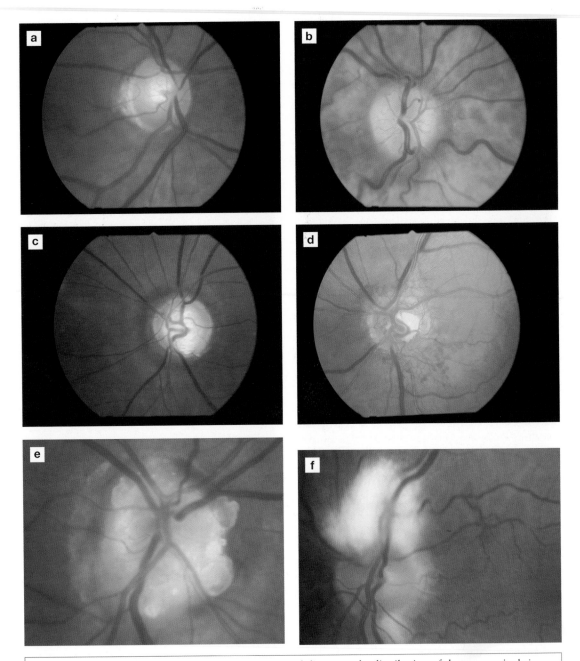

Fig. 5.5 Examples of optic disc abnormalities. **(a)** Normal disc: note the distribution of the neuroretinal rim around the disc. **(b)** A swollen disc: the margin is not clearly demarcated; the patient had papilloedema. **(c)** The cup is enlarged, the neuroretinal rim thinned and the ISNT pattern lost. The patient has glaucoma. **(d)** New vessels are growing at the disc: this patient had diabetes. **(e)** The disc has an irregular lumpy appearance and optic disc drusen. **(f)** Myelinated nerve fibres at the disc margin.

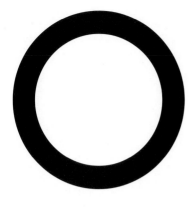

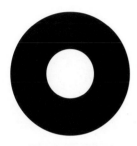

Fig. 5.6 The effect of disc size on cup-to-disc ratio and neuroretinal rim area. These two discs are of different size and have an obvious difference in cup-to-disc ratio. The area of the neuroretinal rim is the same in both, however.

Table 5.1	Systematic examination with the direct ophthalmoscope
Red reflex	
Anterior segment with +10 D lens	
Disc	Shape
	Colour
	Margin
	Cup-to-disc ratio
	Neuroretinal rim
Retinal vascular arcades and surrounding retina	
Macular region and foveal reflex	
Peripheral retinal quadrants	

examine the retina surrounding the vessel. Next move to the macula (by asking the patient to look straight at the light) and note if the foveal reflex appears normal; look for any abnormalities in the macular region. Finally examine the retinal quadrants in turn, asking the patient to look in the appropriate direction. For example, if the examiner wishes to look at the superior part of the retina, the patient is asked to look upwards.

The different filters and illuminators, such as the red-free filter, can be used as appropriate. Figure 5.7 shows some of the abnormalities that may be seen.

The interpretaton of abnormal findings is made in the light of the patient's clinical condition and therefore a history of systemic disease, as well as ocular symptoms, must be taken before the examination

begins. The system of fundus examination is summarised in Table 5.1.

Pitfalls in the use of the direct ophthalmoscope

It is important that the batteries in the instrument are charged or fresh so that adequate illumination is obtained. It is vital to ensure that the examiner's eye is close to the instrument on the examiner's side and that the instrument itself is very close to the patient's eye, usually within 2 cm. The closer to the patient's eye, the wider the angle of view. The commonest cause of difficulty in achieving a good retinal view is being too far away from the patient.

It is quite common for examiners to hold their breath while performing this examination and this limits the length of the examination to about 30 s or so. It is important, therefore, to make a conscious effort to breathe normally and this allows sustained examination of the retina.

It is common for patients to start looking in different directions and therefore necessary for the examiner to reassure them that they are doing well and to maintain their fixation on a particular spot, if possible.

Indications

Virtually every patient's fundus should be examined if possible and certainly when the examiner is a junior ophthalmologist in training. The more patients that are examined in this way, the better one becomes at the technique.

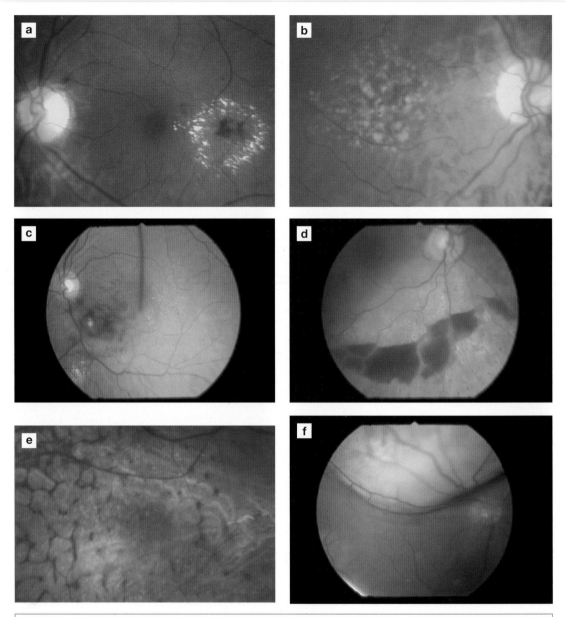

Fig. 5.7 Examples of retinal abnormalities. **(a)** Exudates in a circular (circinate) pattern with a retinal haemorrhage in the centre. **(b)** Drusen at the macula; note the margins are less distinct than those of the exudates. **(c)** The retinal haemorrhage here follows the pattern of the nerve fibre layer. The white lesion on the left is a cottonwool spot, a sign of retinal ischaemia. Note how it differs from the exudates and drusen. The retinal vein appears tortuous and swollen. This patient had a branch retinal vein occlusion. **(d)** A preretinal haemorrhage. **(e)** Pigmentary retinopathy: this patient had retinitis pigmentosa. **(f)** A choroidal melanoma.

Indirect ophthalmoscopy

This term was coined because it was found that, if one looked indirectly over the top of a direct ophthalmoscope, using it simply as a light source, and shone the light through a condensing lens, then a wide-angle inverted view of the fundus was obtained. Thus the original technique of indirect ophthalmoscopy was a monocular one. This was adapted in the 1960s with the development of the indirect ophthalmoscope, which utilises binocular vision and thus gives a very useful stereoscopic view of the fundus. A hat (headband) indirect ophthalmoscope and slit-lamp indirect lenses are available.

Hat (headband) indirect ophthalmoscope

Method of use

For binocular indirect ophthalmoscopy a dilated pupil is essential. The patient should ideally be lying on an examination couch situated so that the examiner is able to move around the patient's head. The patient is warned that the eye is going to be examined with a bright light.

A typical hat indirect ophthalmoscope is shown in Figure 5.8a. This has prisms built into the eyepieces to allow the observer's interpupillary distance to fit within the image of the patient's pupil. A +2 D lens is often built into the eyepiece of the indirect ophthalmoscope, which helps to reduce accommodative effort and is especially helpful to presbyopic surgeons! The headband is tightened and the sliders on the bottom of the eyepieces adjusted to suit the examiner. The illuminating beam is then adjusted so that it can be seen with both eyes and its height is altered so that the beam falls on the examiner's thumb when it is held at the level of the sternum and at arm's length. The brightness of the light is adjusted with the rheostat on the control box, or on the headset itself. The size of the illuminating light can be varied; a small beam is useful when looking through a small pupil. Some indirect ophthalmoscopes will also have a red-free and cobalt blue filter.

The examiner then positions him- or herself so that the eye to be viewed is illuminated by the headset (Fig. 5.8b). The indirect lens is then held at arm's length approximately 2 cm in front of the patient's eye in the path of the illuminating light. The white band on the lens casing should be pointing towards the patient. Moving the lens gently back-

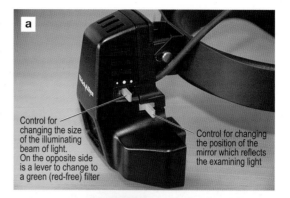

Control for changing the size of the illuminating beam of light. On the opposite side is a lever to change to a green (red-free) filter

Control for changing the position of the mirror which reflects the examining light

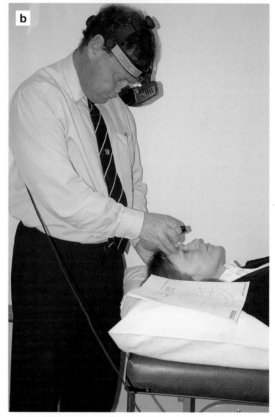

Fig. 5.8 (a) The indirect ophthalmoscope; **(b)** the indirect ophthalmoscope in use.

ward from the patient's eye should bring the retina into view. This takes practice! All movements of the lens should be small; gentle tilting may improve the view and help reduce unwanted reflections. The posterior pole and optic disc are first examined.

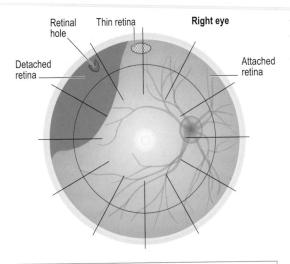

Fig. 5.9 A typical retinal drawing with annotated pathology.

The peripheral retina is viewed by asking the patient to look down and up and to the right and left. It is important that the examiner also moves around the patient to obtain the best view of the retina, making sure that the illumination light enters the eye at the most appropriate angle. The indirect light source and the examining lens must be kept in a straight line with the area of interest in the retina. This may involve bending the knees!

Although the upside-down and laterally inverted image takes some getting used to, if the patient is lying down on an examining couch and examined from the head end, then the view that is seen can be drawn directly on to a retinal diagram placed the right way up with respect to the examiner.

Figure 5.9 shows a typical retinal diagram with annotated pathology. These drawings are very important and useful if accurately drawn. Locating a retinal tear at surgery can be difficult, especially if the eye is gas-filled. Having a drawing to refer to can make locating breaks and other features easier by following vessels and noting relative positions of retinal lesions.

Indentation

A retinal indenter will both increase the peripheral view and throw some retinal lesions into relief (for example, retinal tears) so they are more easily seen. The patient is asked initially to look up or down

to facilitate placement of the indenter through the lower or upper lid respectively (Fig. 5.10). The patient then looks towards the indenter and the examiner gently presses on the indenter; a small indentation should be seen in the peripheral retina. The indenter is gently moved round the eye, and again the examiner needs to move around the patient to maximise the view.

Different-strength indirect lenses can be used under different circumstances and Table 5.2 shows their relative magnification factors. The standard is a 20 D lens but for a wider angle of view a 28 D is available. This latter lens is also useful for viewing the retina in a gas-filled eye. A 14 D is advantageous when examining the macula because of its greater magnification. The lower the power of the lens, the further from the patient's eye it needs to be held. Figure 5.11 shows the three commonly used lenses.

Pitfalls

A lot of practice is needed to ensure that the light source and examining lens are kept in direct line

Table 5.2	Different magnification effects of different lenses	
	Angle of view	**Magnification**
Contact lenses		
Area centralis	70°	0.94×
Transequator	110°	0.7×
Equator pus	114	0.44×
Macular pus 5.5	36°	5.32×
Three-mirror	60°/66°/76°	1.06×
Non-contact lenses		
Super 66	96°	1.0×
Super 90	116°	0.76×
20 D	46°	3.08×
28 D	53°	2.13×
14 D	36°	4.11×
40 D	69°	1.67×

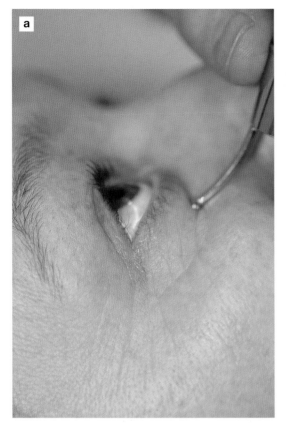
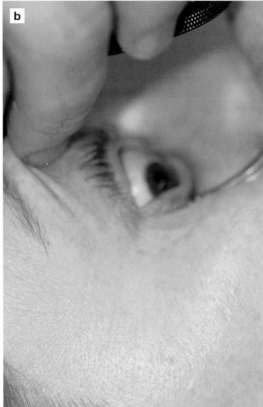

Fig. 5.10 (a) An indenter being used to push a peripheral part of the retina into view whilst using the indirect ophthalmoscope. The patient is asked to look up while the indenter is positioned. **(b)** The indenter is used to bring the inferior retina into view while the patient looks down.

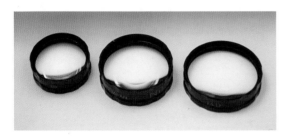

Fig. 5.11 The 28, 20 and 14 D lenses used with the indirect ophthalmoscope.

with the area of interest on the retina. It is common to try to move the examining lens in the wrong direction in order to bring the area of interest into view, because of the laterally inverted and upside-down image. Again, this is overcome fairly easily with regular practice.

Indications

Indirect ophthalmoscopy is used for examining the peripheral retina when looking for retinal holes. With indentation it can access the most peripheral parts of the retina. This form of ophthalmoscopy is also useful in overcoming media opacities such as cataract or vitreous haemorrhage to obtain a view of the retina.

Slit-lamp-based indirect lenses

90 D lens

The 90 D lens can be used to carry out indirect ophthalmoscopy using the slit lamp as a light

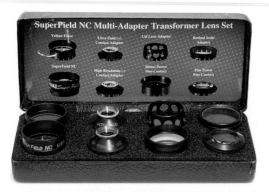

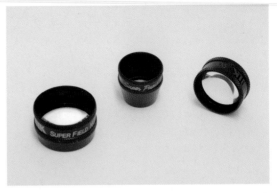

Fig. 5.12 The superfield lens with various attachments for obtaining wider or narrower (more magnified) views of the fundus as well as a graticule for measuring fundus lesions.

Fig. 5.13 Three non-contact fundus lenses: the superfield, the super pupil and the 90 D.

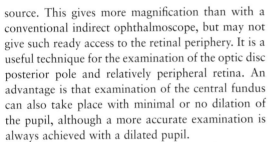

source. This gives more magnification than with a conventional indirect ophthalmoscope, but may not give such ready access to the retinal periphery. It is a useful technique for the examination of the optic disc posterior pole and relatively peripheral retina. An advantage is that examination of the central fundus can also take place with minimal or no dilation of the pupil, although a more accurate examination is always achieved with a dilated pupil.

Other commonly used non-contact lenses are variants of the 90 D such as the 60 D, the superfield NC (non-contact) and the 70 D lens. Table 5.2 shows their relative magnification factors. These must be taken into account when using the lenses to deliver laser energy to the fundus as different spot sizes will result with each lens. Light energy varies in power with the inverse-square law (twice the distance means a quarter of the energy), thus the relative magnification becomes important when trying to deliver a set amount of energy, for example, in photodynamic therapy.

Examples of the different lenses are shown in Figures 5.12 and 5.13.

Method of use (90 D)

The slit beam is positioned vertically and centrally in front of the patient's pupil. The short mirror should be in place. The lens is held as shown in Figure 5.14 parallel to the patient's cornea and close to it. The examiner's fingers can be used to support the eyelids. The slit beam thus passes through the lens and pupil to the retina. The slit lamp is then slowly drawn

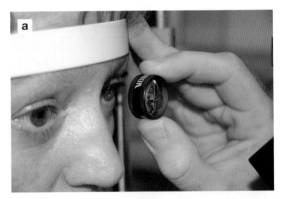

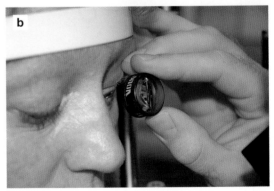

Fig. 5.14 (a) The 90 D lens being held vertically and parallel to the corneal plane with the light from the slit lamp central in the pupil and 90 D lens. **(b)** When the patient looks up the lens is tilted so that the top is moved towards the examiner and when looking down (as here), the lower edge is tilted towards the examiner.

backwards and towards the examiner whilst the examiner maintains a view through the binocular eyepieces until the inverted retinal image comes into focus. The slit beam is manipulated (see Ch. 2) to vary the area of retina being illuminated and the patient asked to look in the relevant direction to view different areas of the retina. The lens is tilted to look at various parts of the peripheral fundus (Fig. 5.14). Adjustment to the focus also allows the vitreous to be seen.

The system of examination is similar to that outlined for the direct ophthalmoscope.

Pitfalls

It must be remembered that the image obtained at the slit lamp through these lenses is upside down and laterally inverted. It is easy to get confused when drawing the fundus on a record card. The best way to ensure the correct representation of the fundus is to place the record sheet upside down on the slit-lamp table and draw the image as it is seen through the lens. When the record card is turned the correct way round, the picture will be correctly oriented.

Indications

This is a useful method of examination for patients in a general clinic to obtain a view of the fundus, even when the pupil is not dilated. It gives a reasonably magnified image and a good field of view. The optic disc is well seen and the stereoscopic view is useful in analysing the neuroretinal rim. It is also a useful method for delivering laser energy to the fundus, for it does not disturb the corneal surface, giving a clear image.

The Hruby lens

The Hruby lens used to be supplied with Haag–Streit slit lamps and comprises a −58.6 D lens (thus negating the optical strength of the eye) mounted on a manoeuvrable arm (Fig. 5.15). It is placed in the mounting hole of the slit lamp and positioned with its plano surface towards the examiner and close to the patient's eye. The slit is used as an illumination source and the slit lamp is drawn back or forwards from the eye until focus is obtained. The ridge on the bottom of the mounting spike slots into the central groove on the base plate. This keeps the lens within the working range automatically as the slit lamp is manoeuvred during the examination. It produces a right-way-round life-size image of the fundus.

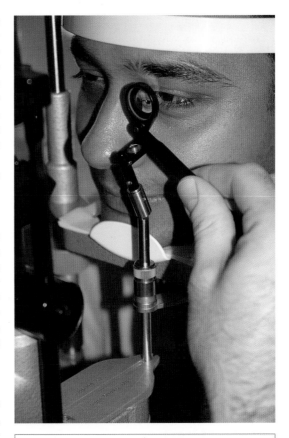

Fig. 5.15 The Hruby lens, now largely superseded by other non-contact lenses, in use with the slit lamp.

Contact lenses for retinal examination

A number of contact lenses can be used to view the fundus and periphery of the retina. The traditional lens used in the clinic is the Goldmann three-mirror lens, which has a central viewing portion for looking at the disc and macula and three differently angled mirrors for viewing the retinal periphery and also the anterior-chamber drainage angle. The mirrors are usually set at 60, 66 and 76° (Fig. 5.16). The steeper-set lens is smaller and is used for gonioscopy.

These can give a greater degree of control over the image obtained as they stabilise the eye to a degree. Some, like the Mainster macular lens (Fig. 5.17a), give a high magnification and are useful for diagnosing and treating macular pathology. These lenses use a fluid contact medium to form the

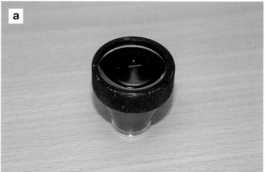

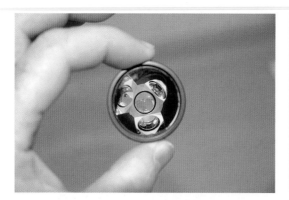

Fig. 5.16 The Goldmann three-mirror lens with three differently angled mirrors and a central clear area for macular and disc examination.

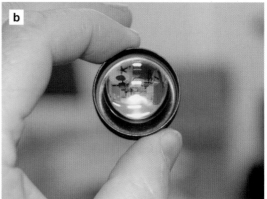

interface between the cornea and the lens. The area centralis lens is also useful for macular work whilst the transequatorial lens (Fig. 5.17b) gives a wide-angle view and is useful for delivering laser to the retinal periphery when applying panretinal photocoagulation or treating a retinal break.

Method of use

Goldmann three-mirror

The cornea is anaesthetised with topical anaesthetic such as proxymetacaine and a coupling agent such as 1% hydroxypropyl methylcellulose is applied to the well of the contact lens (see Ch. 4 for a discussion on the microbiological aspects of diagnostic contact lens use). The lens is carefully applied to the eye: the examiner should inform patients that they may feel it touch the eyelids but not the eye. This must be accomplished quickly if the coupling medium is not to be lost; it may help to ask the patient to look up when the lens is being applied. The patient then looks straight ahead and the slit beam is aimed on to the mirror to be used. The lens is then rotated on the eye to obtain views of different parts of the peripheral retina. The patient can also be asked to move the eye in a particular direction to bring more peripheral retina into view.

Pitfalls

Trapping air between the contact lens and the cornea can degrade the image and this is avoided by using a relatively viscous coupling agent. Corneal abrasions

Fig. 5.17 (a) The Mainster macular contact lens. This gives a magnified view of the macula and allows some control over eye movements during laser treatment. **(b)** The transequatorial lens gives a wide-angle view of the fundus. It is ideal for applying panretinal photocoagulation.

can be caused if manipulations are not gentle, or if there is corneal pathology such as Fuchs' dystrophy, leading to an oedematous corneal epithelium. Care should be taken in patients who are immediately postoperative. The conjunctiva and other tissues may be inflamed and sensitive and infection could be introduced with use of the lens.

Other contact lenses are applied in the same way but the fundus is viewed directly through the lens. Some of these lenses will also provide an inverted view of the fundus.

Indications

The Goldmann three-mirror lens provides an excellent view of the peripheral retina. The disadvantage of the contact lens methods is that they have to touch the eye. They are particularly useful in delivering laser therapy.

Summary

Direct and indirect, contact and non-contact methods are available for viewing the fundus. The choice of techniques depends on the clinical situation. A direct ophthalmoscope is useful for examination of the optic disc and posterior pole, particularly when a slit lamp is not to hand. Indirect techniques allow a better view of the retinal periphery and provide a stereoscopic image. Slit-lamp-based indirect methods also allow an excellent view of the optic disc and macula.

- Examination of the retina is best done in a systematic way so that nothing is missed
- Practice is needed in examining the retina as the images seen are often inverted, laterally and vertically
- Magnification factors must be taken into account with the various lenses used, especially where the size of lesions or laser spot size for treatment is important
- Non-contact lenses are a useful alternative for postoperative patients – avoiding the possibility of transferring infection and manipulation of inflamed tissue

Further reading

Kanski J. Clinical ophthalmology. Oxford: Butterworth-Heinemann; 2003.

Mainster MA, Crossman JL, Erickson PJ et al. Retinal laser lenses: magnification, spot size and field of view. Br J Ophthalmol 1990; 74: 177–179.

Ryan SJ, Hinton DR, Schachat AP, Wilkinson CP. Retina. St Louis, MO: Mosby; 2005.

Spalton DJ, Hitchings RA, Hunter PA et al. Atlas of clinical ophthalmology. St Louis, MO: Mosby; 2004.

Varma R, Spaeth GL. The optic nerve in glaucoma. Philadelphia: JB Lippincott; 1993.

Optical and anatomical assessment of the cornea

LARRY BENJAMIN

Introduction

The cornea accounts for two-thirds of the refractive power of the eye. Small changes in corneal curvature can have a dramatic effect on image formation. Changes in corneal clarity also have a dramatic effect on visual acuity. This chapter examines how the refractive power of the cornea can be measured (keratometry) and how the anatomical structure of the eye can be quantified (pachymetry and specular microscopy) and looks at new techniques for assessing the optical properties of the eye as a whole (wavefront aberrometry).

Keratometry

Keratometry is used to assess corneal shape, curvature and regularity, giving information about its refractive power. Just as small changes in corneal curvature cause a large change in corneal power, so small errors in measurement can affect the accuracy of calculations based on them, for example biometry (see Ch. 13).

Keratometry is possible because the cornea acts as a convex mirror as well as a lens. The keratometer measures the reflection of an illuminated image of known size and position. This allows the radius of curvature of the mirror (or the anterior surface of the cornea) to be calculated. These measurements assume a refractive index of between 1.332 and 1.3375 for the cornea; different machines use different values.

Most of these instruments are designed to assess the central 3 or 4 mm of the cornea, as this is optically the most important part. However, in modern refractive surgery the asphericity of the peripheral cornea can have an important bearing on optical outcomes.

Instruments

Placido disc

A Placido disc comprises a plate of alternate black and white rings concentrically placed around a convex viewing lens (Fig. 6.1). It enables a qualitative estimate of corneal shape to be made. The central lens allows close viewing of the reflection of the rings from the anterior corneal surface when the examiner holds the disc to his or her eye. It is important to illuminate the disc from behind the patient so that a bright reflection is seen from the cornea (Fig. 6.2). The reflected image will normally show little distortion of the rings, unless the cornea has an irregular shape when the reflection will appear distorted (Fig. 6.3).

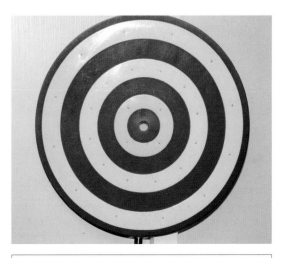

Fig. 6.1 A Placido disc. Illuminated versions are also available. A central 2 D lens aids focusing on the patient's cornea.

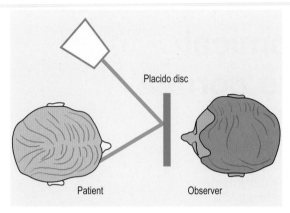

Fig. 6.2 Ilumination of the Placido disc.

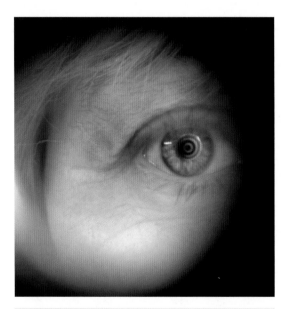

Fig. 6.3 A normal reflection from a Placido disc.

Keratometers

Prior to the introduction of computerised topography, the main types of keratometer in clinical practice were the Javal–Schiotz and the Helmholtz machines. They work on slightly different principles. With the Javal–Schiotz the object size is varied to achieve a standard image size; with the Helmholtz, the object size is fixed and the image size is adjusted.

In theory it would be possible to measure the size of the image reflected from the cornea with a graticule and, if the object size and position were known, calculate the radius of curvature of the cornea. In practice this would be difficult because the eye is constantly moving. This problem has been overcome in the keratometer by incorporating a doubling prism into the system to provide two images of the object or mire. This comprises two prisms joined together so that one moves the image up and the other moves the image down. Altering the position of the prism will alter the size of the doubled image. As the prism moves towards the object the distance separating the two images is reduced, and eventually they can be made to touch. At this point the size of the reflected image and the size of the doubled image are equal. The image size can then be calculated from the relative position of the doubling prism. This is how the Helmholtz keratometer works.

Alternatively the position of the prism is kept constant and the size of the object changed to match that of the doubled image. This method has been adopted in the Javal–Schiotz keratometer.

The doubled image will move with the eye and thus can still be aligned, although significant eye movement will change the area of cornea being measured.

Javal–Schiotz keratometer

The two illuminated objects or mires comprise a rectangular orange box and a green double-staircase shape (Fig. 6.4). There is a 1 D difference in each step of the staircase. The mires can be moved in

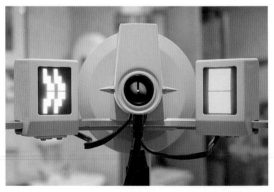

Fig. 6.4 The Jarval–Schiotz keratometer: patient's view during a measurement. The patient is asked to look into the central telescope.

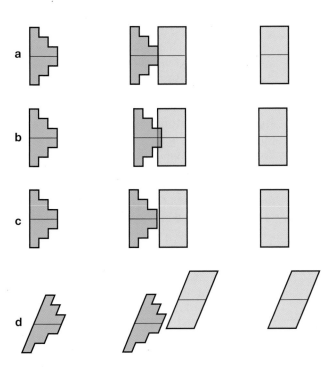

Fig. 6.5 The appearance of the mires to the observer. **(a)** The correct position: the inner images just touch. **(b)** The object (separation of the mires) is not great enough. **(c)** The separation of the mires is too great. **(d)** The axis of the keratometer and the meridian of the astigmatism are not aligned. The lines in the centre of each mire should be level; the keratometer should be rotated until this is so.

equal and opposite directions around an arc with the subject's eye at the centre. Moving the mires apart increases the object size, while moving them closer together decreases the object size. The mires can also be rotated around the optical axis to measure any meridian of the cornea. A fixed Wollaston doubling prism is incorporated behind the objective lens.

The examiner observes the reflection of the images through a telescope. It is important that the images are clearly focused and that the eyepiece has been adjusted for the examiner (see Ch. 13). This ensures that the object distance from the lens is constant. Using the Vernier device to adjust the position of the mires, the doubled image of the two illuminated shapes is made just to touch (Fig. 6.5). The radius of curvature is then read directly from the scale (Fig. 6.6). The units of measurement are dioptres of refractive power or millimetres radius of curvature. The smaller the radius of curvature, the steeper the cornea and the greater the refractive power of the corneal surface.

If keratometry is being performed as part of cataract biometry, it is sensible to take the keratometric measurements first as the use of a contact ultrasound probe can disturb the ocular surface and may make taking keratometry readings difficult. Similarly,

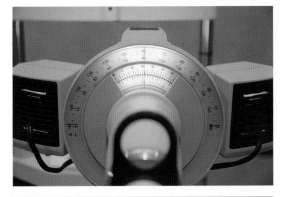

Fig. 6.6 The scale on the Javal–Shiotz keratometer showing the meridian being assessed and the dioptric power measured.

asking the patient to blink just before the readings are taken can aid measurement as the tear film will be refreshed and provide a smooth optical surface.

Helmholtz keratometer

Here the size of the object is fixed but the doubled image is adjusted by varying the position of the prism. The object mire is an illuminated circle with

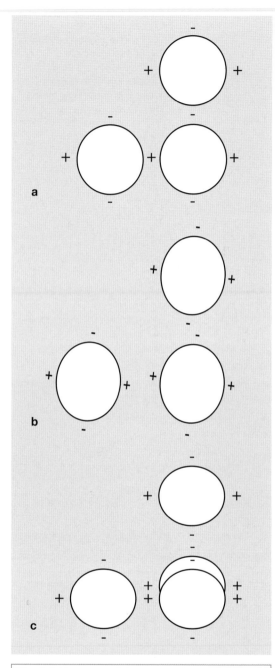

a + and – marker separated by 90° (Fig. 6.7). The vertical and horizontal position of the prisms are adjusted until the images are correctly aligned (Fig. 6.7a). The radius of curvature is read from the dials used to adjust prism position.

Recording keratometry results

Most corneas are toric, that is, they show some degree of astigmatism. Toric surfaces have maximum power running in one direction (meridian) and minimum power, usually but not always, at right angles to the first meridian. The analogy commonly used to explain this concept to patients is that of a rugby ball, which has similar properties. For any toric surface it is important to record not only the power or curvature of the principal meridians, but also the direction (axis) in which they lie. Returning to our example of the rugby ball, it can lie on its side, on end, or anywhere in between. Figure 6.8 shows the standard axis notation used to record the direction of astigmatism.

Keratometry results should be recorded as corneal curvature or power *along* a given meridian direction. The @ symbol is often used to denote 'along', for example, 7.35 mm @ 140 or 45.17 D @ 140. The degree symbol (°) should be omitted. Unless the cornea is perfectly spherical, there will be two readings, for example:

7.35 mm @ 140	or	+45.17 D @ 140
8.05 mm @ 50	or	+41.24 D @ 50

Some keratometers have two axis scales running in opposite directions. The user is strongly recommended to estimate the approximate axis of the meridian that is being measured by inspecting the position of the mires, using a trial frame or Figure

Fig. 6.7 Alignment of the mires with a Helmholtz-type keratometer. **(a)** The mires are correctly aligned: the + of the horizontal images overlap and the – of the vertical images overlap. **(b)** The axis of this patient's astigmatism is not aligned with the axis of the keratometer. **(c)** The focus of the keratometer is incorrect.

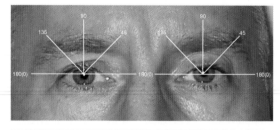

Fig. 6.8 Axis notation. Note that the same notation is used for both eyes, and that 180 rather than zero is used for horizontal.

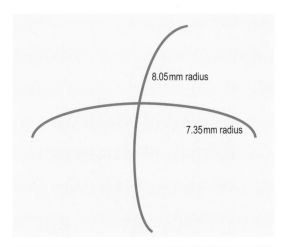

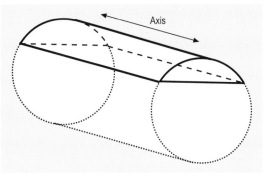

Fig. 6.10 An optical cylinder.

Fig. 6.9 Example toric surface showing two surface powers running perpendicular to each other.

6.8, and to ensure that it agrees with the scale that is used to read the result.

There is more than one way to record the power of a toric surface, and this is a common source of confusion even for experienced surgeons. The term *axis* is particularly troublesome unless its meaning is clear.

Take for example the surface in Figure 6.9. Assuming a refractive index of 1.332 it has keratometry readings of:

| 7.35 mm @ 180 | or | +45.17 D @ 180 |
| 8.05 mm @ 90 | or | +41.24 D @ 90 |

The same surface can be written in a notation called crossed-cylinder. A cylinder such as a drink can is curved in only one direction, the other being flat. Figure 6.10 shows a section cut from a glass cylinder. In similar fashion to a toric surface, it has power in one direction, but zero power at right angles to that. The direction along which a cylinder has zero power is known as the cylinder axis.

A section cut from a cylinder of radius 7.35 mm and stood on its end, i.e. with its axis vertical, would have a power of +45.17 dioptres of cylinder power (DC) horizontally, and zero along its axis. This would be written as +45.17 DC axis 90 or +45.17 DC × 90. A second cylinder of radius 8.05 mm with its axis horizontal would have a power of +41.24 DC × 180. If we placed those two

cylinders back to back, perpendicular to each other, the resultant power would be:

+45.17 DC × 90
+41.24 DC × 180

There is yet another way to write this same surface power, and that is in sphere-cylinder notation, commonly used for spectacle prescriptions. Writing the first power as a sphere, and the difference between the two as the cylinder, we get:

$$\frac{+45.17 \text{ DS}}{-3.93 \text{ DC} \times 180}$$

Alternatively, we can write the second power as the sphere, and again, the difference between the two gives the cylinder power:

$$\frac{+41.24 \text{ DS}}{+3.93 \text{ DC} \times 90}$$

All these notations describe exactly the same surface power, but note that the *axis* has changed compared with the keratometry readings. For this reason, the × symbol used in crossed-cylinder or sphere-cylinder notation should never be used in recording keratometry results.

Hand-held keratometers

These devices are invaluable for bed-bound patients or those who cannot sit upright at the slit lamp (Fig. 6.11). They are also useful for children who are having cataract surgery and who cannot cooperate with normal measurements as they can be used on anaesthetized patients.

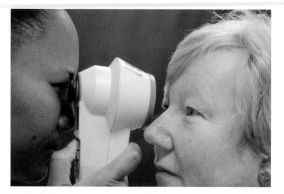

Fig. 6.11 The hand-held keratometer in use.

Hand-held keratometers have an inbuilt mechanism for measuring tilt and will be accurate within 15° of the horizontal plane.

Computerised topography

Modern topography is used to map the surface of the cornea accurately (Fig. 6.12). The maps so produced, unlike a contour map of the land, do not show the physical elevation of the cornea, but the distribution of its power in dioptres. This is related to corneal curvature. Most devices measure the central 3–4 mm and thus often miss important data relating to corneal asphericity at the periphery. The principle used for measurement is the same as for the Placido disc but the image of the rings is captured by a video

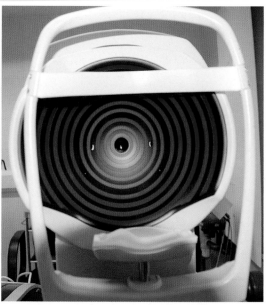

Fig. 6.12 A computerised corneal topography machine.

capture card and stored and interpreted by the computer. A typical corneal map is shown in Figure 6.13. The main image shows the distribution of corneal power. A bowtie shape is usual. The steepest and flattest meridians are also shown with their relevant axes and power.

Fig. 6.13 A typical normal bowtie configuration from a corneal topography machine. Also shown are the steepest and flattest meridians.

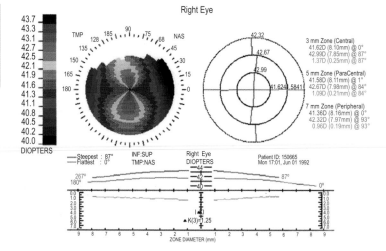

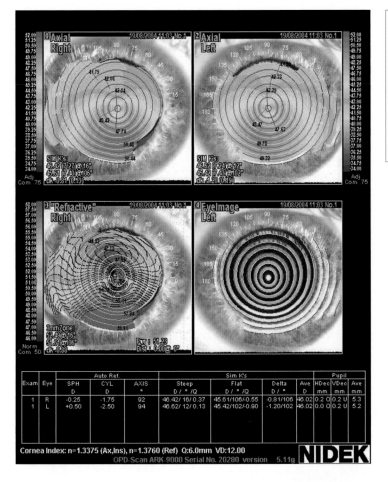

Fig. 6.14 Multiple results printed out from a single corneal topography reading. The topography rings reflected from the cornea are seen in the lower right frame with coloured rings drawn by the computer which allow analysis of the distance between the rings and thus effective corneal power.

Additional measurements are available on different machines and these can include the video image of the corneal reflections, a contact lens fitting map and superimposition of the map on the rings (Fig. 6.14).

The Orbscan topographer simultaneously scans the anterior and posterior surfaces of the cornea, thus giving additional clinical and optical information which may be useful for refractive surgery.

Intraoperative keratometry

It may be necessary to assess corneal curvature during surgery, for example to help adjust the tightness of sutures during a corneal transplant. Microscope-mounted light-emitting diodes are available for this purpose, as is an intraoperative vertically mounted keratoscope. These options are, however, relatively expensive. More economical is the use of either a Maloney keratoscope (Fig. 6.15) or the circular end

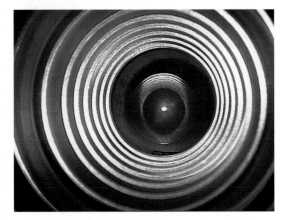

Fig. 6.15 The Maloney keratoscope. A version for the slit lamp is also available. It gives a qualitative assessment of corneal curvature.

of a safety pin. These can be held in the light path of the microscope above a wetted corneal surface and the reflection of the circular end used to assess to regularity of the corneal surface. A modification of this has been developed into a quantifiable device (Morlet and Lindsay, 1995).

Sources of error

As with all instruments, it is important that the keratometer is looked after and regularly serviced and calibrated. It must be correctly set up and focused, if applicable. In addition to errors that may result from a poorly serviced instrument the following problems may occur:

- An irregular or dry corneal surface can give inaccurate readings or at least make it difficult to take readings. The presence of scars or previous surgery (corneal transplantation, trauma repair, old keratitis) can also cause problems. Sometimes the application of 0.3 or 1% hypromellose to the ocular surface gives a smoother surface for measurements, although interpreting data obtained in this way must be done cautiously.
- If the patient looks off-axis an erroneous reading will result. Misalignment of the viewing telescope or capture system will cause similar errors.

- Previous laser refractive surgery can lead to erroneous readings with a marked difference between central and peripheral readings. The curvature of the posterior corneal surface may also be affected, as may the refractive index of the cornea itself.
- Recording results '90° off': as mentioned earlier, reading the wrong scale will result in the two meridians being reversed. If these results were used to place a corneal incision so as to reduce astigmatism, the effect would be to increase the astigmatism instead.

Application of keratometry

Biometry

An essential part of modern cataract and refractive surgery practice, keratometry combined with axial length measurements forms preoperative biometry. For each change in radius of curvature of 1 mm of the anterior corneal surface, the corneal power changes by 6 D. Accurate measurements are therefore essential (see Ch. 13).

Monitoring disease progression

Keratometry is a useful method of recording and monitoring corneal changes in keratoconus (Fig. 6.16).

Fig. 6.16 Corneal map of a patient with keratoconus showing the typically downwardly displaced cone.

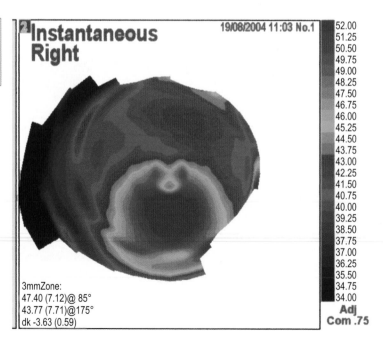

Instantaneous Right

19/08/2004 11:03 No.1

52.00
51.25
50.50
49.75
49.00
48.25
47.50
46.75
46.00
45.25
44.50
43.75
43.00
42.25
41.50
40.75
40.00
39.25
38.50
37.75
37.00
36.25
35.50
34.75
34.00

3mmZone:
47.40 (7.12)@ 85°
43.77 (7.71)@175°
dk -3.63 (0.59)

Adj
Com .75

Contact lenses

Accurate lens fitting requires careful assessment of the corneal curvature and axes of astigmatism. However, it should be borne in mind that keratometers only measure the central 3 mm or so, while a soft contact lens typically has a diameter of 14 mm. Contact lenses should be left out of the eye for at least 2 days (soft lenses) or for a minimum of 2 weeks (hard lenses) before keratometry is performed if the results are to be used for laser refractive surgery on the cornea. Wearing lenses can temporarily alter corneal shape and therefore refractive power.

Refractive surgery

Keratometry or corneal mapping is essential as part of the preoperative assessment for laser or incisional refractive surgery, including cataract surgery. The corneal power map so produced is useful for following changes as the cornea heals and also for determining the steep axis around which incisional surgical manoeuvres are made.

Assessing corneal aberrations

Wavefront aberrometry

Although keratometry can be used to assess some abnormalities of corneal shape, it is becoming evident that some visual symptoms are better analysed and described by the effect that the optical systems of the eye have on the quality of vision. Although in its infancy in terms of understanding, wavefront analysis or aberrometry is fast becoming popular in assessing the optical properties of the eye. Increasingly, research is being directed at the use of the technique in modifying treatments such as corneal reshaping with excimer laser by using wavefront-guided treatment algorithms that may give 'better' results. This has yet to be substantiated with a controlled clinical trial.

Essentially wavefront machines (Fig. 6.17) send a pulse of infrared light into the eye and analyse the front of the waveform that is reflected back out of the eye (the wavefront), thus deducing what effect the eye's optical characteristics have had on the initial wave sent in. Various algorithms are used to analyse the wavefront, including Zernicke polynomial equations and Fourier analysis. By estimating the relative contribution of different aberrations caused by the eye's optical surfaces, attempts can be made to

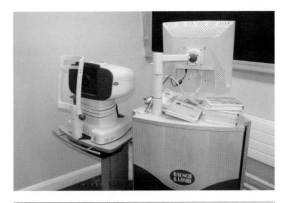

Fig. 6.17 Picture of the Bausch and Lomb wavefront analyser. This utilises Zernicke polynomial equations to analyse the emitted wavefront aberrations.

iron these out by treating the eye with, for example, the excimer laser.

The technique may help explain some postoperative problems following cataract surgery. The following case serves as an example. After cataract surgery a patient complained bitterly that the vision was 'not right': she was seeing 'sheets of light' and had other visual symptoms. Wavefront analysis showed a significant amount of spherical aberration (Fig. 6.18a, b). Her implant was swapped for one with an aspheric front surface, relieving her of her symptoms.

The aberrometer allows the various higher-order optical aberrations such as spherical aberration, coma and trefoil to be 'switched off' by the software to examine the effect on the wavefront. Once a wavefront map has been generated and is displayed on screen, the software allows the examiner to 'remove' higher-order aberrations one at a time by clicking on a screen icon (Fig. 6.18). The software then shows a modified wavefront map without that particular aberration or group of aberrations present to see which particular aberration is potentially a cause of disturbed vision. Thus it can be a useful technique when diagnosing optical symptoms in pre- and postoperative patients. It must be stressed however that there still remains much work to be done on what are and what are not important higher-order aberrations in terms of quality of vision.

Fig. 6.18 (a) The preoperative wavefront analysis showing spherical aberration.
(b) Removing spherical aberration from the wavefront picture shows the resulting image to be significantly changed, suggesting that the major contribution came from spherical aberration.

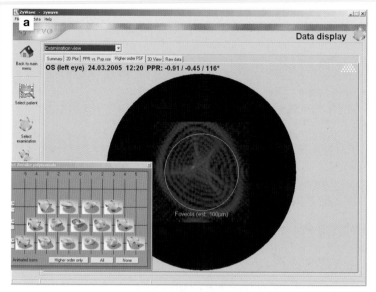

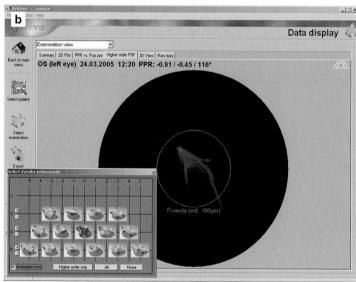

Specular microscopy

This technique allows an estimation of endothelial cell density. The corneal endothelium is responsible for dehydrating the cornea and keeping it clear.

Specific specular microscopes are available; alternatively there are adaptors for slit lamps and photo slit lamps (Fig. 6.19). They allow a small area of corneal endothelium to be imaged and the cell density estimated by using the sampled area as representative of the whole cornea.

The usual cell density at birth is around 4000 cells per square millimetre and during a normal lifetime around half this number is lost. When the count drops below about 1000 cells/mm^2 then function starts to be affected and increased diurnal variation in vision occurs, as the cornea absorbs water from the eyelids at night, resulting in significant thickening of the stroma.

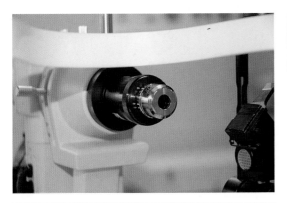

Fig. 6.19 The specular microscope attachment on a photo slit lamp for examining endothelial cells.

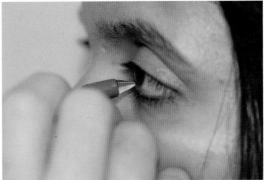

Fig. 6.20 The ultrasonic pachymeter being used to assess regional corneal thickness.

Pachymetry

Pachymetry is used to measure the thickness of the cornea. It provides an indirect means of assessing corneal endothelial function. As indicated above, if the endothelium is damaged, stromal thickening occurs. It is a useful method of assessing corneal function and recovery after a corneal transplant. Optical pachymetry is described in Chapter 2 and is often used to measure the central corneal thickness. It is also important to know what the central corneal thickness is in patients with glaucoma as this can affect the measurement of intraocular pressure (see Ch. 3).

Regional pachymetry, measurement of multiple points on the cornea, is part of the work-up for refractive surgery. For example, the peripheral corneal thickness must be known before embarking on arcuate keratotomy so that penetration into the anterior chamber does not occur.

This is readily and easily achieved with an ultrasonic pachymeter (Fig. 6.20). Beware, however, of measurement artefact, as if the cornea is thickened by increased corneal water content, the velocity of the ultrasonic wave will be altered.

- Structure and function are closely related in the cornea
- Small changes in corneal curvature cause significant optical effects
- Careful measurements of corneal curvature are essential to avoid large errors arising from the examination technique used
- An adequate tear film is important for measurements relying on reflection from the anterior corneal surface – lid disease can thus disturb such measurements by upsetting the regularity of the corneal surface

References and further reading

Corbett MC, Rosen E, O'Brart D, Stevenson R. Corneal topography: principles and applications. London: BMJ Books; 1999.

Elkington AR, Franks HJ. Clinical optics. Missouri: Blackwell Scientific; 1984.

Leyland M, Benjamin L. Clinical assessment of a hand-held automated keratometer in cataract surgery. Eye 1997; 11: 854–857.

Morlet N, Lindsay PA. Intraoperative semiquantitative keratometry using the keratoscopic astigmatic ruler. J Cataract Refract Surg 1995; 21: 616–619.

Testing the visual field

BRUCE JAMES

Introduction

The mapping of the extent of the visual world is important in the diagnosis of disorders affecting the optic nerve and visual pathway. It may also give information about some retinal conditions such as retinitis pigmentosa. The visual field is not flat: smaller or dimmer objects can be detected in the centre of the field, corresponding to the fovea, than in the periphery of the field. This produces a 'hill of vision' (Fig. 7.1). The blind spot on the temporal aspect of the field corresponds to the optic nerve where there are no photoreceptors.

Visual fields may be tested simply at the bedside by confrontation tests and more comprehensively on manual and automated perimeters. Two major strategies for testing fields are available: static and kinetic perimetry. In static perimetry the brightness or size of an object within the field is increased until patients can see it. In kinetic perimetry patients indicate when they first see an object of fixed size or

brightness as it is slowly moved from outside the visual field centrally. Newer forms of perimetric testing assess the patient's ability to detect the movement of a stimulus within the visual field.

The visual field

The field of vision in each eye extends from the visual axis approximately superiorly to 60°, inferiorly to 75°, temporally to 100° and nasally to 60° (Fig. 7.2). Over some 120° centrally objects can be seen by both eyes (Fig. 7.3). The visibility of a spot within the field will depend on its size, the intensity of the light, movement, colour of the object and the duration of stimulus presentation. The background illumination against which the object is seen is also important. Within each visual field is the blind spot. This lies at 10–15° temporally. It measures 6° horizontally and 8° vertically.

The threshold of a stimulus indicates the brightness of a static object of fixed size against a stable

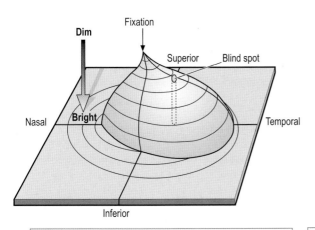

Fig. 7.1 The hill of vision.

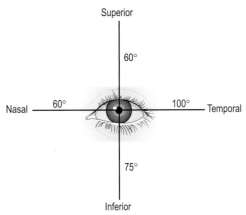

Fig. 7.2 The extent of the visual field.

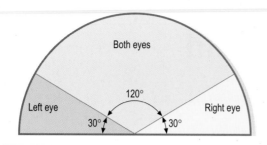

Fig. 7.3 The binocular visual field.

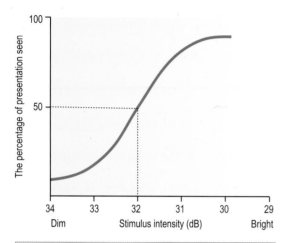

Fig. 7.4 The frequency-of-seeing curve. The threshold is the intensity of the stimulus which gives a 50% chance of it being seen at that point in the visual field. In this example it is 32 dB.

background that, when presented to a subject a number of times, would be identified 50% of the time. A suprathreshold stimulus would be seen 95% of the time. This is graphically represented on a frequency-of-seeing curve (Fig. 7.4). Parts of the visual field with the same threshold can be linked with a line, termed an isoptre. These resemble contour lines and thus enable the three-dimensional hill of vision to be represented in two dimensions (Fig. 7.5). In automated perimetry the individual threshold of each point tested is reported, usually in decibels. The greater the number, the *dimmer* the stimulus.

Confrontation field testing

These techniques are useful in examining for gross defects. They can be performed at a number of levels. Carefully executed, with a thorough explanation to the patient beforehand, they can reveal much important information.

Light projection

This is useful in those with very poor vision. A bright light is shone into the eye in each quadrant and switched on and off; the patient has to say when the light is seen. Each quadrant of the eye is tested in turn. It is important to ensure that the fellow eye is completely occluded.

Hand identification

The examiner asks the patient to cover one eye. Both of the examiner's hands are held in front of the other eye at a distance of 50 cm (Fig. 7.6). The patients fixes on the examiner's nose which is visible between the two hands and is asked to report whether the two hands appear identical. Patients with a temporal or nasal hemisphere defect will report that one hand appears absent or indistinct. Those with an altitudinal hemispherical defect will report that the palm or fingers of both hands are missing or faint.

Finger-counting

The patient covers one eye and fixes on the examiner's nose. The examiner holds a varying number of fingers in each quadrant of the patient's visual field at a distance of about 1 m and at 45° from fixation. Points at 1.30, 4.30, 7.30 and 10.30 clock-hours are then tested (Fig. 7.7). The patient reports how many fingers are seen. If the fingers are not seen correctly they are moved towards fixation until they are identified – this is a simple form of kinetic perimetry. Alternatively they can be brought into view from the examiner's fist in stages closer to fixation – static perimetry.

Testing with a neurological pin

This is essentially a more refined version of finger-counting using a smaller object, usually a red or white neurological pin. The patient covers an eye and fixes on the examiner's nose. The object, held at arm's length from the patient, is slowly introduced into the visual field from the periphery. The patient is asked to say when the object is seen (kinetic

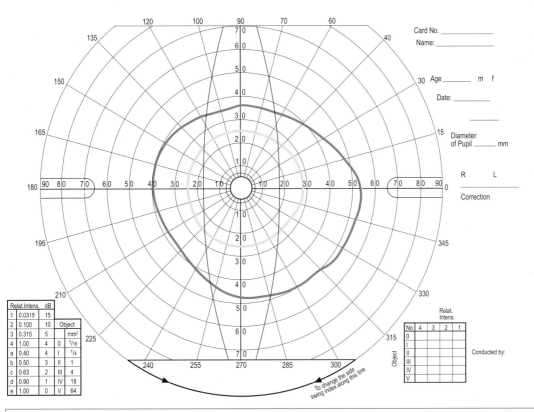

Relat.Intens.		dB
1	0.0315	15
2	0.100	10
3	0.315	5
4	1.00	4
a	0.40	4
b	0.50	3
c	0.63	2
d	0.90	1
e	1.00	0

	Object	
		mm²
0		¹/₁₆
I		¹/₄
II		1
III		4
IV		18
V		64

To change the side swing index along this line

Object	Relat. Intens.				
	No	4	3	2	1
	0				
	I				
	II				
	III				
	IV				
	V				

Conducted by:

Fig. 7.5 Contour mapping of the hill of vision with isoptres. The lines link parts of the field with the same threshold. The colours represent the threshold to different intensities of stimulus. The red, a very dim light, is only seen at the very top of the hill of vision by the fovea. The blue, a bright light, can be seen over a much wider area.

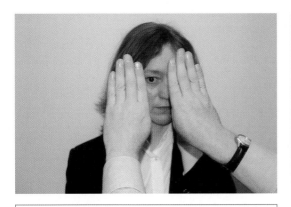

Fig. 7.6 Hand identification, testing the visual field.

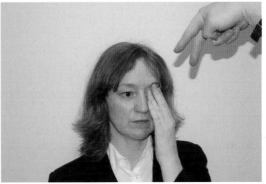

Fig. 7.7 Finger-counting testing of the visual field.

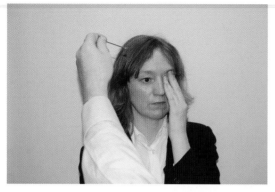

Fig. 7.8 Testing the visual field with a neurological pin.

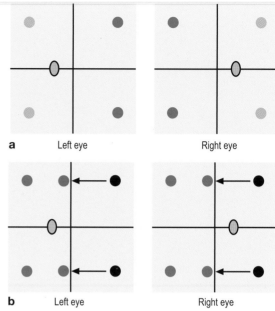

a   Left eye   Right eye

b   Left eye   Right eye

Fig. 7.9 (a) Red desaturation on a patient with a bitemporal hemianopia. The red in the temporal field is perceived as being 'less red' than in the normal nasal field. **(b)** This patient has a left homonymous hemianopia. Static testing shows that red is only appreciated on the right hemifield of both eyes. On crossing the midline from the affected to the unaffected field the patient suddenly perceives the red object.

testing) (Fig. 7.8). It is possible to use this test to compare the patients's field to that of the examiner. Facing one another the test object is held equidistant between the two, both occluding the untested eye. The patient and examiner should be at the same level.

A red pin is particularly useful in looking for neurological defects. Here patients must understand that they have to indicate when they see the pin as a red object. This will occur after they can identify an object entering the visual field.

Red desaturation

A red object of some 1–2 cm of any sort can also be used to compare quadrants of the visual field to check for colour desaturation, again a sign that is particularly useful in detecting a neurological field defect (Fig. 7.9). The nasal and temporal halves of the field or superior and inferior halves of the field are compared, asking patients to say if they note a difference in the quality of the colour in different parts of the field. For example a patient with a bitemporal hemianopia should report that the object appears less red, or washed out in the temporal half of the field of each eye (Fig. 7.9a). This can be confirmed kinetically by asking the patient to indicate when the colour appears to change as the object is moved from the normal to the abnormal field. In a temporal hemianopia this should occur at the vertical midline.

Colour desaturation can also be used to test for differences between the two eyes in the appreciation of red, which is useful if a patient is thought to have an optic neuropathy.

Goldmann perimetry

Although largely replaced by automated perimeters, the Goldmann perimeter still has a place in testing patients for neurological field defects (Fig. 7.10). Essentially a spot of light, the size and intensity of which can be adjusted by the perimetrist, is projected into a large bowl of uniform background illumination. The test must be fully explained to the patient. One eye is tested at a time; the other eye is comfortably occluded. The chin is supported on a rest and the patient is asked to observe a central fixation target. A near-vision correction, if required, is placed in the lens-holder. This is positioned as close to the eye as possible. The position of the patient's eye and

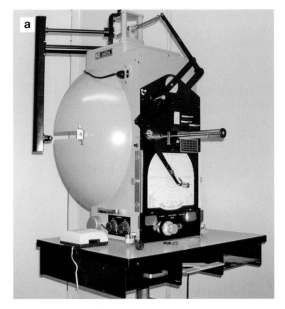

the reliability of fixation can be observed by the perimetrist through a telescope.

Kinetic perimetry

The size and intensity of the light stimulus are selected. This is then moved slowly from the periphery to the centre of the field of vision, at 3–5°/s, by means of a pantograph arm. Patients indicate that they can see the object by pressing the buzzer on a hand piece. The perimetrist records this point on the chart positioned in the chart-holder of the machine. The light source is occluded with a shutter on the right of the machine so that the patient is unable to see the stimulus move to another segment of the field and the test is repeated. In this manner an isoptre for the stimulus can be constructed. A second isoptre with a different size and intensity can then be plotted (Fig. 7.5).

Illuminating the target within the expected position of the blind spot (10–15° from fixation, just below the horizontal meridian) and then moving it until observed by the subject allow the size of the blind spot to be plotted.

Static perimetry

The patient is positioned as for kinetic perimetry but instead of moving a visible target into the visual field, the target is brought into the position to be tested, held stationary and then illuminated for approximately half a second by releasing the shutter lever. If the patient fails to respond the illumination is occluded, the intensity of the target light increased and the process repeated until the patient sees the target. This is taken to be the threshold intensity for that point in the visual field. Additional points are then tested in a similar way.

Types of field defect

The type of field defect present is of obvious diagnostic significance. A scotoma is a focal region of decreased sensitivity surrounded by an area of normal sensitivity (Fig. 7.11). It is absolute if the brightest stimuli cannot be seen within it. For example, the blind spot is an absolute scotoma. If a brighter than expected stimulus can be perceived then it is termed a relative scotoma. A depression is an area of reduced sensitivity without a surrounding area of normal sensitivity. It may appear on the

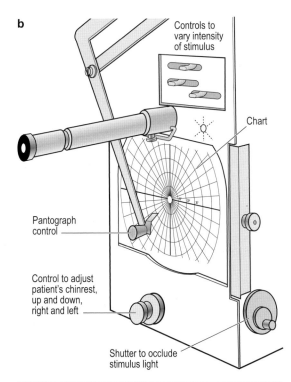

Fig. 7.10 (a) A Goldmann perimeter. **(b)** The main controls of the perimeter.

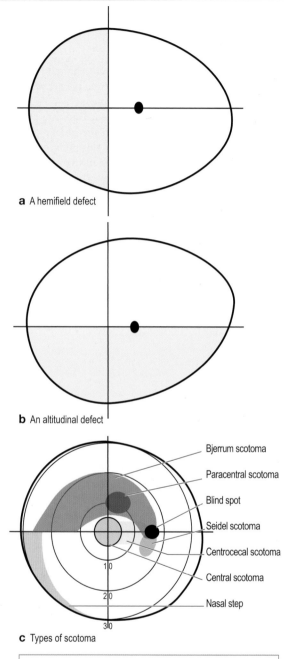

a A hemifield defect

b An altitudinal defect

Bjerrum scotoma
Paracentral scotoma
Blind spot
Seidel scotoma
Centrocecal scotoma
Central scotoma
Nasal step

c Types of scotoma

Fig. 7.11 (a) A hemifield defect. **(b)** An altitudinal defect. **(c)** The types of scotoma.

Goldmann perimeter as a denting of the isoptres. On automated perimeters the actual threshold values are determined and related to a normal database, thus making a depression more readily appreciated.

Generalised depression

There is no focal area of loss but the patient generally requires a brighter stimulus in all locations than might be expected for a patient of that age. On a Goldmann field the isoptres move inward. This might be seen in a patient with a cataract.

Contraction

There is a generalised depression of the field and also loss of peripheral visual field.

Hemifield defect

One-half of the visual field is depressed or absent. This is typically seen in neurological disease.

Altitudinal defect

The superior or inferior hemifield is depressed or absent.

Central scotoma

There is a depression of the central field, involving fixation, but the peripheral field appears normal. This is typical of optic nerve disease. *Centrocaecal scotomas* extend to the blind spot.

Arcuate scotomas

These are caused by defects in the temporal nerve fibre layers. A Bjerrum scotoma is a complete arc-like defect superiorly or inferiorly around fixation. A Seidel scotoma appear as an extension from the blind spot. A paracentral defect appears as a small scotoma within the Bjerrum area. These are typically seen in normal (low)-tension glaucoma.

Nasal step

A relative or absolute scotoma of the superior or inferior nasal field is seen around the midline.

Central island

This is seen in severe glaucoma. Only a small area of central field is present. A peripheral temporal island may accompany this.

Split fixation

There is loss of one-half of the small central island.

Assessing the visual field

It is important to assess both fields and to examine the eye fully to find other clinical signs that will corroborate the cause of the field defect. First decide whether the field loss is unilateral or bilateral. If it is unilateral, decide what sort of defect is present; this will often suggest a particular pathology, as some of the examples detailed above suggest. If the field defect respects the vertical meridian (i.e. a hemianopia is present), look very hard at the other field to ensure that a slight defect is not also present there, which might suggest optic pathway disease. If both fields are involved *one must always consider the possibility of disease affecting the optic pathway*, although it is not unusual for ocular disease to affect both eyes, as with glaucoma. Examples of neurological field defects produced by lesions of the visual pathway are shown in Figure 7.12. A classical junctional scotoma presents with a central scotoma on one side and a superior temporal quadrantanopia in the other. It is caused by damage at the junction between the optic nerve and the chiasm. A loop of fibres from the nasal retina of the opposite eye

may loop into the optic nerve as it crosses at the chiasm, although recently this has been questioned. A homonymous hemianopia or quadrantanopia is always post-chiasmal. The vertical midline is respected. A left-sided field loss results from damage to the right side of the brain. If the temporal lobe of the brain is affected, inferior fibres of the optic radiation are damaged, causing a superior quadrantanopia. Parietal lobe lesions affecting the superior fibres may cause an inferior quadrantanopia. Similarly, lesions above the calcarine fissure of the visual cortex cause inferior field defects and those below the fissure cause inferior defects. Incongruous defects (that is, dissimilar defects in each eye in terms of size and shape) suggest a more anterior defect affecting the optic tract.

Automated perimeters

Automation of target presentation has enhanced the accuracy of perimetry. It also allows for a comparison with a normal data bank so that differences between an individual patient and a normal population

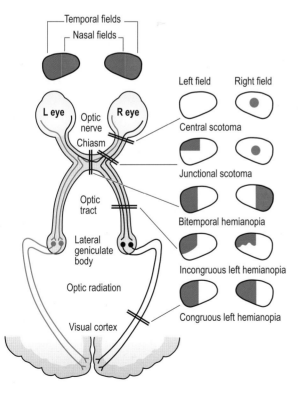

Fig. 7.12 The pattern of neurological field loss linked to the area of damage to the visual pathway.

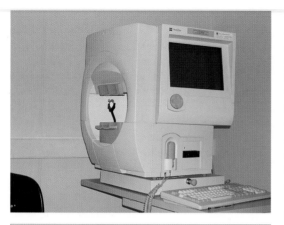

Fig. 7.13 A Humphrey automated perimeter.

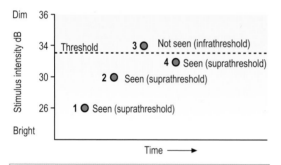

Fig. 7.14 The staircase method for finding threshold. A brighter than threshold light is first seen; the stimulus is dimmed by 4 dB, and it is still seen. On dimming the light by a further 4 dB the patient fails to see it. The intensity of the light is then increased by 2 dB and it is again seen by the patient. The threshold lies between this and the previously unseen (infrathreshold) stimulus, shown by the blue line.

can be highlighted. The Humphrey field analyser (Fig. 7.13) will be used to illustrate the principles of automated perimetry; most commonly, static visual fields are measured. Conventionally a staircase process is used to determine threshold (Fig. 7.14). On Humphrey standard testing the last-seen stimulus is taken as the threshold value. More recent programs use the Swedish interactive testing algorithm (SITA).This makes use of additional information about the visual field to determine threshold

values with fewer steps, speeding up the performance of the test. This algorithm uses the results of the test as it progresses and threshold values of surrounding points and information about typical patterns of field loss to adjust the process of threshold determination. It also paces the test according to the patient's response time. SITA standard uses a conventional 4 and 2 dB step pattern; the SITA fast, which is quicker, uses a 4 dB step pattern. The threshold is calculated at the end of the SITA examination and represents the 50% value on a frequency-of-seeing curve, as previously described (Fig. 7.4).

Using threshold values from a previous visual field can also speed up full-threshold testing.

Test strategies

Automated perimeters can perform a number of different test strategies. Threshold tests are commonly used in diagnosing and monitoring glaucoma patients. These concentrate on the central 24 or 30° of the visual field; each extends slightly further nasally to detect a nasal step field defect. 24-1 and 30-1 programs have points on the horizontal and vertical meridians. The 24-2 and 30-2 tests have points located on either side of these two meridians (Fig. 7.15). There is a 6° interval between each test location. This means that the test should be able to pick up a scotoma the size of the blind spot.

In some patients, for example those with severe glaucoma, the central 10° of the field may be of particular interest. This can be measured with a 10-2 test. This is particularly useful in examining glaucoma patients with severe field loss and possibly split fixation.

Additionally screening tests using various threshold-related and suprathreshold tests can be performed. These use a stimulus that is bright enough to be seen in the peripheral field by most people. These may be useful in screening for disease or examining the more peripheral visual field. It is also possible to test both eyes together to obtain a binocular field, which is important in occupational and fitness-to-drive assessment. A more refined version of the suprathreshold test is the threshold-related test where a stimulus of brightness greater (often by 5 dB) than the expected threshold level of each point to be tested throughout the visual field is used. This adapts the stimulus to the hill of vision rather than using a uniform suprathreshold stimulus across the visual field.

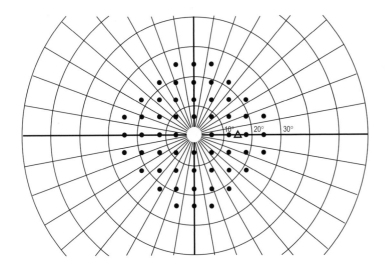

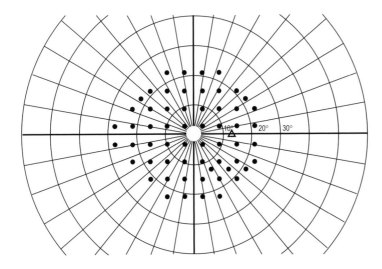

Fig. 7.15 The difference between a 24-1 and a 24-2 visual field test.

Performing the test

Setting up

Perimetry must be performed in a quiet room, comfortably heated or cooled with subdued lighting at a constant level where the test will not be interrupted by distractions (Box 7.1).

It is important to select the correct test to ensure both that the result obtained will help answer the clinical question being asked and that the patient will be able to perform the test with reasonable accuracy. This may mean using a faster strategy on a patient who is only able to concentrate for a short period.

A full explanation must be given to the patient. It is useful to run a demonstration test first for novice patients so that they know what to expect. It is important to reassure patients that on threshold tests not all the spots will be seen and that there may be pauses between groups of stimuli (obviously as the machine is detecting threshold, some of the spots cannot be seen). The need to maintain fixation must be emphasised; the subject must not look round the bowl trying to spot lights. It is also essential to let patients know that they can have a rest by holding down the button of the response switch. For patients

Box 7.1

Success with automated perimetry

- Select the type of field test according to the clinical question to be answered and the patient's ability to perform the test
- Ensure the proper environment for the test. A darkened quiet room with a comfortable temperature is ideal
- The patient should be comfortably seated at the machine and the chair and chinrest should be correctly positioned
- Fit the correct lenses for near correction
- Explain the test to patients and run the demonstration module if this is the first time that they have done the test
- Position the eye correctly using the video monitor
- Explain that not all the lights will be seen and that the test can be paused by holding the response button down

with poor central vision a large fixation diamond is available just below the central fixation spot. The patient looks at the apparent centre of the four lights making up the diamond pattern. If a patient finds that the stimuli are appearing too quickly the presentation rate can be reduced.

Patient positioning

The patient is comfortably seated at the perimeter, a near correction if needed is placed in the lens-holder, and the patient is asked to look at the fixation target. Reading glasses can be used if they can be accommodated comfortably and have a large enough lens. The chinrest is adjusted by means of the video camera to centralise the eye. The other eye is comfortably occluded. The test is started when the patient is happy and understands what they have to do.

Problems during the test

The machine monitors fixation during the test by checking the position of the blind spot. The perimetrist can also check for poor fixation on the video monitor showing the position of the eye. Occasionally patients may appear to have good fixation on the video image of the eye but the machine

indicates that there are excessive fixation losses. Rechecking the blind-spot position and further instruction to the patient will usually cure the problem. An anxious or new patient will benefit from reassurance given during the test. Allow a short break before testing the second eye.

Interpreting the results

The Humphrey 24-2 will be used to illustrate how to interpret an automated visual field (Fig. 7.16). First check that the name and date of birth on the print-out are correct. Next look at the reliability indices.

Reliability indices

Fixation losses. The lower the figure, the better the patient maintained fixation throughout the test. The value should normally be below 20%: greater values than this and small defects in the field may be missed and the size and depth of larger defects will be inaccurate.

False positives occur when the projector moves but fails to illuminate; nevertheless patients indicate that they have seen a light. On more modern perimeters without noisy motors the machine deliberately inserts a long pause, and a response indicates a false positive. A high score suggests that the patient is trigger-happy.

False negatives occur when a stimulus much brighter than that already seen is re-presented and not seen by the patient. This suggests inattention or tiredness.

Gaze-tracker. This monitors eye movement, comparing the centre of the pupil to the position of the first Purkinje reflection from the cornea which changes if the eye moves. Ideally the eye should be completely still and the trace, found at the bottom of the field print-out, should be flat.

Threshold plot

Look at the figures. They represent the raw data or the actual threshold level in decibels for each point tested: the higher the number, the dimmer the light. Do they appear reasonable? Is there a gradual reduction towards the periphery? At fixation the threshold is usually in the low 30s dB and at 24–30° from fixation in the mid to upper 20s dB. The sensitivity decreases with age. The slope between is usually quite smooth.

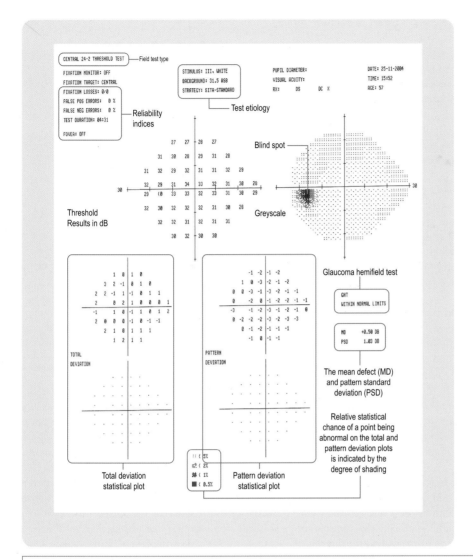

Fig. 7.16 The features of a Humphrey Swedish interactive testing algorithm standard field print-out.

The grey-scale plot

This is simply a pictorial representation of the threshold data. It is only useful to direct the observer to where defects in the field may lie or to discuss a field defect with a patient but otherwise is of limited use. It does not compensate for the age of the patient.

Total deviation plot

This compares each threshold point on the subject's field with a database of normal age-matched subjects.

It shows how much the subject's threshold values for each test point differ from that of the normal group. Below it is a statistical plot showing how likely any difference is to be statistically significant, with a probability ranging from 5 to 0.5%.

Pattern deviation plot

The threshold of the visual field may be globally reduced if, for example, there is a cataract or a small pupil. The presence of a scotoma may be obscured by this general reduction in sensitivity. The pattern deviation plot removes any general reduction in sensitivity to reveal the scotoma. Again, as with the total deviation plot, a statistical print-out below the plot shows the likelihood of the 'corrected' value being abnormal. This plot is probably the best to use when looking for progression in a glaucomatous visual field. It will rapidly provide information about any increase in the depth or size of the scotoma. It is also the best plot to use when comparing a standard threshold field with the newer SITA threshold field.

The glaucoma hemifield test

This compares groups of points in the superior field with mirror-image groups in the inferior field (Fig. 7.17). If there is a difference it is marked as being outside normal limits. It is particularly useful in detecting glaucoma where a field defect is often present or more marked in one half of the field.

The mean defect and pattern standard deviation

These are figures that provide an overall measure of the hill of vision and any scotomas that might be present. The hill of vision might be depressed in a patient with cataract. In this patient the mean defect will be a negative figure (Fig. 7.18). The mean defect may not be significantly altered by a small scotoma, however. The pattern standard deviation measures the extent of a scotomatous deficit in the hill of vision (Fig. 7.19).

Performing a field test is an arduous task for a patient and there may be a fluctuation in the threshold on retesting a point during the same examination. On full-threshold tests this is measured as short-term fluctuation and is derived by measuring the threshold of a number of points twice. The greater the differ-

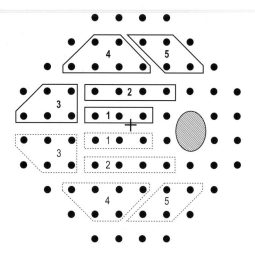

Fig. 7.17 The glaucoma hemifield test compares a mirror image of groups of points in the superior and inferior visual field. In glaucoma the field damage is often worse in either one half of the field or the other. The test helps to indicate subtle degrees of asymmetry.

ence in threshold on the first and second occasion, the greater is the short-term fluctuation. A measure of this short-term fluctuation is given in the numerical print-out of the full-threshold field. Furthermore the pattern standard deviation is corrected for this threshold fluctuation and appears as the corrected pattern standard deviation. It effectively reduces the pattern standard deviation if a significant short-term fluctuation is present. The greater the fluctuation in threshold, the less sure one can be that an apparent scotoma is due to a true deficit rather than a large variation in measured threshold.

Fig. 7.18 The mean defect.

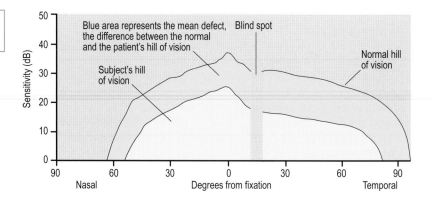

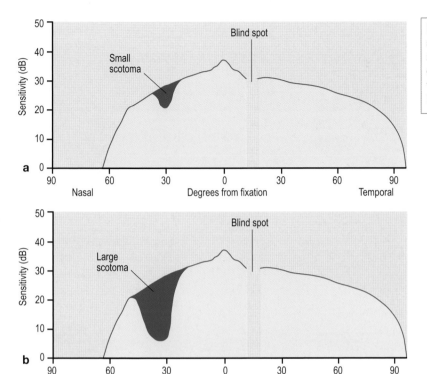

Fig. 7.19 The pattern standard deviation is a measure of the depth and extent of the scotoma. It would be greater in case b than case a.

Once the field has been analysed in this manner the defect itself is then considered in exactly the same way as the Goldmann field detailed before (Fig. 7.20).

Common artefacts on automated fields

A visual field is seldom performed in isolation. Results may occur which are at variance with other clinical signs. It is important to ask whether an artefact may have caused an anomalous visual field test.

Obstructions

If a lens or a patient's glasses are used to perform the test the frame of the lens can cause an apparent peripheral scotoma. This usually affects the marginal or edge points and may occur in a complete ring. The patient's eye should be as close as possible to the corrective lens.

An apparent superior scotoma with a sharp cut-off may result from ptosis; taping the lid may help prevent this.

An angioscotoma results if a test point lies on the course of a blood vessel. It is a feature of static perimetry and usually occurs around the blind spot.

Corneal, lenticular and vitreous opacities may all cause field defects that may be misinterpreted. A thorough examination of the eye is necessary if the field is to be interpreted correctly.

Missed blind spot

This does not necessarily indicate poor fixation. It may simply be that the blind spot fell between test locations.

Threshold abnormalities

A very high value for threshold, that is, an ability to see a very dim light, suggests that the patient is just constantly pressing the button. This is usually associated with a high false-positive score.

A clover-leaf field suggests that the patient has lost concentration after a short while (Fig. 7.20d). The central field in each quadrant appears normal; points here are tested first to determine the likely threshold value. As testing proceeds the patient loses interest and fails to respond to the stimuli. A faster test may help overcome this.

Small variations in retinal shape may cause refractive scotoma as the stimulus becomes blurred.

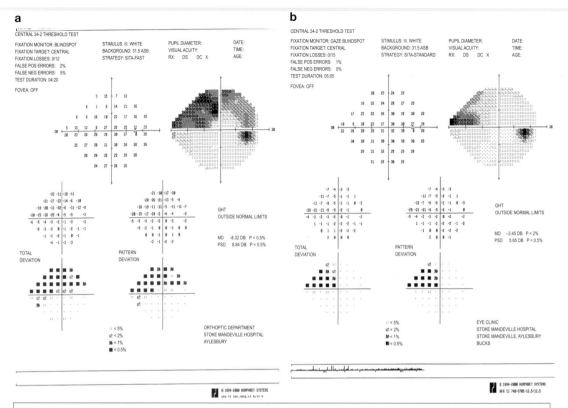

Fig. 7.20 Examples of field defects detected on automated perimetry. **(a)** A superior arcuate scotoma. **(b)** A nasal step.

A small pupil (for example, if the patient is applying pilocarpine) or incorrect corrective lenses may cause an apparent scotoma.

Assessing progression

The print-out from an automated perimeter contains a large amount of information. Viewed in a logical manner, this information can be rapidly assimilated and a judgement made as to whether or not a defect is present. Assessing field for change, which is important in the management of glaucoma, is a harder task, complicated by the inevitable between-occasion fluctuation. A variety of different methods, largely created for clinical trials in glaucoma, have been used to try and make this assessment easier (Birch et al. 1995) but each yields significantly different results. Some may form part of the perimeter software. Glaucoma progression analysis is available for the Humphrey field analyser. This flags up a

reduction in sensitivity in three or more points on two consecutive follow-up tests. In clinical practice the judgement remains largely a visual one, trying to assess whether a scotoma has deepened or enlarged. In most glaucoma patients at least five fields are really necessary before a judgement on progression can be made with any confidence. The pattern deviation plot is the most useful for assessing progression.

Short-wavelength automated perimetry (SWAP)

This replaces a white light stimulus with a blue light stimulus and a yellow light for background illumination. The yellow background reduces the sensitivity of the green and red cones, thus it is predominantly the blue cones, and the ganglion cells to which they are connected, that are stimulated. It appears that

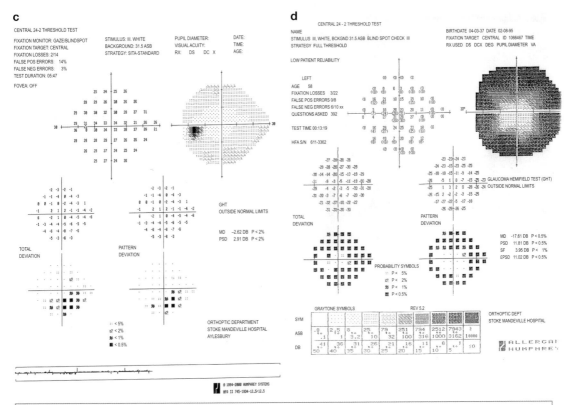

Fig. 7.20, *cont'd* Examples of field defects detected on automated perimetry. **(c)** An early inferor scotoma: note how it is emphasised on the total and pattern deviation statistical plots. The glaucoma hemifield test is also abnormal. The defect might be missed if only the grey-scale was used. **(d)** A clover-leaf field defect. The subject has given up during the last part of the test, having seen the central stimuli at the start.

this test is able to detect glaucomatous visual field defects at an earlier stage. This might be because this pathway is selectively damaged in glaucomatous optic neuropathy or because one is selectively testing a part of the visual system and thus the effect of redundancy (it is suggested that part of the visual pathway represents spare capacity) is minimised. There is however a greater variability in testing between subjects and within subjects than with white-on-white perimetry and as yet the technique has not become clinically well established.

Frequency-doubling technology (FDT)

This is a novel form of perimetry that developed from the frequency-doubling illusion (Fig. 7.21). In the original device the central 20° of the visual field

was divided into 17 test areas (Fig. 7.22). The patient looks at a screen through an eyepiece (Fig. 7.23). A 0.25 cycle per degree sinusoidal grating with a 25 Hz counterphase flicker (that is, the blacker part of the grating is changed to the whiter part of the grating 25 times a second) is presented in each of the test areas and the contrast of the grating required for the subject to see the flicker is recorded. The illusion is mediated by the M-cell pathway (accounting for some 10% of optic nerve axons), which responds to low-contrast, high-temporal-frequency motion stimuli. FDT is effectively producing a motion stimulus. The other pathway, the P-cell pathway, accounts for 90% of the axons and responds to high-contrast, low-temporal-frequency, static stimuli. This test may again detect glaucomatous defects at an earlier stage than conventional perimetry. It may

Fig. 7.21 Switching between two low-frequency counterphases (left) produces the illusion that a grating of twice the frequency is seen (right).

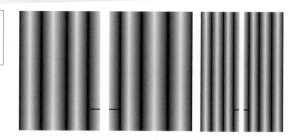

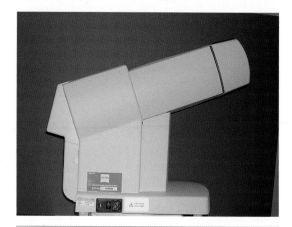

Fig. 7.23 The frequency-doubling technology perimeter.

RIGHT EYE

Test Duration 00:53 mm

Deviation

0°

FIXATION ERRS   0/3
FALSE POS ERRS   0/3

LEFT EYE

Test Duration 02:02 min

Deviation

30°

FIXATION ERRS   0/3
FALSE POS ERRS   0/3

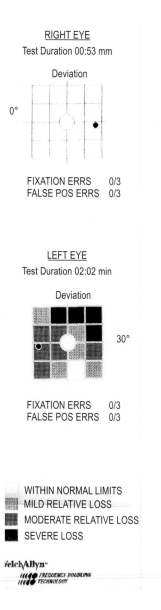

WITHIN NORMAL LIMITS
MILD RELATIVE LOSS
MODERATE RELATIVE LOSS
SEVERE LOSS

WelchAllyn
FREQUENCY DOUBLING
TECHNOLOGY

Fig. 7.22 The print-out from the frequency-doubling technology perimeter. Seventeen areas within the central 20° of the visual field are tested.

be that the M-cell pathway is preferentially lost in glaucoma. Alternatively, by testing a smaller number of nerve fibres one may, as with SWAP, be minimising the effects of redundancy. The test can be run in a screening mode which is fast (usually just over a minute) or a longer threshold mode. Comparisons between this perimeter and the Humphrey perimeter have been promising.

A newer version of the machine allows a similar pattern of points to be tested as the 24-2 (55 points) and 30-2 (69 points) Humphrey field analyser. This is obviously at the expense of an increased test time.

The Amsler chart

The Amsler chart was designed as a test of macular function. It can be used to measure the central field and detect scotomas but also gives information about metamorphopsia (distortion) attributable to macular disease, for example macular degeneration. The standard chart is a square of white lines against

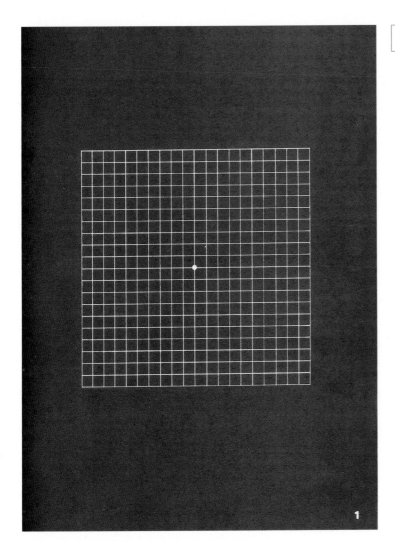

Fig. 7.24 The Amsler chart.

a black background with a white fixation spot centrally (Fig. 7.24); the reporting sheet with black lines and a white background is often used instead. It corresponds to an area of approximately 10° around the centre of the visual field. The chart is held at approximately 30 cm from the eye to be tested. The patient wears glasses and the chart is well illuminated. The central white spot is fixated and the following questions asked. The patient indicates the area of the chart that appears abnormal.

- Can you see all the corners and sides of the large square?
- Are there any interruptions in the network of squares?

- Do you see all the lines, both horizontal and vertical, as straight and parallel or do any appear distorted?

The answers direct the examiner to the part of the macula that is likely to be abnormal.

Summary

Mapping of the visual field can be accomplished simply with confrontation tests or using more complex perimeters. In deciding which test to perform it is important to know what questions are to be answered about the visual field and to consider whether or not the patient is going to be capable of performing the test. Correct performance of the correct test in an appropriate environment is the only way of ensuring a meaningful result. When interpreting the field, always consider both right and left together. If you ask the following questions you are unlikely to make a serious mistake:

- Could this be a neurological field defect?
- What additional clinical findings support the presence of this field defect?
- Are there other clinical findings (for example, early disc cupping in glaucoma) that are sufficient to suggest a diagnosis despite an apparently normal field?

- A variety of methods are available to test the field of vision, no matter how poor the visual acuity
- The field can give information about retinal and optic nerve function as well as the visual pathways between the chiasm and the occipital cortex
- The nature and pattern of the field loss can give valuable clues to the underlying causative pathology
- Appropriate testing in an appropriate environment to match the ability of the patient to cooperate is essential for reliable and useful test results

---

References and further reading

Aung T, Foster PJ, Seah SK. Automated static perimetry: the influence of myopia and its method of correction. Ophthalmology 2001; 108: 290–295.

Birch MK, Wishart PK, O'Donnell NP. Determining progressive visual field loss in serial Humphrey visual fields. Ophthalmology 1995; 102: 1227–1235.

Budenz DL, Rhee P, Feuer WJ. Comparison of glaucomatous visual field defects using standard full threshold and Swedish interactive threshold algorithms. Arch Ophthalmol 2002; 120: 1136–1141.

Casson R, James CB, Rubinstein A, Ali H. A clinical comparison of FDT and Humphrey perimetry. Br J Ophthalmol 2001; 85: 360–362.

Gardiner SK, Crabb DP. Frequency of testing for detecting visual field progression. Br J Ophthalmol 2002; 86: 560–564.

Heijil A. The Humphrey visual field analyser, construction and concepts. Doc Ophthalmol Proc 1985; 42: 77–84.

Heijl A, Bengtsson B, Patella M. Glaucoma follow-up when converting from long to short perimetric threshold tests. Arch Ophthalmol 2000; 118: 489–493.

Johnson CA, Adams AJ, Casson EJ, Brandt JD. Blue-on-yellow perimetry can predict the development of glaucomatous field loss. Arch Ophthalmol 1993; 111: 645–650.

Quigley H. Identification of glaucoma-related visual field abnormality with the screening protocol of frequency doubling technology. Am J Ophthalmol 1998; 125: 819–820.

Vesti E, Johnson CA, Chauban C. Comparison of different methods for detecting glaucomatous visual field progression. Invest Ophth Vis Sci 2003; 44: 3873–3879.

Examination of the orbit and ocular adnexae

RAMONA KHOOSHABEH and LARRY BENJAMIN

Introduction

In this chapter the clinical macroexamination of the orbit, eyelids and lacrimal drainage system will be covered. These structures are associated with a significant amount of ophthalmic disease and morbidity. Although modern imaging techniques have had a significant impact on diagnosis, the clinical tests described in this chapter are still important and help determine the correct investigations to perform.

The orbit

The orbit is the bony socket containing the globe, the extraocular muscles, Tenon's fascia, the orbital fat, the lacrimal gland, nerves and blood vessels.

The examination of the orbit is guided by a full and detailed history of the presenting complaint. This should include the nature, duration and severity of symptoms as well as any associated pathology gained from systemic enquiry. Symptoms related to sinus disease should be sought because of the close proximity of the sinuses to the orbits.

Orbital examination may require a number of different tests to be performed. A blow-out fracture, for example, may produce a plethora of orbital signs such as enophthalmos, a step in the inferior orbital margin, decreased sensation in the distribution of the infraorbital nerve and restriction of extraocular movements and possibly altered vision. A careful and systematic examination routine is essential.

Examination of the orbit

The examination begins with observation of the two orbits, particularly looking for symmetry and asymmetry. Asymmetry of the orbits may indicate bony disease or skull suture anomalies such as unicoronal synostosis (premature fusing of one coronal skull suture).

The position of the globe is next assessed to see if proptosis (exophthalmos) is present. It is useful to observe patients from behind, asking them to extend their neck. Viewing the eyes from the top enables the examiner to see if any proptosis present is symmetrical or unilateral (Fig. 8.1). It is very important to distinguish between proptosis and a contralateral enophthalmos. Similarly, an ipsilateral lid retraction can be mistaken for a proptosis.

Proptosis may be axial or non-axial. Axial proptosis, a displacement of the globe horizontally forward from its usual position, suggests retro-ocular pathology such as an orbital apex mass or muscle swelling. Non-axial proptosis, where the globe is displaced not only forwards but also away from its usual axis, suggests a mass arising from elsewhere in the orbit (usually anteriorly) such as a lacrimal gland tumour.

A change in proptosis associated with exertion (exercise or a Valsalva manoeuvre) may indicate a venous anomaly in the orbit. The patient should be

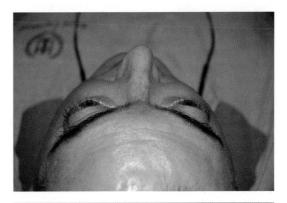

Fig. 8.1 Assessing proptosis from behind the patient in dysthyroid eye disease.

asked to perform a Valsalva's manoeuvre to look for an increase in proptosis.

Measurement of proptosis

An exophthalmometer is used to measure proptosis objectively. This works by measuring the forward projection of each cornea compared to a fixed landmark, the outer bony orbital rim against which the instrument rests.

The intercanthal distance is first measured on the front scale of the instrument. This is used to ensure repeatability of measurements over time (Fig. 8.2). Small changes, which may indicate progressive orbital pathology, can then be recorded accurately. The fixation point taken up by the patient should be the same for every measurement. The position of the apex of the corneal reflection in the sloping mirror of the exophthalmometer is measured against the scale on the bottom of the mirror. It is important for accurate recording to ensure that the measurement is made when the examiner has lined up the down-pointing mark on the mirror scale with the small dome in front of the mirror. This ensures that the angle at which the examiner makes the reading is always constant. Normally, the corneal apex is less than 20 mm from the lateral bony orbital margin and there is usually 2 mm or less difference between the two eyes (Fig. 8.3).

The protrusion of the corneal apex can also be measured with a plastic ruler placed on the lateral orbital margin but this is not very accurate.

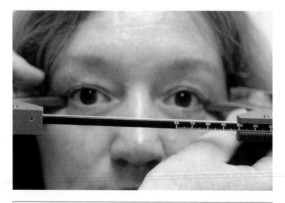

Fig. 8.2 An exophthalmometer held against each lateral canthal margin, allowing the intercanthal distance to be read for repeatability of measurements.

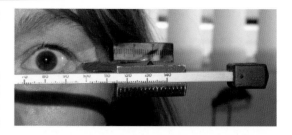

Fig. 8.3 The forward protrusion of the cornea is read with the blue conical marker and down-pointing line on the exophthalmometer mirror scale aligned.

Additional clinical examination of the orbit

Lid position and movement can give clues to orbital pathology. Lid erythema or swelling may accompany infective and inflammatory conditions. The orbital margins should be carefully palpated to examine for masses or areas of induration, tenderness or structural abnormality. Orbital emphysema can be palpated (crepitus). It suggests a communication between the sinuses and the orbit, particularly after trauma or surgery.

If pulsation of the globe is present auscultation with a stethoscope should be performed. Bruits may be heard in the presence of a carotid-cavernous sinus fistula.

Sensation of the skin in the distribution of the infraorbital, supraorbital and supratrochlear nerves should be tested both for light touch and pinprick. After trauma with a suspected blow-out fracture of the orbital floor, the infraorbital nerve is often damaged (Fig. 8.4).

Special attention should be paid to the area of the lacrimal gland to exclude enlargement. The upper lid should be everted as part of this procedure.

Examination in the orbital apex syndrome

This syndrome is caused by any pathology affecting the apex of the orbit. Figure 8.5 shows the structures involved as they enter or exit the orbital foramina.

Examination must therefore be performed to test the function of each of these structures.

This includes assessment of visual acuity (see Ch. 1), colour vision (see Ch. 1), pupil function (see Ch. 10), ocular motility (see Ch. 9) and orbital region sensation.

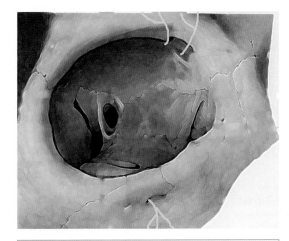

Fig. 8.4 The supraorbital, supratrochlear and infraorbital nerves exiting from their respective notches supplying sensation to the skin of the brow forehead and cheek.

Summary

A proper clinical examination of the orbit relies on a number of specific and more general techniques to make a diagnosis and assess the effect of any pathological change. It should also help direct the clinician to the most appropriate investigations, for example, blood tests or scans, to confirm the diagnosis.

Clinical evaluation of Blepharoptosis (Ptosis)

Classification of ptosis

The traditional classification of acquired and congenital ptosis is not clinically useful apart from timing the onset of ptosis. A classification based on the mechanism that causes ptosis rather than the moment when the deficit developed is much more appealing. It helps establish a clinical diagnosis and a surgical management plan.

The aetiology of ptosis ranges from an innocent contact lens-related aponeurotic ptosis, where unnecessary neurological referral and imaging investigation can be avoided, to fatal conditions such as lung carcinoma and dissecting carotid aneurysm presenting as a ptosis associated with Horner's syndrome.

The following subgroups are traditionally considered.

- Dysgenesis: This is either a simple ptosis or one associated with extraocular muscle deficits such as a double elevator palsy and miswiring syndromes such as the Marcus Gunn jaw-winking phenomenon and superior rectus levator synkinesis.
- *Myogenic:* The levator muscle complex is not working.
- *Myoneural:* This involves an abnormality of the neuromuscular junction.
- *Neurogenic:* The nerve supply to the levator complex is damaged.

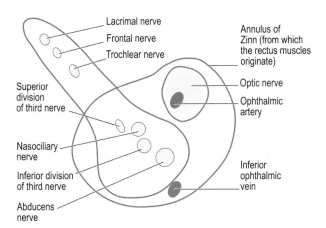

Lacrimal nerve
Frontal nerve
Trochlear nerve
Annulus of Zinn (from which the rectus muscles originate)
Superior division of third nerve
Optic nerve
Ophthalmic artery
Nasociliary nerve
Inferior division of third nerve
Inferior ophthalmic vein
Abducens nerve

Fig. 8.5 The structures at the orbital apex.

- *Aponeurotic:* The insertion of the levator into the lid is deficient.

Pseudoptosis

Here the levator complex is normal in its anatomy and function, yet the eye appears to be ptotic. Mechanical ptosis from a tumour, enophthalmos, upper lid retraction of the other eye or asymmetric faces are examples of such causes. Patients with a past history of facial palsy may develop aberrant regeneration and a spastic ptosis which is the result of orbicularis spasm rather than a levator muscle defect. In pseudoptosis, therefore, the underlying problem should be addressed first.

Examination

Particular attention to the following measurements helps determine into which aetiological group the ptosis is likely to fall.

Margin reflex distance 1 (MRD1)

This is the distance between the corneal light reflex and the upper lid margin. Patients with ptosis use their frontalis muscle to elevate the eyelid, so it is very important to prevent the eyebrow elevation by stabilising the brow while performing measurements for ptosis. The examiner does this by applying pressure over the frontalis muscle with the fingers (Fig. 8.6).

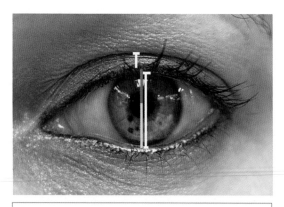

Fig. 8.6 Measurement of margin reflex distance 1 (MRD1: red), MRD2 (yellow) and interpalpebral aperture (white). The short white line superiorly indicates the measure of eyelid show.

Margin reflex distance 2 (MRD2)

This is the distance between the corneal light reflex and lower lid margin (Fig. 8.6).

Palpebral aperture

This is the distance between the upper and lower lid margin (Fig. 8.6). Again, it is very important to stabilise the brow. The palpebral aperture is dependent on the position of the lower lid and therefore is not as useful as MRD1. The palpebral aperture should be noted when the patient is looking down with the neck slightly extended. The presence of ptosis in downgaze is an important sign in a patient who might otherwise have a normal aperture in the primary position. Changes in the palpebral aperture should also be noted when the patient is chewing, eating or jaw-thrusting as it might indicate a miswiring problem such as the Marcus Gunn syndrome.

Eyelid show

This is the distance between the lash margin and the lower end of the upper lid fold as the patient looks straight ahead (Fig. 8.6). The eyelid show is dependent on the insertion of the septum and the volume of the pre-aponeurotic fat pad.

Levator function

The brow is again fixed. A transparent ruler is held in front of the eyelid and the patient is asked to look as far down and then as far up as possible. The maximal excursion of the upper eyelid is then measured with the ruler. A levator function less than 4 mm is generally an indication for brow suspension rather than levator surgery.

Skin crease

This is the distance between the lash line and the first crease as the patient looks down (Fig. 8.7). The normal skin crease is between 5 and 8 mm, although it is lower in orientals. A recessed skin crease in the presence of ptosis is a good indication of an aponeurotic defect. An absent skin crease is normally suggestive of poor levator function.

Extraocular movement

The presence of motility abnormalities such as a double elevator palsy, third-nerve palsy or reduced movement suggesting a myopathy should be excluded. Their presence will obviously aid diagnosis.

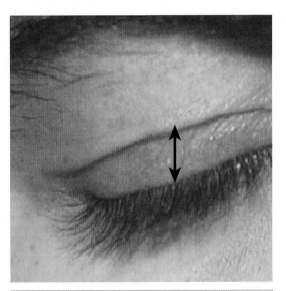

Fig. 8.7 Measurement of the skin crease.

The position of the lids should be noted in different position of gaze. Variability of ptosis in different position of gaze is an indication of aberrant re-generation after a third-nerve palsy. Note also the speed of saccades: slow saccades are indicative of myopathic muscles. In myasthenia gravis the saccades have an initial high velocity. The preservation of high-velocity saccades in myasthenia, even in the presence of severe ophthalmoplegia, suggests that the muscle fibres generating rapid movements (twitch fibres) can be relatively spared even when the muscle fibres responsible for the maintenance of eccentric (tonic fibres) are severely affected. This gives rise to the clinical appearance of 'quiver' movements, so characteristic of myasthenia.

Cogan's twitch

The patient is first asked to look down for 15 s. A small upshoot of the eyelid is noted as a myasthenic patient then moves back to the primary position. This is not dissimilar to the preservation of twitch fibres in myasthenic extraocular movements.

Bell's phenomenon

Ask the patient to close the eye forcibly. The examiner then lifts the patient's upper eyelid manually. In a patient with a normal Bell's phenomenon the globe will rotate upwards and the cornea will be covered by the eyelid. If a patient does not have a good Bell's phenomenon, a cautious ptosis correction should be undertaken to prevent subsequent corneal exposure. In some patients with a very poor Bell's phenomenon, surgery is contraindicated.

Pupil

A small pupil might indicate a Horner's syndrome and a large pupil might be a sign of a third-nerve palsy. Occasionally in aberrant third-nerve palsy the size of pupil will change in different position of gaze.

Contralateral upper lid retraction

Note any contralateral upper lid retraction, which may occur as a manifestation of Hering's law (see Ch. 9).

Fatigability

Ask the patient to look up and down for about 1 min to induce fatigue. Sustained upgaze for 1 min will achieve the same result. Progressive ptosis will ensue in a myasthenic patient. Measure MRD1 before and after these fatigue tests. Note that myasthenic patients might also develop diplopia with this test. Patients with aponeurotic defects also complain of worsening ptosis in the evening or when they are tired. This is thought to be due to a general reduction in sympathetic tone.

Rest test, heat test and ice test

The rest test, heat test and ice test are easily performed. Apply an ice-filled glove to the affected eye for 10 min. In a myasthenic patient the ptosis improves by 2 mm or more (Fig. 8.8). Heat applied in similar manner (using warm water) as well as simply closing the eyes for 10 min also improves a myasthenic ptosis. The common denominator of all these tests, rest, seems to be the relevant factor. However the ice test appears to improve the ptosis more dramatically than rest alone. The activity of the acetylcholinesterase enzyme is reduced by the cold in addition to the effect of rest. This is thought to be the cause of the disparity between the tests.

The ice test is easy to perform and has 95% sensitivity and 100% specificity. This non-invasive test, as well as a positive acetyl-cholinesterase antibody (100% specificity), has now almost replaced the Tensilon test in the diagnosis of myasthenia gravis.

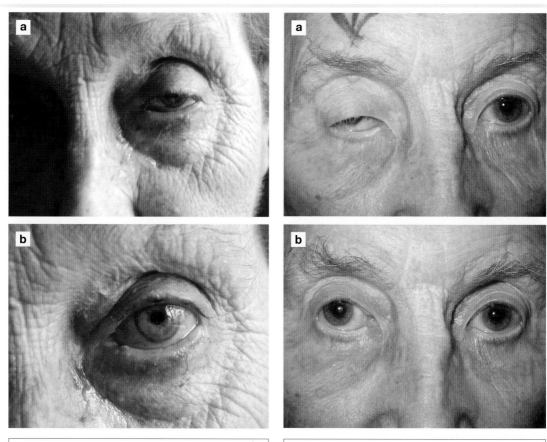

Fig. 8.8 Ptosis in a myaesthenic patient **(a)** improving with the ice test **(b)**.

Fig. 8.9 Improvement in ptosis **(a)** following administration of phenylephrine **(b)**.

Phenylephrine test

The use of phenylephrine drops should be an integral part of the routine assessment of any ptosis patient. Although in the original description phenylephrine 10% was used, equally good results can be obtained with phenylephrine 2.5%, which may also cause fewer systemic complications.

One drop of phenylephrine 2.5% is instilled in the upper fornix. Phenylephrine is an alpha-agonist that stimulates the alpha-receptors in Müller's muscle, causing its contraction and hence lid elevation (Fig. 8.9). It is possible to demonstrate the potential outcome of surgery to a patient with a positive response to phenylephrine. One can also unmask a coexisting ptosis in the so-called normal eye which appeared normal due to increased levator stimulation (Hering's law).

Laboratory testing

Single-fibre electromyogram (EMG: 100% sensitivity) repetitive EMG and muscle biopsy are other more invasive tests that are very helpful in identifying the site of pathology in myopathic and myasthenic ptosis.

Myasthenic ptosis can also have a paraneoplastic origin. Myasthenia gravis may be associated with lung carcinoma. Lambert–Eaton syndrome is also commonly associated with lung carcinoma. Although there is a certain overlap between the two, auto-antibodies can be used to distinguish paraneoplastic myasthenia serologically from the Lambert–Eaton syndrome.

Summary

Ptosis is a common condition presenting to ophthalmologists. A complete clinical examination should place the ptosis in the correct diagnostic category. The ophthalmologist can then save the patient unnecessary investigation by identifying, for example, a simple aponeurotic ptosis.

Clinical evaluation of Epiphora

Epiphora (watering eye) is one of the most common complaints encountered in ophthalmic departments. Tearing can result from three causes: (1) anatomical obstruction of the drainage system from the puncta to the nose; (2) function block; and (3) hypersecretion. Tears are produced by the lacrimal gland at a rate of 1 µl/min. The volume of tears in the eye is about 7 µl and tear drainage capacity is 50 µl/min. This reduces to 30 µl/min in patients older than 45.

Causes of epiphora

Anatomical obstruction of the drainage system from the puncta to the nose

The obstruction may be partial or complete. It is usually caused by occlusion of the nasolacrimal duct. The paradox of epiphora and a dry eye may fall in this group as well. Patients who have to use artificial tears find it difficult that they are troubled by epiphora upon exposure to stimuli such as heat, sun and wind. The reduced flow of tears through the tear drainage system in a dry-eye patient may result in stricture formation at some point, causing this paradoxical effect.

Function block

This results from a deficiency of the lacrimal pump in an otherwise patent drainage system. Although an absolute functional block only occurs in facial palsy, inadequacy of the lacrimal pump can result from a number of causes. Involutional changes in the orbicularis in and around the canaliculi and sac lead to pump deficiency. A lax lid or lid malposition, for example punctal ectropion or entropion, are important to note. A prominent conjunctival fold (conjunctivochalasis), enlarged plica semilunaris or a hypertrophied caruncle can easily obstruct the punctum and give rise to epiphora in the presence of an otherwise anatomically patent system. Conjunctivochalasis is not restricted to the lower bulbar conjunctiva, and can equally contribute to the pathogenesis of dry eye by obliterating the lower and upper tear meniscus, causing an unstable tear film and irritation, particularly in downgaze.

An abnormal blink in blepharospasm or contact lens wear can also give rise to a so-called functional block. A peculiar tear overflow of a functional type also occurs in patients with meibomian gland dropout. A healthy oily layer is necessary to 'hold' the aqueous layer of the tear film in place. Inadequacy of this oily layer results in the tears spilling over the lid margin. These patients usually say that 'my eyes are always wet', although there is not much overflow of tears over their cheeks.

Hypersecretion

A reflex hypersecretion by the lacrimal gland is seen in ocular-surface disease. Blepharitis causes a disturbance of the tear film associated with meibomian gland drop-out and increased evaporation that may result in hypersecretion.

It is apparent that epiphora is a very complex symptom and its investigation requires thorough consideration and understanding of all these possible causes. For example, patients with a partial anatomical block or functional epiphora may be discharged as a patent syringing of the lacrimal drainage system has been taken as a measure of normality. This group of patients are the most difficult to manage and treat.

Investigation of epiphora

History

A full history recording the onset of symptoms, exacerbating or provoking factors, associated eye disease and a history of any facial trauma is important. Patients might not correlate their symptoms to a past facial palsy unless this is directly enquired into. Asking patients to blow up their cheeks can demonstrate a residual weakness of facial muscles. Induced eyelid ptosis indicates aberrant regeneration after a facial palsy in the past (Fig. 8.10).

Slit-lamp examination

Pay particular attention to the presence of lid margin disease: if present, it needs to be treated. Look too for any lid malposition such as entropion, ectropion or lower-lid retraction. Similarly, note an enlarged caruncle or redundant plica or redundant conjunctival folds inferiorly, affecting the distribution of the tear film as well as disturbing lacrimal pump action. A simple excision of a redundant fold or subtotal excision of an enlarged caruncle is a very simple surgical procedure with a high success rate

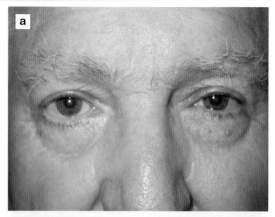

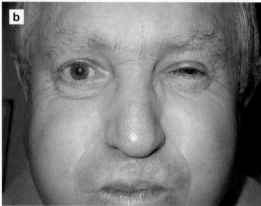

Fig. 8.10 Aberrant inervation following a facial nerve palsy **(a)**. Blowing up the cheek causes ptosis **(b)**.

in appropriate patients. Look for any superficial punctate staining of the cornea, which might indicate surface dryness and point to hypersecretion in a dry eye.

Tear meniscus level

The absolute tear meniscus level and the ratio between the two eyes are an excellent diagnostic indicator of nasolacrimal duct deficiency. Its reduction after lacrimal surgery is an indication of success.

The height is measured at the slit lamp with a narrow straight vertical beam set at 0.2 or 1 mm. The tear meniscus height is measured from the lid margin to the top of the meniscus along the globe surface. The 1 mm beam is used first. In cases where the tear meniscus is less than half of the height of

the 1 mm beam, the 0.2 mm beam is used. Gentle vertical manipulation of the lower lid with a finger is helpful in detecting the top of the tear meniscus. The measurements are expressed to the nearest 0.1 mm. The ratio between the two eyes is then calculated. The median normal tear meniscus height is 0.2 mm.

The reflux and microreflux test

To perform a reflux or regurgitation test, apply finger pressure directly over the lacrimal sac. The test is considered positive if purulent material regurgitates from the upper punctum. This is normally seen in infected nasolacrimal duct obstruction (mucocoele).

In the microreflux test, two drops of 0.25% sodium fluorescein dye are instilled in the inferior cul-de-sac and the patient is made to blink five times to activate the lacrimal pump. Excess fluorescein dye is blotted away using tissue paper. The skin over the lacrimal sac is massaged with moderate pressure using an index finger. The test is considered positive, that is, the system is blocked, if there is continuous reflux of fluorescein-stained tears from the inferior punctum. It has a sensitivity of 97% and specificity of 95% in detecting nasolacrimal duct obstruction.

Jones 1 and 2 tests

The Jones test is one of the most physiological, with close to 100% specificity. The sensitivity, however, is lower as detection of dye in the nose can be difficult. Sensitivity can be increased to 97% if an endoscope is used to examine the nose.

Jones 1 (as described by Jones). A small wire nasal applicator with a small amount of cotton wound around its end is bent into a gentle curve and moistened with cocaine (5%) and adrenaline (epinephrine) chloride (1:1000) and passed into the anterior part of the inferior nasal meatus as high and as far forward as possible. A drop of fluorescein 2% is instilled into the inferior cul-de-sac of the eye. After 12 min in patients over 45 and 3–6 min in patients under 45, in a completely normal drainage system, fluorescein should be found staining the cotton in the nose. Modification to this test as originally described by Jones will make a difference to the timing of the results.

Jones 2. If fluorescein is not recovered after a Jones 1 test, one then proceeds to a Jones 2 test. The remaining dye is first irrigated from the conjunctival sac. The patient's head is tipped forward to allow fluid to run out of the anterior nares. Normal saline is then injected slowly through a lacrimal cannula inserted as far as the common canaliculus. If no fluid is retrieved from the nose it indicates a complete blockage distal to the common canaliculus. Detection of fluorescein-stained fluid is indicative of incomplete block and the presence of clear fluid is an excellent indication of canalicular pump failure. Although Jones 1 and 2 are excellent qualitative tests, they are not quantitative and will not demonstrate different degrees of obstruction.

Fluorescein dye disappearance test (FDDT) (fluorescein clearance test)

One drop of 2% fluorescein is instilled into the lower fornix and its disappearance from the tear film after 5 min is noted as a measure of tear drainage. The individual is instructed not to squeeze or rub the eyes. This test is particularly useful when there is a significant residual dye at 5 min (0.8 mm or more of tear lake). The degree of residual dye is graded between 0 and 4. A modification of the test using a Schirmer strip at 3 and 10 min further quantifies the degree of obstruction. Here the colour on the strips is compared to a standard scale. Clearance of fluorescein from the eye is also dependent on the volume of tears produced. The intensity of residual fluorescein in the lower meniscus after 5 min is compared to a standardised visual scale (0–6). This is a quantitive measurement of tear secretion and therefore a very sensitive test for dry eyes.

The drop test

Drops of 10 μl lukewarm saline solution are repeatedly instilled into the conjunctival sac for 3 min. Excessive saline solution is then removed from the medial lacrimal lake with a micropipette and measured. The difference between the volume instilled into the fornix and the volume removed by micropipette gives a measure of the volume of tears drained by the tear duct (Fig. 8.11). The drop test provides a quantitative measurement of lacrimal drainage function.

Syringing and probing

A well-performed syringing gives excellent information about the anatomy of the lacrimal drainage system. Anaesthetic drops are instilled in the fornix. The punctum is dilated if indicated with a Nettleship dilator or, if a small punctum is present, a punctal

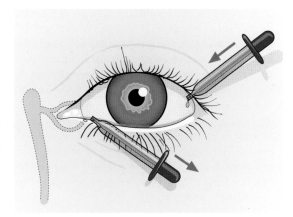

Fig. 8.11 The drop test. The drainage capacity is the difference between the amount of fluid instilled and removed by the examiner.

seeker. A lacrimal cannula is then advanced through the lower canaliculus for about 8 mm. The lid should be held taut to avoid intracanalicular mucosal folds obstructing the passage of the cannula. Saline is then injected through the cannula with a syringe. The degree of regurgitation from the upper punctum is noted and the patient is asked to report any taste of saline in the nose or throat. The degree of regurgitation from the upper punctum is directly related to the degree of obstruction in the system beyond the common canaliculus.

Regurgitation through the same canaliculus indicates canalicular obstruction. The canaliculi are then probed individually and any partial or complete resistance is noted. The probe is advanced into the sac until it meets a bony hard stop. This indicates that the obstruction, if present, is below the sac. A soft stop at any distance from the punctum is a stricture within the canaliculi or sac, depending on its distance from the punctum.

Tests of tear secretion

Dry eye may result from reduced tear production, for example in lacrimal gland disease, or increased evaporation, as may occur in meibomian gland disease. The tear layer comprises an outer lipid layer, a middle aqueous layer and an inner mucin layer (which may in part be mixed with the aqueous layer). The lipid layer helps to stabilise the tear film and spread it over the eye.

Dry eye is a common problem in an eye department. History is important to assess what symptoms a patient has, what makes them worse and when they occur. It is important to enquire about any associated ocular or systemic disease. Examination of the eye will reveal any eyelid malposition (see below). The meibomian glands should be observed. The tear meniscus is measured as in a patient with epiphora. Secondary effects of dryness on the cornea and conjunctiva are sought. The application of fluorescein and rose Bengal stain will aid this examination (see Ch. 2). In addition the following tests may help quantify tear production.

Schirmer's test

This test is for deficiencies in the aqueous layer of the tear film. A small 5 mm wide strip of filter paper is placed on the unanaesthetised lower tarsal plate and the eye closed for 5 min. The paper is removed and the amount of wetting recorded. It should be more than 10 mm at 5 min. If the test is repeated with the eye anaesthetised with a drop of topical anaesthetic, the effect of reflex secretion is removed and a measure of basal secretion is thus obtained.

Tear break-up time

This gives a measure of the quality of the tear film. Fluorescein dye is applied to the eye and the patient is asked to blink. The lids are held apart, or the patient is told not to blink, and the time taken for the smooth layer of the tear film to break up into dry spots is recorded. With a normal tear film this should exceed 10 s.

Summary

In summary, a thorough knowledge of the different causes of epiphora, one or two well-performed physiological clinical tests and accurate syringing and probing are often adequate for arriving at a correct diagnosis without the need for imaging.

Evaluation of eyelid malposition

The eyelids must:

- mechanically protect the cornea and eyeball. This requires the eyelids to meet effortlessly upon eyelid closure vertically and to wrap around the globe horizontally between the medial and lateral canthus

- provide an effective blink to renew the tear film
- provide an effective pump for lacrimal drainage. This in turn requires the punctum to rest in the lacrimal lake (anywhere between the plica and the limbus) and for the eyelids to have adequate orbicularis tone to pump tears away towards the lacrimal sac.

It therefore becomes apparent that an abnormal position of the eyelids, for example entropion, ectropion, upper or lower lid retraction as well as lid laxity of different grades, will affect one or more of the above functions. The tarsus forms the skeleton of the eyelid. The lower eyelid tarsus is about 4 mm in height and the upper about 10 mm. The smaller tarsus of the lower eyelid gives less stability than the upper eyelid, thus malpositions such as entropion and ectropion are more frequently seen in the lower lid.

The tarsus is held in position by a balance of the following forces:

- medial and lateral canthal ligaments
- upper and lower lid retractors
- outer lamella (skin)
- inner lamella (conjunctiva)
- orbicularis tautness and the position of the orbital fat.

Any disturbance of these factors will move the lid to an abnormal position. For instance, if there is conjunctival shrinkage the lid will turn in (cicatricial entropion). In any form of skin deficiency, the lid will be pulled out (cicatricial ectropion). If the pull of the retractors is greater than normal the lid is pulled down or up (upper and lower lid retraction in dysthyroid eye disease). If the retractors are dehisced or the lid is lax, its position depends on the balance of skin or conjunctival forces and the size of the tarsus.

There are also anatomical and involutional factors in the tarsus itself that give rise to entropion or ectropion in a given individual. The tarsal plates become smaller with age: this is a factor in the increasing frequency of lid malposition in the elderly. Patients with an entropion have smaller than average tarsal plates when compared to a normal age-matched population. Patients with ectropion have larger tarsal plates. Males have larger tarsal dimensions than females and thus a greater incidence of ectropion.

The histological differences are also interesting. There appear to be significantly more orbicularis

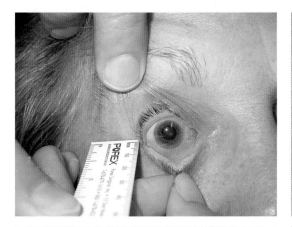

Fig. 8.12 Assessment of lower-lid laxity.

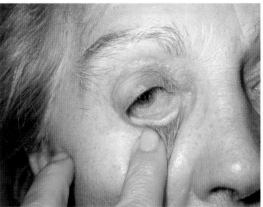

Fig. 8.13 Assessment and measurement of lateral canthal laxity.

and Riolan's muscle ischemia, atrophy and collagen fragmentation with ectropion than with entropion. Entropion shows more septal and tarsal atrophy. In both conditions, the skin and conjunctiva show chronic inflammation and scarring as a constant feature.

Understanding the mechanism of these different elements is of great importance in deciding the correct surgical procedure.

Examinination of a patient with malposition of the eyelids

General laxity

One should not be able to pull the eyelid away from the globe by more than 8–9 mm (Fig. 8.12). Horizontal laxity is probably one of the main pathological factors in age-related entropion and ectropion; it is doubtful whether surgical correction without horizontal shortening of the eyelid will be adequate.

Snap test

This detects subclinical laxity, which is important in assessing eyelid pump efficiency. Pull the eyelid away with the index finger while viewing the lid with the slit lamp and let go. A normal eyelid snaps back without the need for a blink.

Lateral canthal laxity

Rounding of the lateral canthus is usually a sign of laxity. In the absence of laxity the lid will not move medially from its attachment to the lateral orbital rim (Fig. 8.13).

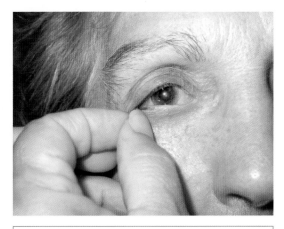

Fig. 8.14 Assessment of medial canthal laxity.

Distraction test for medial canthal laxity

Medial canthal tendon laxity is assessed first by noting the position of the punctum at rest and second by measuring the amount of lateral displacement of the punctum with the distraction test (Fig. 8.14). The normal position of the lower punctum is just lateral to a perpendicular line drawn from the upper punctum. In the distraction test the lower lid is pinched medially and then pulled laterally and the amount of lateral movement of the punctum in relation to the corneal limbus is graded from 0 to 6. Any grade of 4 or above requires medial canthal stabilisation (Olver, 2001).

Lower-lid retractor assessment

Ask the patient to look up and then down. Note the excursion of the lower lid; similarly, assess the elevation of the upper lid. The presence of a lower-lid skin crease is also an indicator of good retractor function. Note that upper-lid retraction together with upper-lid entropion indicates retractor scarring, for example, in trachoma. Surgical intervention requires lengthening of the retractor layer as well as lid eversion.

Prolapse of orbital fat

Prolapse of orbital fat produces a mechanical force to induce or exaggerate an entropion. Because of the normal more anterior position of the orbital fat in orientals, they may be more predisposed than Caucasians to the development of involutional entropion rather than ectropion. Removal of lower eyelid fat should be considered in entropion repair in such patients.

Adequacy of skin

Pinch the lower lid in the middle and pull it upwards. Adequate skin is present if the lower eyelid can reach the upper limbus (Fig. 8.15). Skin shortage is particularly important in ectropion and, if it is not addressed, will lead to failure of the surgical procedure.

Tarsal height

Note the height of the tarsus. If it is less than 4 mm in the upper lid or 2 mm in the lower lid, one might

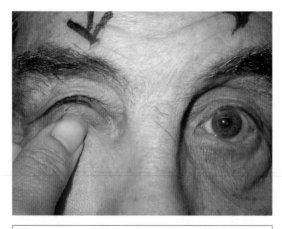

Fig. 8.15 Assessment of the adequacy of the lower-lid skin.

need to add additional material such as hard palate in any surgical procedure.

Summary

Surgical treatment of all eyelid abnormalities should be custom-made to the individual. Often more than one factor needs to be addressed to achieve effective and long-lasting results. This requires a detailed examination of the lids to understand the mechanism of the eyelid malposition.

- Structure and function are very closely related, so an intimate knowledge of orbital anatomy is essential
- Appropriate testing gives vital clues as to causal pathology or, at least, the site of the pathology
- Accurate measurements are vital to be able to monitor progression or stability of disease processes convincingly

Further reading

Bashour M, Harvey J. Causes of involutional ectropion and entropion-age-related tarsal changes are the key. Ophthalm Plast Reconstr Surg 2000; 16: 131–141.

Burkat CN, Lucarelli MJ. Tear meniscus level as an indicator of nasolacrimal obstruction. Ophthalmology 2005; 112: 344–348.

Camara JG, Santiago MD, Rodriguez R et al. The micro-reflux test: a new test to evaluate nasolacrimal duct obstruction. Ophthalmology 1999; 106: 2319–2321.

Carter SR, Chang J, Aguilar GL, Rathbun JE, Seiff SR. Involutional entropion and ectropion of the Asian lower eyelid. Ophthalm Plast Reconstr Surg 2000; 16: 45–49.

Danks JJ, Rose GE. Involutional lower lid entropion: to shorten or not to shorten? Ophthalmology 1999; 106: 85–89.

Di Pascuale MA, Espana EM, Kawakita T, Tseng SC. Clinical characteristics of conjunctivochalasis with or without aqueous tear deficiency. Br J Ophthalmol 2004; 88: 388–392.

Harrad RA, Shuttleworth GN. Superior rectus-levator synkinesis: a previously unrecognised cause of failure of ptosis surgery. Ophthalmology 2000; 107: 1975–1981.

Jones LT. An anatomical approach to problems of the eyelids and lacrimal apparatus. Arch Ophthalmol 1961; 66: 111–124.

Lertchavnakul A, Gamnerdsiri P, Hirunwiwatkul P. Ice test for ocular myasthenia gravis. J Med Assoc 2001; 84 (suppl. 1): S131–S136.

Macri A, Rolando M, Pflugfelder S. A standardized visual scale for evaluation of tear fluorescein clearance. Ophthalmology 2000; 107: 1338–1343.

Movaghar M, Slavin ML. Effect of local heat versus ice on blepharoptosis resulting from ocular myasthenia. Ophthalmology 2000; 107: 2209–2214.

Olver JM, Prabhati JS, Wright M. Lower eyelid medial canthal tendon laxity grading: an interobserver study of normal subjects. Ophthalmology 2001; 108: 21–25.

Sahlin S, Chen E. Evaluation of the lacrimal drainage function by the drop test. Am J Ophthalmol 1996; 122: 701–708.

Sisler HA, Labay GR, Finlay JR. Senile ectropion and entropion: a comparative histopathological study. Ann Ophthalmol 1976; 8: 319–322.

Toprak AB, Erkin EF, Kayikcioglu O et al. Fluorescein dye disappearance test in patients with different degrees of epiphora. Eur J Ophthalmol 2002; 12: 359–365.

Wojno TH. Down gaze ptosis. Ophthalm Plast Reconstr Surg 1993; 9: 83–88.

Zappia RJ, Millder B. Lacrimal drainage function: 2. The fluorescein dye disappearance test. Am J Ophthalmol 1972; 74: 160–162.

Ocular motility examination

MANOJ V. PARULEKAR

Introduction

Examination of eye movements is an important part of any neurological examination. The third, fourth and sixth cranial nerves supply motor fibres to the extraocular muscles, the seventh nerve innervates the orbicularis oculi and the second (optic) and fifth (trigeminal) nerves carry sensation from the eye.

Examination of eye movements is also an integral component of examination of the eyelids and pupils.

Binocular vision is the ability of the higher visual centres in the brain to process the visual signals from both eyes simultaneously to produce a single image. It is a function of higher-evolved species. It is important for both eyes to point in the same direction to produce a similar image on both retinas. Coordinated eye movements are therefore essential for binocular vision.

There are six extraocular muscles. The superior rectus, inferior rectus, medial rectus and inferior oblique are innervated by the oculomotor (third) nerve, the superior oblique by the trochlear (fourth) nerve and the lateral rectus by the abducens (sixth) nerve. The extraocular muscles are striated voluntary muscles.

Three muscles control eyelid movements. The levator palpebrae superioris is supplied by the third nerve, the orbicularis oculi is supplied by the seventh nerve and Müller's muscle is under sympathetic control.

Overview

Ocular motility examination must be carried out in a well-lit room. The room must be large enough to allow a fixation target to be ideally positioned at 6 m (20 ft), or at least 3 metres (10 feet) with a mirror to project the image at 6 metres (20 feet).

It is important to test the visual acuity of both eyes before commencing the examination (see Ch. 1).

Good visual acuity in both eyes is essential for performing the cover tests. This is because a poorly sighted eye will not take up fixation on the target and the test is invalidated. In such cases, other tests such as the Hirschberg and prism reflex test can be used, as described later.

The refractive error of the subject must be determined before commencing examination. One must ascertain if the subject wears spectacle correction or contact lenses, and whether it is for distance or near or both. The power of the glasses can be determined by neutralisation or focimetry.

A significant proportion of the population with strabismus are children. It is important to win their confidence first and to use child-friendly targets such as a toy or a funny-face sticker on a fixation stick (Fig. 9.1).

Other essential equipment includes accommodative targets for distance and near, an occluder and a pen torch.

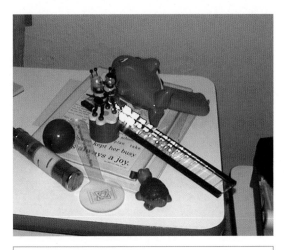

Fig. 9.1 Some of the simple equipment used to examine a child.

History

It is important to obtain an accurate history where possible.

Ascertain what patients are most bothered by, how troublesome the symptoms are, and what are their expectations.

The symptoms may be visual or non-visual. Visual symptoms include double vision (diplopia), photophobia/glare and oscillopsia (sensation of object moving/spinning).

Non-visual symptoms may be related to the appearance of the eyes (cosmetic) or abnormal head posture.

Examination

Head posture

Examination of patients begins almost as soon as they enter the room. Abnormal head posture should be noted. This is the hallmark of incomitant squints. A deviation is described as concomitant when it measures the same in various positions of gaze, and incomitant if it varies with change in gaze. The greater the underaction of the muscle, the more marked the head posture. The head is turned in the direction of action of the underacting muscle. This

is to move the eye out of the field of action of the underacting muscle, thus relieving diplopia. For example, the face turned to the left indicates underaction of the left lateral rectus or right medial rectus (Figs 9.2 and 9.3).

The presence of a head posture is an indirect clue to the presence of binocular vision; there would be no diplopia without binocular vision, and as a result no head posture.

It is important to remember that chin elevation or depression may also occur with pattern strabismus (A, V or Y pattern) in the absence of obvious muscle underaction. For example, chin depression will occur with underaction of the inferior rectus or the superior oblique of either eye or V-pattern esotropia or A exotropia. This reduces the angle of squint, making it easier to control.

Head tilt occurs with underaction of the oblique muscles. The head is tilted to the opposite side with an underacting superior oblique and to the same side with underaction of the inferior oblique (rare).

Abnormal head posture also occurs in certain forms of nystagmus, particularly when the nystagmus varies with the position of gaze. Adopting a head posture rotates the eyes in the direction where the nystagmus is dampened.

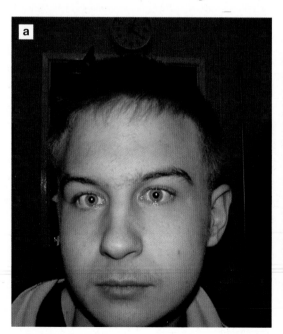
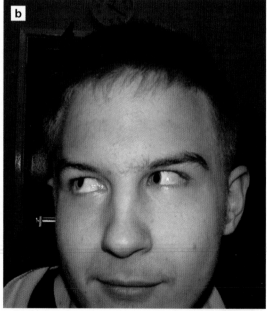

Fig. 9.2 Face turned to the right **(a)** to prevent the right hypertropia that develops in right gaze **(b)**.

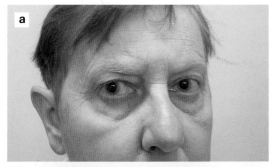

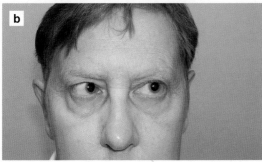

Fig. 9.3 Face turned to the left **(a)** due to left lateral rectus palsy **(b)**.

Causes of abnormal head posture
Ocular

Ocular misalignment (squint): seen in incomitant strabismus

■ Paresis of third, fourth or sixth nerve

■ Restriction of eye movements as in thyroid eye disease, Brown's syndrome, blow-out fracture

■ Pattern strabismus: A- or V-pattern

■ Cranial dysinnervation syndromes, such as Duane's syndrome

Nystagmus

Non-ocular

Muscular: due to sternocleidomastoid shortening (congenital or acquired) or spasm (may be due to sinusitis, mastoiditis, cervical adenitis)

Skeletal: Klippel–Feil anomaly, other cervical spine/scapular deformities

Habitual (Fig. 9.4)

It is important to remember that abnormal head posture can also be due to non-ocular causes (Box 9.1).

Examination of the eyelids

Examination of the eyelids is an important part of an ocular motility examination. Obvious lid malposition should be noted.

True ptosis may occur with a third-nerve palsy. It can also accompany monocular elevation deficiency (double elevator palsy).

Pseudoptosis may occur with superior rectus underaction. The lid is droopy on the same side as the hypotropic eye. It disappears when the hypotropic eye is forced to take up fixation (by covering the other eye).

Lid retraction may accompany strabismus when there is mechanical restriction of elevation of the fixing eye, for example due to a tight/tethered inferior rectus. When the hypotropic eye attempts to take up fixation, the superior rectus on that side has to work harder to overcome the mechanical restriction. This results in a greater number of impulses flowing to both the superior rectus and the levator on that side, resulting in lid retraction.

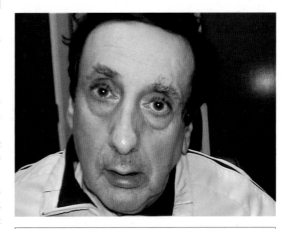

Fig. 9.4 Habitual head tilt to the left with a degree of facial asymmetry.

Change in position of eyelid with eye movement

The position of the eyelid may change with the direction of gaze in certain forms of strabismus.

Third-nerve palsy due to trauma may be followed by partial recovery with aberrant regeneration. The

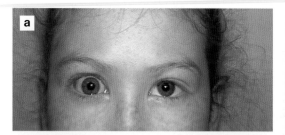

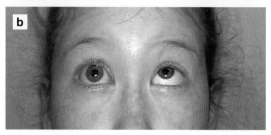

Fig. 9.5 Right upper-lid retraction **(a)** due to mechanical restriction of the right superior rectus **(b)**.

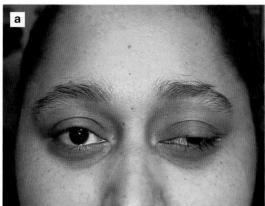

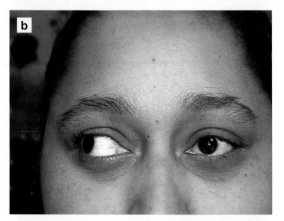

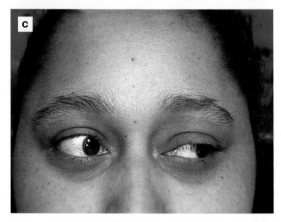

Fig. 9.6 Changes in palpebral fissure with eye movement. The ptotic left upper lid **(a)** elevates in adduction **(b)** and droops in abduction **(c)**. This is due to abnormal medial rectus levator synkinesis following third-nerve palsy with aberrant regeneration.

fibres grow back but may be misrouted to supply structures not previously innervated by these fibres (Fig. 9.6). A common pattern seen is medial rectus levator synkinesis, where the fibres supplying the medial rectus also innervate the levator. This results in elevation of the eyelid on attempted adduction, and ptosis on abduction.

In Duane's syndrome, depending on the type, there may be widening of the palpebral fissure on looking in one direction, and narrowing in the other.

Mechanical restriction of the superior rectus may also cause upper-lid retraction (Fig. 9.5).

Other points to be noted are the presence of an epicanthal fold, and an excessively wide bridge of the nose causing the eyes to appear too close together (pseudo-convergent squint).

Examination of the pupils

The size of the pupils must be noted as part of the initial assessment.

Any change in relation to eye movements must be noted (again, this may be seen with third-nerve palsy with aberrant regeneration).

Examination of eye movements

Ocular motility examination should start initially with the subject fixating at 6 m (distance) followed by examination with a near (30 cm) target.

Examination must be carried out initially with and later without glasses.

Certain observations can be made while talking to the patient. These include:

- Is there any misalignment of the eyes looking straight ahead?
- If so, which eye is deviating? Is it turning in or out?
- Is it consistently one eye that squints, or do they alternate?
- Is it intermittent or constant?
- Does the squint break down easily?

Measuring ocular deviation

Light reflex tests

Hirschberg corneal light reflex test. This test relies on observing the light reflected off the cornea – Purkinje I image – from a light source positioned at 30 cm. The reflex should normally be central and symmetrical in both eyes. It will be displaced nasally in divergent squints and temporally in convergent squints.

One millimetre of displacement corresponds to approximately 7° or 15 prism dioptres (PD) of misalignment. Assuming a 3.5 mm diameter pupil, this would give a deviation of 15° (30 PD) if the reflex were at the pupillary margin, 45° (90 PD) at the limbus and 30° (60 PD) between the two (Figs 9.7–9.10).

While this is not a very accurate test, it is nevertheless a useful test in young children. It is also very useful in estimating the deviation if one eye is blind (non-fixing) as the cover test cannot be performed in this situation.

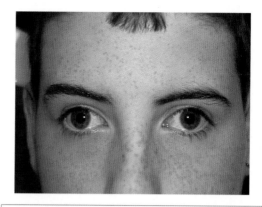

Fig. 9.8 Nasally displaced corneal reflex suggests an exodeviation measuring approximately 30 PD.

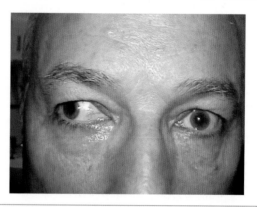

Fig. 9.9 Hirschberg test: corneal reflex at the limbus suggests deviation of approximately 90 PD.

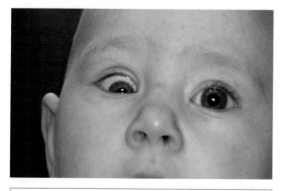

Fig. 9.7 Hirschberg test with vertical deviation of approximately 45 PD.

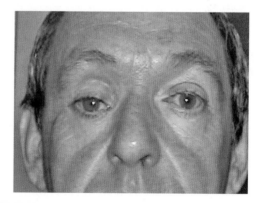

Fig. 9.10 Symmetrical Hirschberg reflexes despite apparent ocular misalignment confirm the absence of squint. The eyes appear misaligned due to displacement of the right orbit following a fracture.

The cover test

This is a very important test in assessing any ocular deviation. It must be performed for both distance and near, with and without glasses.

The principle. When attempting to fix on an object (either in the distance at 6 m or near at 30 cm), if both eyes are aligned, they will fix simultaneously on the object. In the presence of an ocular deviation, however, one eye (the fixing eye) will fixate on the object while the other eye (the deviating eye) will deviate outward (divergent squint) or inward (convergent squint).

If the fixing eye is covered, the deviating eye will make a corrective movement to take up fixation on the object. This corrective movement will be *opposite to the direction of the squint*. The deviating eye will move outwards if it was previously turned in (convergent), and conversely will move inwards with a divergent squint.

In order to perform the cover test, each eye must have sufficient vision to see the chosen fixation target (generally the top letter on a Snellen visual acuity chart, or an object on the far wall at eye level). It is essential to cover each eye and check this before performing the cover test.

There are two types of cover test: (1) the unilateral cover–uncover test; and (2) the alternate cover test.

The unilateral cover–uncover test

In this test, one eye is covered and then uncovered. Each eye is tested in turn. The subject is asked to look at the fixation target and one eye is covered with an occluder for approximately 3 s, and then uncovered. This is done twice, initially looking at the uncovered eye for any corrective movement when the cover is brought in, and then observing the occluded eye as the cover is removed to see whether it makes a corrective movement to take up fixation (Fig. 9.11).

Alternate-cover test

In this test each eye is covered alternately. The subject is asked to observe the fixation target and the occluder is moved from one eye to the other, each eye being covered for approximately 3 s. Both eyes are observed and any corrective movement is noted. There will be a corrective movement outwards with a convergent squint and an inward movement with a divergent squint. With vertical deviations, there will be a corresponding upward or downward

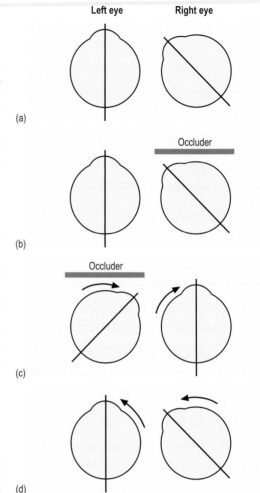

Fig. 9.11 The unilateral cover–uncover test. **(a)** The right eye is esotropic. **(b)** The cover is placed over the right eye; there is no movement. **(c)** The left eye is then covered, the right eye moves out to take up fixation, the left eye moves in. **(d)** The left eye is uncovered and moves out to take up fixation, with the right eye moving in once again.

movement. This is accompanied by a corresponding movement of the eyelid. If the vertical deviation is small, the corrective movement of the eye may not be easily seen and the movement of the eyelids may be a useful clue. The eye making the corrective downward movement is the hyperdeviating eye.

The deviation may be manifest (present without dissociation, also termed tropia) or latent (only seen when the eyes are dissociated, also termed phoria). The alternate-cover test is more dissociative than the cover–uncover test and reveals the total (latent plus manifest) deviation. The cover–uncover test on the other hand only shows the manifest deviation.

Primary and secondary deviation

Primary and secondary deviations occur in incomitant squints resulting from mechanical restriction or paralysis. The deviation observed with the unaffected eye fixing is the primary deviation. The secondary deviation occurs when the subject fixes with the affected (paralytic/restricted) eye. The secondary deviation is always larger than the primary deviation. This results from increased stimuli flowing to the paretic/restricted eye to take up fixation, and as a result more stimuli also flow to the yoke muscle of the contralateral eye (Hering's law: see below) producing a larger deviation.

The primary deviation is measured with a prism over the non-fixing eye while the secondary deviation is measured with the prism over the fixing eye.

Nine positions of gaze

The nine diagnostic positions of gaze (Fig. 9.12) are looking:

- up, up and to the right and up and to the left
- right, straight and left
- down, down and to the right, and down and to the left.

The cover test can be performed in the nine positions of gaze. This information is very useful, particularly in incomitant squints (paralytic or restrictive) to identify the underacting muscle(s). It is often useful to perform the cover test with the subject looking in the direction of maximum diplopia. This can help identify the offending muscle if the deviation is very small. The eye with the underacting muscle will make a corrective movement in the direction of gaze when uncovered.

If the movement is subtle, it may be difficult to interpret the results. In this situation, the subject's responses can be used to identify the underacting muscle. When one eye is covered, one of the images will disappear. The underacting muscle projects the outer of the two images and the contralateral agonist produces the inner image. Each eye is covered in turn and the subject is asked to report when the outer image disappears – the covered eye is the side with the affected muscle.

Range of eye movements
Ductions, versions and vergence

Ductions are uniocular eye movements. They are tested by observing monocular eye movements with the opposite eye covered.

Versions are binocular eye movements in the same direction, i.e. both eyes looking right, or both looking left.

Vergence is also a binocular eye movement but the two eyes move in opposite directions. Convergence

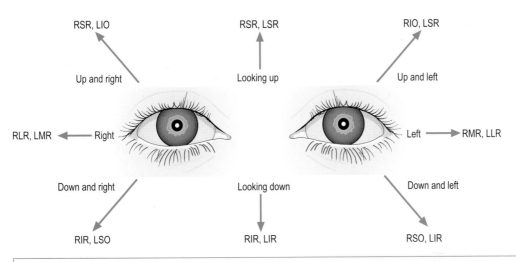

Fig. 9.12 The eight diagnostic positions of gaze.

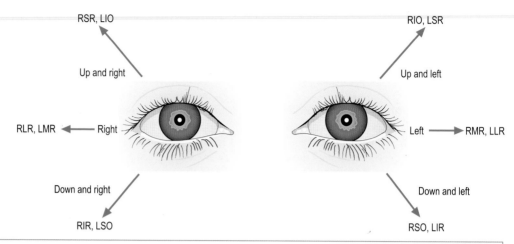

RSR, LIO

Up and right

RLR, LMR ← Right

Down and right

RIR, LSO

RIO, LSR

Up and left

Left → RMR, LLR

Down and left

RSO, LIR

Fig. 9.13 Pictorial depiction of the six cardinal positions and the muscles exerting maximum effect in each position.

describes a bilateral inward movement while divergence is a bilateral outward movement. In practice, only convergence is tested (described later).

If versions are normal, testing ductions does not provide any additional information and is unnecessary. If however, the versions are abnormal, monocular ductions must be tested, especially in the direction of limited eye movement.

Ductions and versions are tested in the six cardinal (diagnostic) positions of gaze (Fig. 9.13). These are looking: (1) right; (2) up and right; (3) down and right; (4) left; (5) up and left; and (6) down and left. These positions are chosen because they represent the sites of maximum action of the six extraocular muscles. Any over- or underaction in these positions can isolate and identify the offending muscle.

Ductions and versions are governed by Hering's and Sherrington's laws.

Hering's law states that, when the impulse for movement is initiated, the same amount of innervation flows to the yoke muscle in the other eye.

Sherrington's law of reciprocal innervation states that, whenever a muscle receives an impulse to contract, its antagonist will receive an equal amount of inhibitory input to relax.

Underaction of a muscle on version testing may be due to muscle paresis, mechanical restriction, inhibitional palsy or a large underlying deviation.

Inhibitional palsy is part of the chronic changes seen in long-standing paralytic squints. There is overaction and contracture of the ipsilateral antagonist, overaction of the contralateral agonist and inhibitional palsy of the contralateral antagonist in accordance with Sherrington's law of reciprocal innervation.

The action of any muscle can be graded on a scale of –4 to +4. Zero is considered normal; –4 represents maximum underaction and +4 maximum overaction (Fig. 9.14).

Convergence

Testing for convergence is a very important part of ocular motility examination. Poor convergence may be seen in divergent strabismus, especially near exotropia. Overactive convergence may be seen in accommodative esotropia, and in infantile esotropia. Convergence may be lost in some forms of internuclear ophthalmoplegia and may be of localising value (it is preserved in posterior lesions of the medial longitudinal fasciculus).

Locating the approximate position of the near point of convergence in centimetres from the eye is the simplest way of assessing adequacy of convergence. It is measured by bringing a fixation target progressively closer to the eyes in the midline and recording (with the help of a scale) the distance at which the subject reports diplopia and/or one of the eyes fails to adduct and diverges. It should be no greater than 15 cm.

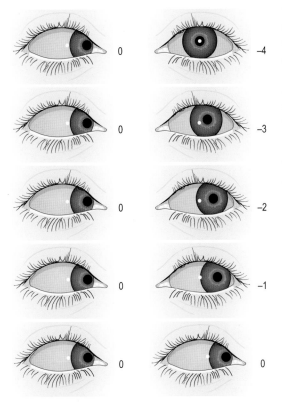

Fig. 9.14 Pictorial depiction of grading of left lateral rectus muscle underaction of varying degrees. Zero is normal and −4 is maximum underaction.

The amplitude and range of convergence can be measured using the Royal Air Force (RAF) rule but this is of limited clinical value.

Forced duction test

This test is usually performed in the operating theatre before or during surgery but may also be performed on cooperative adult patients in clinic under topical anaesthesia. It is useful in detecting mechanical restriction of a muscle, thus differentiating paresis from tethering/adhesions as a cause of muscle underaction.

The conjunctiva and episcleral tissues are grasped with toothed forceps and the eye is rotated into the field of action of the muscle being tested. The test can be performed on any extraocular muscle. When testing the recti, the eye is pulled slightly anteriorly, and when testing the obliques, the globe is pushed back into the orbit to maximise tension on the tendon. The superior oblique is tested by rotating the eye into maximum adduction and the inferior oblique by rotating it inwards and down.

The forced duction test is observer-dependent and as a result prone to errors. The results may vary depending on patient apprehension, anaesthetic and operator technique.

Force generation test

This test requires the patient to be actively cooperative and awake. The subject is instructed to look in the direction of the muscle being tested, for example abduction when testing the lateral rectus. The conjunctiva is grasped near the opposite limbus with forceps and the examiner exerts traction in the opposite direction and evaluates the resistance. The greater the resistance, the stronger the action of the muscle. This test is useful in assessing the action of the muscle but cannot differentiate between mechanical and paralytic underaction.

Saccades

Saccades are rapid eye movements between two points in space. The purpose of saccades is to re-establish fixation on another object. The classic example is the eye movement that occurs during fixation pauses when reading.

Saccades can be horizontal, vertical or oblique. The rectus muscles are believed to be mainly responsible for generating saccades.

When testing saccades, the subject is instructed to look alternately at two separate objects such as a hand and a fist held far apart – horizontally for horizontal saccades and vertically for testing vertical saccades.

The speed of saccadic movement (saccadic velocity) noted and compared for the two eyes and in both directions. A reduction in horizontal saccades indicates weakness of the muscle generating the saccades. Absence of saccades could be due to saccadic palsy caused by involvement of the brainstem centres.

Saccadic velocity is reduced in paralytic strabismus but is unaffected in mechanical restriction.

Smooth pursuit

Smooth pursuit movement is a slow, steady eye move-ment to follow a moving object in the field of vision. It is less useful than saccades in diagnostic evaluation.

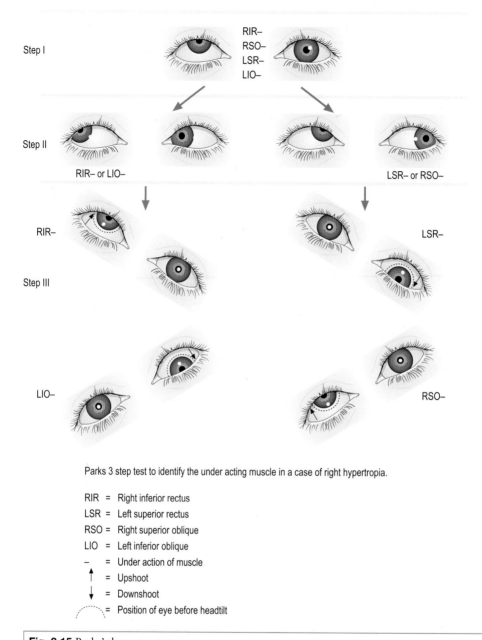

Parks 3 step test to identify the under acting muscle in a case of right hypertropia.

RIR = Right inferior rectus
LSR = Left superior rectus
RSO = Right superior oblique
LIO = Left inferior oblique
– = Under action of muscle
↑ = Upshoot
↓ = Downshoot
⌒ = Position of eye before headtilt

Fig. 9.15 Parks' three-step test.

Doll's-head manoeuvre

The range of ocular movements can be tested by passively rotating the head from side to side and observing eye movements (after ascertaining there is no neck trauma or instability). This test is very useful in children and unconscious patients. Under normal circumstances, the eyes lag behind and should exhibit a full range of ocular rotation. A full range of movement on this test excludes mechanical and infranuclear causes of limited eye movements.

Conditions with limited range of voluntary eye movements that can be improved by the doll's-head manoeuvre include gaze palsy and progressive supranuclear palsy.

Parks' three-step test

The three-step test is the key to diagnosing isolated cyclovertical (vertical rectus or oblique muscles) muscle palsy (Fig. 9.15). It was described by Marshall Parks. The three steps are:

1. Cover test in primary position: this identifies the hypertropic eye. The underacting muscle could be one of the two depressors (inferior rectus and superior oblique) of the hypertropic eye or one of the two elevators (superior rectus and inferior oblique) of the hypotropic eye. For example, with right hypertropia, it could be the right inferior rectus or superior oblique, or left superior rectus or inferior oblique.
2. Cover test in right and left gaze: this tells us if the hyperdeviation increases in right or left gaze. The obliques have maximum vertical action in adduction and the recti in abduction. Depending on where the diplopia is maximum, the underacting muscle can be narrowed down from four muscles to the two acting in that position of gaze. For example, if the diplopia worsens on right gaze, it narrows it down to right inferior rectus or left inferior oblique.
3. Bielschowsky head tilt test (Fig. 9.16): this is based on the observation that tilting the head results in intorsion of one eye and extorsion of the other to maintain a single image. The superior rectus and superior oblique are intorters and inferior rectus and inferior oblique are extorters.

Bielschowsky head tilt test

If the superior oblique (intorter) on one side is underacting, that eye will be excyclorotated (12 o'clock position is rotated outward) in the primary position due to unopposed action of the ipsilateral antagonists (inferior rectus and inferior oblique).

The other intorter of that eye (the superior rectus) will overact to try and correct the extorsion. The superior rectus is chiefly an elevator, and the overaction will result in elevation of the affected eye relative to the other unaffected eye.

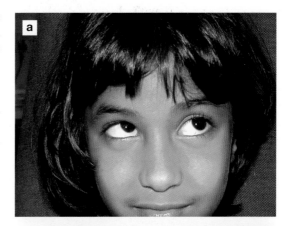

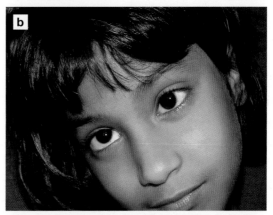

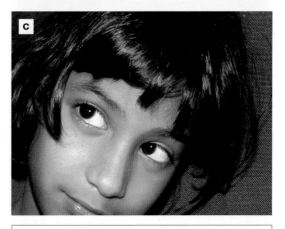

Fig. 9.16 Bielschowsky head tilt test in a case of right superior oblique weakness. **(a)** Secondary right inferior oblique overaction; **(b)** right eye elevates on tilting the head to the right shoulder; **(c)** Right hypertropia reduces on head tilt to the left shoulder.

This phenomenon may not be readily apparent in the primary position but will become more manifest if the head is tilted towards the shoulder on the same side as the affected eye. This manoeuvre will result in excyclorotation of the affected eye and incyclorotation of the fellow eye. Both eyes will attempt to make a corrective movement in the opposite direction by recruiting the superior rectus and superior oblique of the affected eye and inferior rectus and inferior oblique of the fellow eye. For reasons mentioned above, the superior rectus will overact and the affected eye will elevate.

The opposite will happen when the head is tilted towards the unaffected side and, as the superior rectus does not have to overact any more, the hyperdeviation of the affected eye becomes smaller or disappears.

In the above case, we have narrowed down the underacting muscle to the right inferior rectus (extorter of the right eye) or left inferior oblique (extorter of the left eye).

If, on performing the Bielschowsky head tilt test, it produces a right hypertropia on tilting the head to the right shoulder, the muscles that come into play are the intorters of the right eye (superior oblique and superior rectus) and the extorters of the left eye (inferior rectus and inferior oblique). As we have already narrowed it down to the right inferior rectus or left inferior oblique, this points to the right inferior rectus as the underacting muscle.

Torsion

The two images may not always be parallel to each other. If the cyclovertical muscles (vertical recti or obliques) are involved, the images may be tilted relative to each other. Oblique muscle dysfunction is more likely to cause symptomatic torsion than the vertical recti.

Horizontal rectus muscle involvement will not result in torsion.

Testing for torsion

A simple way to test for torsion is to present a linear object, e.g. a pencil, to the subject. If there is torsion, one of the images will be tilted. One can now perform the alternate-cover test at this point and ask the subject to report when the tilted image disappears. The eye that must be covered to make the tilted image disappear is the affected eye. It is also possible to determine the direction of tilt and

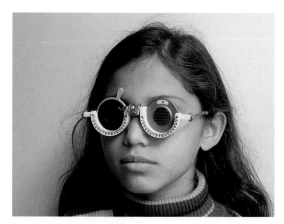

Fig. 9.17 Double Maddox rod test for torsion.

identify the affected muscle. The subject can be given two linear objects and asked to place them in the same position as the two images. We have previously identified the affected eye and, based on the position of the two pencils, one can determine if the tilted image seen is intorted or extorted for the affected eye. For example, if the right eye is affected and the image seen by the right eye is intorted, this means the eye is extorted (the image is always rotated in the opposite direction to the position of the eye). This is due to underaction of the intorters of the right eye (superior rectus or superior oblique).

Another way of testing (and quantifying) torsion is by using two Maddox rods (see below), one in front of each eye (Fig. 9.17). The subject will see two streaks of light at an angle to each other. One of the rods can then be rotated to make the two images coincide and the angle of torsion can be read off the trial frame.

Torsion can also be quantified using the synoptophore (see below).

Prism tests

Simultaneous prism cover test (SPCT)

It is important to check that the fixation target can be seen clearly by each eye before performing the cover tests. The SPCT measures the angle of deviation under binocular conditions (manifest deviation only). The full angle of deviation (latent plus manifest) can be determined by the alternate prism cover test. The SPCT must be performed before the alternate prism cover test to avoid dissociating the two eyes.

Once the deviating eye has been identified on the cover–uncover test and the angle estimated on the Hirschberg test, a prism of estimated strength to neutralise the manifest deviation is selected. The fixing eye is covered with an occluder and the prism is simultaneously placed over the deviating eye, base out for esotropia and base in for exotropia (Fig. 9.18). If no movement is seen, the power of the prism corresponds to the size of the manifest deviation. If there is residual movement, stronger or weaker prisms are used until neutralisation is achieved.

Alternate prism cover test (APCT)

In this test, the prism of approximate power based on Hirschberg testing is placed in front of the deviating eye and the alternate cover test is performed. The prism strength is adjusted until neutralisation is achieved. This test measures the total deviation (manifest plus latent) as it completely dissociates the two eyes.

The Krimsky reflex test

This is based on the same principle as the Hirschberg test. Prisms of increasing strength (base in for exo-deviation, base out for esodeviation) are held in front of the fixing eye to replace the displaced corneal reflex to the centre of the deviating eye. It can be performed even when the visual acuity is very poor in one of the eyes. The disadvantage is that it tends to underestimate larger deviations.

Primary and secondary deviation

Remember that the secondary deviation is always greater than the primary deviation (p. 109). The primary deviation is measured with prisms over the non-fixing eye, and the secondary deviation with prisms over the fixing eye.

Tests for Diplopia

The principle of diplopia testing is to determine whether the images seen by the two eyes coincide or are separated in space.

If both eyes are presented with identical images that must be fused to produce a single image, this is less disruptive to the fusional mechanisms and is described as a non-dissociative test. Non-dissociative tests are less likely to detect latent deviations as the fusional mechanisms can act to control any latent component. If, however, the two eyes are presented with dissimilar images that must be superimposed on each other, it disrupts the fusional mechanisms more completely and is more likely to uncover latent deviations. Such tests are termed dissociative.

Dissociative tests

Maddox rod test

The Maddox rod is a lens system consisting of a series of parallel cylinders (Fig. 9.19). If a point source of light is observed through the lens, it produces a streak of light perpendicular to the direction of the cylinders. The single Maddox rod test is usually used to assess diplopia and detect deviations. The double Maddox rod test is used to assess torsion.

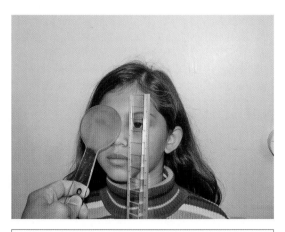

Fig. 9.18 The simultaneous prism cover test.

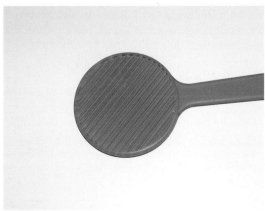

Fig. 9.19 Maddox rod.

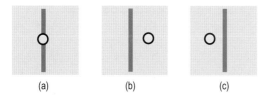

(a)　　　　　　(b)　　　　　　(c)

Fig. 9.20 (a) Maddox rod in front of right eye. The line and spot coincide, indicating the presence of binocular single vision. **(b)** Maddox rod in front of the right eye. The line and spot do not coincide. The response on the left suggests crossed diplopia (exodeviation). **(c)** The response on the right represents uncrossed diplopia due to an esodeviation.

If the cylinders are placed horizontally, the streak produced is vertical, and vice versa.

One eye looks through the rod at a point source of light and sees a streak, while the other sees the point source. Depending on the direction and degree of separation of the images, the diplopia can be characterised and quantified (Fig. 9.20).

By convention, the red Maddox rod is placed horizontally in a trial frame in front of the right eye. The left eye observes the point of light. If the red line bisects the point, it signifies orthophoria (no manifest or latent deviation) (Fig. 9.20a). If there is separation, and the red line is to the left, there is an exodeviation (Fig. 9.20b). If it is to the right of the white light (uncrossed diplopia), it denotes an esodeviation (Fig. 9.20c).

The test is then performed with the cylinders vertically to assess vertical deviations. Prisms of appropriate strength can be placed to move the images to coincide.

Red-glass test

In this test, a red filter is placed in front of one eye and the subject is asked to observe a point source of white light and describe what is seen. Two lights indicate a diplopia response. If the response is a single light, the colour of light is identified. Red or white indicates suppression, while pink indicates fusion.

Worth four-dot test (WFDT)

This test is highly dissociative and may produce a diplopia response in the absence of a manifest

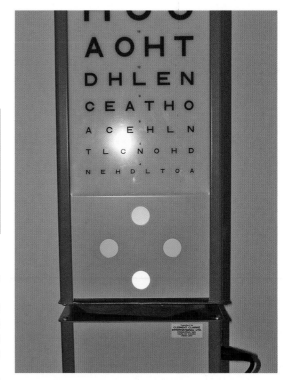

Fig. 9.21 Worth four-dot test (WFDT).

deviation. It involves placing a red filter in front of one eye and a green filter in front of the other and observing four dots – two green, one red and one white (Fig. 9.21).

The normal subject would see four lights – two green, one red and the fourth may be seen as pink or light green depending on which eye is dominant (Fig. 9.22a). Five lights (two red, three green) would indicate a diplopia response (Fig. 9.22b) while seeing only two red or three green lights would indicate suppression (Fig. 9.22c).

Non-dissociative tests
Bagolini glasses
These are lenses with striations that can be placed in the trial frame and rotated into any axis (Fig. 9.23). As the two eyes see a differently oriented image of similar colour and brightness, it is less disruptive to fusion.

Typically the striations are oriented at 45 and 135° in front of the two eyes and a fixation light is held 40 cm away in the midline. The patient is

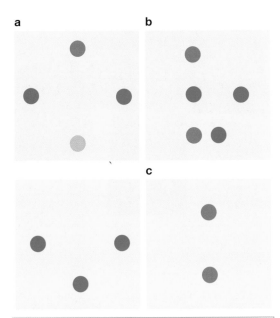

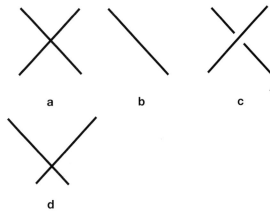

Fig. 9.24 Bagolini glasses. **(a)** Normal response. **(b)** Suppression response. **(c)** Foveal suppression scotoma. **(d)** Ocular deviation.

Fig. 9.22 (a) Normal response with the Worth four-dot test (WFDT). **(b)** Diplopia response with the WFDT. **(c)** Suppression response with the WFDT. The patient sees either three green lights or two red.

indicates a foveal suppression scotoma (Fig. 9.24c). If the lines cross asymmetrically, it indicates an ocular deviation (Fig. 9.24d).

Concept of sensory and motor fusion

Motor fusion is the ability to bring the two eyes into alignment and maintain eye position. It is a function of the extraocular muscles.

This could be fusional convergence (bringing the eyes in to correct exodeviations) or divergence (moving the two eyes out to correct esodeviations) or vertical. The range of fusional convergence is greatest, followed by divergence, while vertical fusional range is very small.

While there is an innate fusional ability, it is possible to extend the range of motor fusion either with orthoptic exercises or as an adaptive response to a long-standing deviation, e.g. following congenital fourth-nerve palsy.

The physiological role of motor fusion is to correct for minor misalignments (very commonly seen in normal individuals).

Sensory fusion on the other hand is the ability of the higher visual processing centres to superimpose the two images seen by the two eyes (each eye sees a slightly different image from the other as they are set apart in space) and produce a single image.

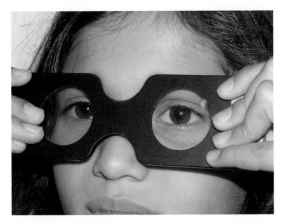

Fig. 9.23 Bagolini striated glasses.

then asked to describe the position of the lines seen. If the lines bisect each other, this indicates normal bifoveal fusion (Fig. 9.24a). If one of the lines is missed entirely, it indicates suppression (Fig. 9.24b), while if the central portion of the line is missed, it

Reasons for assessing binocular single vision (BSV)

- Duration and magnitude of squint: absence of BSV indicates a long-standing, poorly controlled or uncontrolled deviation
- Prognostic value: presence of BSV is a good prognostic sign and indicates the subject may derive functional benefit from squint correction. Absent or weak BSV indicates increased risk of recurrence of the deviation over the long term. Such cases may benefit from adjustable suture squint surgery
- Diplopia: the subject may complain of diplopia if BSV is present. It also indicates the risk of postoperative diplopia if the ocular misalignment remains incompletely corrected after surgery

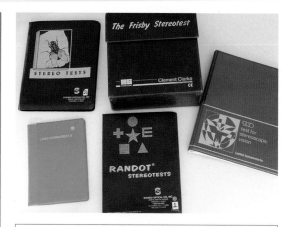

Fig. 9.25 Tests for stereopsis.

There are three degrees of sensory fusion:

1. first degree or simultaneous perception
2. second degree or flat fusion
3. third degree or stereopsis.

Sensory fusion provides the stimulus and impetus to bring the eyes into alignment, while motor fusion helps maintain the alignment. Both are thus important for binocular single vision (BSV).

Sensory assessment
Tests of binocular single vision
Testing for BSV yields information that is useful both diagnostically and in planning treatment (Box 9.2). It is essential to have reasonable visual acuity in both eyes to enable BSV.

When testing for fusion, it is important to correct any manifest deviation with appropriate prisms.

Testing can be performed using the synoptophore in closed space (see below) or in free space.

Tests for first- and second-degree fusion. The principle of testing for first- and second-degree fusion is to present the two eyes simultaneously with non-identical stimuli and determine whether the images seen by the two eyes coincide.

The WFDT, red-glass test and Bagolini striated lens test can all be used to assess first- and second-degree fusion.

Tests for third-degree fusion (stereopsis). Stereopsis is the highest order of binocular vision. The principle of testing for stereopsis is to present the two eyes with two slightly dissimilar images (Fig. 9.25). When viewed together they produce a three-dimensional image due to the disparity.

It may be tested with the synoptophore or using book charts of stereoscopic images for near (Fig. 9.25). These include:

- The Lang stereotest
- Randot stereogram (Fig. 9.26)
- TNO test
- Frisby test.

It is possible to grade stereopsis on the degree of disparity (seconds of arc). The smaller the disparity perceived, the higher the grade of stereopsis.

4,10 and 20 Δ prism test
This test is very useful in assessing uniocular vision and also binocularity in children. It is also used as a test for malingering.

The test involves placing a loose 4 Δ prism base out in front of one of the eyes with the patient fixing on a distant accommodative target and observing for any version or vergence movement (Fig. 9.27). Normally one would expect movement of both eyes away from the eye being tested (conjugate version

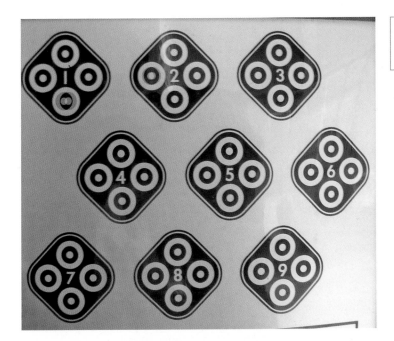

Fig. 9.26 Randot stereogram. Note the slightly dissimilar images to produce disparity.

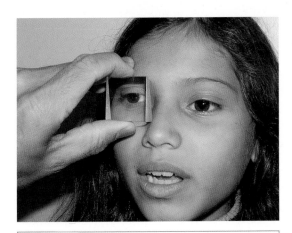

Fig. 9.27 The 20 prism dioptre test.

The test can also be used with a 10 or 20 Δ prism placed base-up or down in front of each eye in turn. This will produce a large vertical conjugate version movement if the eye being tested has good central vision. There is no corrective vergence movement as the vertical fusional range is not adequate to overcome such a large prism. The movement is greater with the stronger prism. Lack of response would indicate poor vision or suppression of the eye being tested. It is thus a very useful test in children, and also as a test for malingering.

The synoptophore

The synoptophore is a very useful instrument in assessing and quantifying ocular deviations (Fig. 9.28). It is also used to assess and grade binocular vision. It is a closed-space assessment as opposed to the cover test performed for distance and near, which is a free-space assessment. Free space assessment is now believed to replicate more accurately the real-life motility disturbances; the synoptophore is less commonly used as a result. It is however very useful in assessing incomitant squints (measurements in nine positions of gaze) and in assessing torsion. It is also used to grade binocular vision and for orthoptic exercises (to improve control of the ocular deviation by improving the fusional reserve).

movement), followed by a corrective vergence movement inwards of the eye without the prism. The test is repeated with the prism over the other eye.

If there is no movement, this could indicate poor vision or suppression in the eye being tested. If the initial version is seen but not followed by the corrective vergence, this indicates suppression in the fellow eye or weak fusion.

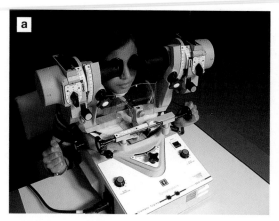

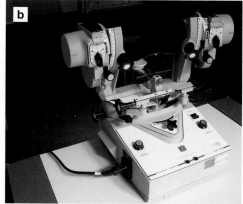

Fig. 9.28 (a, b) The synoptophore.

Hess chart

The Hess chart is used to assess incomitant strabismus, differentiating between paralytic and restrictive deviations and in following incomitant squints when looking for stability before considering surgery.

The Hess chart is rarely used in practice. The Lee screen is more commonly used and is based on the same principle. It is a dissociative test where the two eyes are tested in turn. The eye being tested is presented with a stimulus at a defined location on a grid. The subject will perceive two images if there is diplopia and will be asked to point to the position of the second image on the grid. This is plotted on a chart and the points on the grid are joined to give two charts, one for each eye (Fig. 9.29).

Assessment of the field of binocular single vision

This is usually performed in the orthoptic department on a manual perimeter. The subject views the target with both eyes and follows it around the arc of testing until diplopia is experienced. This is repeated in various meridians and plotted to give the field of BSV.

Additional tests in patients with oculomotor problems

Cycloplegic refraction

This is an essential part of assessing any child with strabismus as there is often a refractive component to the strabismus.

Fundus examination

Fundus examination is very helpful in determining the cause of poor uniocular vision which may be an impediment to binocular vision and result in ocular deviation. It is also useful in objectively assessing torsion by noting the position of the fovea relative to the disc in the two eyes.

Nystagmus

Nystagmus is a rhythmic repetitive to-and-fro movement of the eyes. Nystagmoid (searching) movements on the other hand are random, non-repetitive movements. Nystagmoid movements indicate extremely poor visual function of central origin (posterior visual pathway).

Examination of the patient with nystagmus

It is important to characterise the nystagmus as it may help with diagnosis and prognosis and in planning treatment.

Visual acuity

Assess the uniocular as well as binocular visual acuity. Any latent component of the nystagmus will be uncovered on covering one eye. Binocular visual acuity may be better than uniocular acuity, and of more relevance to daily activities if there is a significant latent component.

Determine the type of nystagmus

Latent or manifest nystagmus. Manifest nystagmus is present all the time while latent nystagmus is seen

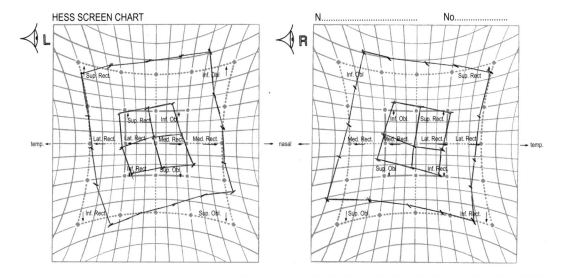

Fig. 9.29 A Hess chart showing bilateral (right more than left) superior oblique paresis.

only when one eye is covered (binocularity is disrupted).

Uni- or multiplanar. If the plane of movement of the eyes (horizontal or vertical) remains constant in all directions of gaze, it is described as uniplanar, and if it varies with gaze, it is termed multiplanar. Uniplanarity is suggestive of idiopathic congenital motor nystagmus. Multiplanar nystagmus is acquired and may need further investigation.

Pendular or jerk. The nystagmus is described as pendular when the to-and-fro movements are of equal amplitude and speed in either direction.

Jerk nystagmus on the other hand is asymmetric with respect to fixation and is faster in one direction than the other. It thus has a fast and slow component. The direction of jerk nystagmus is conventionally described as being in the direction of the fast component.

Direction. The direction of the nystagmus must be noted and may be of diagnostic value.

- Horizontal: the commonest cause is congenital idiopathic motor nystagmus. It can also occur with internuclear ophthalmolplegia
- Vertical: movements may be pendular or jerk (down-beating in cerebellar lesions or up-beating in midbrain lesions)
- Rotary: the eye moves in a circular pattern
- Cyclorotatory: the nystagmus is torsional, and the eye rotates about its own axis

- Seesaw: one eye elevates and intorts and the other depresses and extorts, followed by the opposite corrective movement. This is typically seen in chiasmal lesions, e.g. craniopharyngioma.

Dissociated nystagmus. If the speed and amplitude of nystagmus are different between the two eyes, it is described as dissociated. The classic example of dissociated nystagmus is the abducting nystagmus seen in internuclear ophthalmoplegia. Rarely, nystagmus may be uniocular. Although this may be congenital, it is important to exclude a unilateral optic nerve glioma.

Null point and head posture. Jerk nystagmus is often associated with a certain position of the eyes where the nystagmus is dampened (lowest intensity). The best visual acuity is achieved with the eyes in this position. This point is called the null point and is usually in or near the straight-ahead position. If the null point is to either side of the midline, the subject may adopt an abnormal head posture. This is typically a face turn in horizontal jerk nystagmus away from the null point, thus rotating the eyes towards the null point where the nystagmus is dampened. The null point position is usually adopted only when performing fine visual tasks and may not be readily apparent.

A null point is typically seen with congenital idiopathic motor nystagmus.

Fatigability. The nystagmus may be persistent or rapidly fatigable. Rapidly fatiguing nystagmus is of less clinical significance.

Large or small amplitude (fine or coarse). The amplitude (degree of excursion of the eyes in each nystagmus cycle) must be noted. The greater the amplitude, the poorer the visual acuity.

Fast or slow. This refers to the speed of movement of the eyes. It is not of great clinical significance.

Dampening on convergence. Certain forms of nystagmus dampen on convergence. This is typically seen in congenital idiopathic motor nystagmus.

- Eye movement disorders occur from a wide variety of causes, including:
  Neuro-ophthalmic disorders
  Congenital and acquired strabismus
- Examination must involve the head position, pupils and eyelids as well as the eye movements themselves
- When examining children, winning their confidence is important
- Degree of control of eye movement disorders may influence management
- Access to accurate and repeatable orthoptic testing is essential

---

Further reading

Bielschowsky A. Lectures on motor anomalies: II. The theory of heterophoria. Am J Ophthalmol 1938; 21: 1129.

Brodie SE. Photographic calibration of the Hirschberg test. Invest Ophthalmol Vis Sci 1987; 28: 736.

Goldstein JH. The intraoperative forced duction test. Arch Ophthalmol 1964; 72: 5.

Helveston EM. Diagnostic and surgical techniques for strabismus with restrictions. In: Surgical management of strabismus: an atlas of strabismus surgery, 4th edn. St Louis, MO: CV Mosby; 1993: 257.

Kushner BJ. Ocular causes of abnormal head postures. Ophthalmology 1979; 86: 2115.

Kushner BJ. Errors in the three step test in the diagnosis of vertical strabismus. Ophthalmology 1989; 96: 127.

Metz HS. Restrictive factors in strabismus. Surv Ophthalmol 1983; 28: 71.

Metz HS. Quantitative evaluation of the strabismus patient. Int Ophthalmol Clin 1985; 25: 13.

Parks M. Sensorial adaptations in strabismus. In: Ocular motility and strabismus. Hagerstown, MD: Harper and Row; 1975: chapter 8.

Pratt-Johnson J, Tillson G. Sensory evaluation of strabismus. In: Management of strabismus and amblyopia: a practical guide. New York: Thieme; 1994: chapter 4.

Simons K. A comparison of the Frisby, random-dot E, TNO, and Randot circles stereotests in screening and office use. Arch Ophthalmol 1981; 99: 446.

von Noorden GK. Paralytic strabismus In: Binocular vision and ocular motility: theory and management of strabismus, 5th edn. St Louis, MO: CV Mosby; 1996: p 52.

Wright KW, Walonker F, Edelman P. 10-Diopter fixation test for amblyopia. Arch Ophthalmol 1981; 99: 1242.

CHAPTER 10

The pupils

BRUCE JAMES

Introduction

Examination of the pupils provides information about the eye as well as the afferent and efferent pathways controlling pupillary reaction. It is important when examining the pupils not to forget to search for ancillary signs, for example, abnormalities in lid position or an abnormality of eye movements which may assist in making a diagnosis. The size of the pupils in healthy individuals may vary not only as a result of changes in light and accommodation but also with factors such as fatigue and sleep (constriction or miosis) or emotional arousal (dilation or mydriasis). The pupils are under the control of the autonomic nervous system. The sympathetic nervous system innervates the dilator muscle of the iris (Fig. 10.1). Disorders of this pathway produce a Horner's syndrome by allowing unopposed action of the parasympathetic system which, by way of the third cranial nerve, innervates the sphincter muscle. A third-nerve palsy is the commonest cause of interruption to this pathway.

Both pupils normally constrict when a light is shone in either eye, mediated by the direct and consensual light reflex (Fig. 10.2).

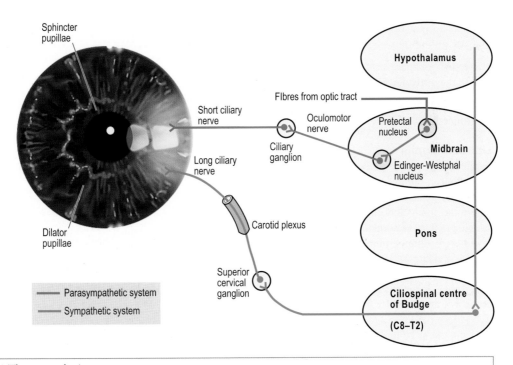

Fig. 10.1 The sympathetic nervous system.

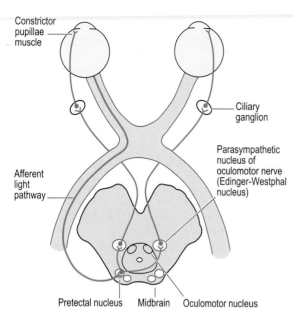

Constrictor pupillae muscle

Ciliary ganglion

Parasympathetic nucleus of oculomotor nerve (Edinger-Westphal nucleus)

Afferent light pathway

Pretectal nucleus   Midbrain   Oculomotor nucleus

Fig. 10.2 The direct and consensual light reflex.

Initial examination of the pupils

First, in normal room lighting, examine the shape and size of both pupils:

- Are they of equal size?
- Are they irregular in shape?

If the pupils are different in size the next step is to determine which is abnormal.

Unequal pupils

Inequality of pupil size may not necessarily be pathological. Some 11% of normal people have an anisocria greater than 0.3 mm. The best way to determine if an abnormality is present and if so, which pupil is abnormal is to examine the pupils in different illumination. In dim lighting a normal pupil will dilate but not a pathologically constricted pupil (for example, miosis associated with Horner's syndrome). In bright light a pathologically dilated pupil will not constrict (mydriasis associated with a third-nerve palsy).

A unilateral Holmes–Adie's pupil may initially be larger than its normal fellow but with time may become smaller. It will react slowly, if at all, to changes in illumination. It is due to an inflammation

of the ciliary ganglion which denervates the iris and the ciliary body.

Irregular pupils may be caused by purely ocular disease (Box 10.1). Examples include ocular inflammation (iritis), with the formation of adhesions between the iris and the lens (posterior synechiae), trauma and intraocular surgery (Fig. 10.3). Previous acute angle-closure glaucoma with associated ischaemia of the iris may leave the patient with a dilated and unreactive pupil. Developmental abnormalities of the anterior segment, as in Reiger's mesodermal dysgenesis or colobomata of the iris, may also cause pupillary irregularity and displacement (correctopia). It may also be seen in the irido-corneal-

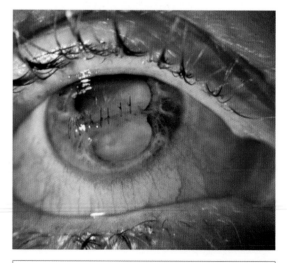

Fig. 10.3 Posterior synechiae and an irrgular pupil following penetrating trauma to the eye.

endothelial (ICE) syndrome. Iris tumours may result in a distorted pupil. Neurosyphilis, diabetes and encephalitis can cause a small irregular pupil (Argyll Robertson pupil).

Response to light

Next examine the light response. Remember that in the very young and the elderly the pupil response is reduced. First test each pupil separately. The patient looks at a *distant target* and a uniform bright light is used to illuminate the eye. Assess the speed of pupillary reaction. This will be delayed (or tonic) in a Holmes–Adie's pupil (see above). If suspected, close examination, preferably with a slit lamp, may show a spiralling or vermiform (worm-like) movement in response to light-induced constriction. A tonic pupil may also be an indication of ocular disease, such as acute iritis (look for associated circumcorneal injection or slit-lamp signs of inflammation) and chronic ocular ischaemia, where mydriasis may also be present. An absent or reduced light reflex with preservation of the near reflex is seen in an Argyll Robertson pupil and Parinaud's syndrome (caused by a lesion in the pretectal nuclear complex which disrupts the retinotectal fibres but preserves the supranuclear accommodative fibres). It may also be seen in diabetic patients and those with myotonic

dystrophy. A range of topical and systemic drugs may paralyse pupillary movement.

Testing for a relative afferent pupillary defect (Marcus Gunn Pupil)

The response of both pupils is now observed when a light is shone into the left eye. Normally, both should constrict. With the patient continuing to fixate a distant object the light is moved smoothly and fairly quickly to the right eye, while the light is kept perpendicular to the pupil. The reaction of both pupils is again observed. Normally the pupils will remain constricted, although an initial slight miosis may be seen associated with the loss of stimulus and consequent mydriasis as the light moves from one eye to another. If the right optic nerve is damaged dilation of both pupils will be seen. The consensual and direct light reflexes are interrupted because of the damage to the optic nerve (the afferent limb of both reflexes, see Fig. 10.2). Returning the light to the left eye, where the optic nerve is intact, results in constriction of both pupils (Fig. 10.4).

This phenomenon is termed a *relative afferent pupillary defect* (RAPD). It is a powerful test of optic nerve disease. It is not seen in patients with cataract nor in retinal disease, unless it is very severe in nature. It may very occasionally be seen in severe amblyopia.

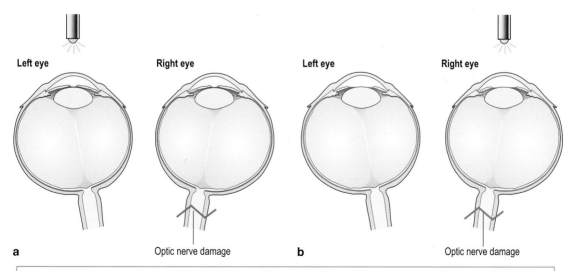

Left eye **Right eye** **Left eye** **Right eye**

a Optic nerve damage **b** Optic nerve damage

Fig. 10.4 Testing for a relative afferent pupillary difference. **(a)** The right optic nerve is damaged. The light is shone in the left eye; both pupils constrict (the direct and consensual light reflex). **(b)** The light is moved to the right eye and there is no afferent limb to the reflex, thus both pupils dilate.

The near response

The near response is really a triad of accommodation, pupillary constriction and convergence. It is not technically a reflex as such because each part of the response relies on separate nerve cells within the oculomotor nucleus which are themselves coordinated by supranuclear mechanisms.

To examine the pupillary part of the response the patient is asked initially to observe a distant object and then a near target. The pupils are observed for the miosis accompanying accommodation. Clinically the importance of the near pupillary response is when it is greater than the response associated with the light reflex. This light-near dissociation may be seen in diabetes, multiple sclerosis, neurosyphilis and in Parinaud's syndrome. It is also a feature of the Argyll Robertson pupil.

Pupillary abnormalities associated with eye movement disorders

Third-nerve palsies are associated with dilation of the pupil, although this may not always be the case; in some third-nerve palsies the pupillomotor fibres are spared. Subsequent regeneration of the third nerve may result in misdirection of fibres, thus nerve fibres from ganglion cells responsible for eye movements may grow back to the ciliary ganglion and hence innervate the iris sphincter muscle. This may be seen following damage to the nerve at any point and is usually seen after 9 weeks following injury. Carefully observe the pupils for constriction when the patient is adducting, elevating in adduction and depressing the eyes in a uniformly lit room. The effect has also been termed a pseudo Argyll Robertson pupil because of the poor light response due to the third-nerve palsy but the constriction of the pupil on adduction is caused by the aberrant regeneration. Eye movements may also be accompanied by elevation of the eyelid resulting from aberrant regeneration of nerve fibres to the levator muscle. This oculomotor synkinesis is rare after ischaemia to the nerve; a compressive lesion should be suspected. It may occasionally be seen without the signs of an acute third-nerve palsy, for example in meningiomas affecting the cavernous sinus.

A patient with Parinaud's syndrome shows convergence retraction nystagmus; this is best demonstrated with an optokinetic drum. This is rotated downwards so that the fast saccades occur upwards; the eyes are seen to converge and retract into the orbit. These patients may also have poor upgaze.

Pupillary abnormalities associated with eyelid abnormalities

Horner's syndrome is associated with a ptosis of the affected eye caused by interruption of the sympathetic supply to Müller's muscle. A third-nerve palsy usually presents with a more profound ptosis due to the levator muscle being paralysed. Trauma around the eye may also result in an irregular pupil and an altered lid position.

Other causes of pupillary abnormality

Miosis may be seen in comatose patients (but beware those on pilocarpine for glaucoma or patients who have taken morphine). In a comatose patient with a unilateral expanding supratentorial mass such as a haematoma, a dilated pupil may be caused by pressure on the third nerve.

Pharmacological examination of the pupils

Diagnosis of pupillary dysfunction can be further refined with pharmacological tests (Table 10.1). These are particularly useful in establishing the affected neuron in Horner's syndrome.

Box 10.2

Examination of the pupils

- Compare pupil size: if abnormal, look at the effect of changing illumination
- Look for an irregularity in the shape of the pupil
- Assess the direct and consensual reaction to light
- Look for a relative afferent pupillary difference
- Assess the near reaction
- Examine the patient for any associated features (abnormality of eye movements, asymmetry of lid position)
- Consider pharmacological testing

Table 10.1	Pharmacological tests for pupillary dysfunction		
Pharmacological test	**Looking for:**	**Comments**
Pilocarpine 0.125% Read response after 40–60 min	Suspected Adie's pupil Suspected atropine in eye	Constriction due to denervation hypersensitivity No effect
Cocaine 4% Read response after 40–60 min	Horner's syndrome	No effect, normal pupils dilate. Blocks noradrenaline (norepinephrine) uptake, little is released by Horner's pupil
Hydroxyamphetamine 1% 48 h after cocaine test Read after 40–60 min Perform when Horner's syndrome has been present for at least 1 week	To differentiate pre- and postganglionic Horner's	Preganglionic Horner's and normal pupils dilate; postganglionic Horner's, no effect. It releases noradrenaline from nerve endings. Postganglionic lesions result in the death of the nerve so no noradrenaline is available for release
Phenylephrine 1% Read after 40–60 min Can be used immediately after cocaine test	To differentiate pre- and postganglionic Horner's	Dilates postganglionic Horner's due to denervation hypersensitivity

- Pupil testing gives information about local ocular pathologies as well as the afferent and efferent pathways controlling the pupil responses
- Eyelid abnormalities may be associated with pupil signs
- The relative afferent papillary defect (RAPD) is a very important sign and should be tested for in all patients with reduced vision on one or both sides before pupil dilatation. Make it a routine for all patients, or it may be forgotten

Further reading

Loewenfeld IE. Simple central anisicoria: a common condition, seldom recognised. Trans Am Acad Ophthalmol Otolaryngol 1977; 83: 832–839.

Wilhelm H. Neuro-ophthalmology of pupillary function – practical guidelines. J Neurol 1998; 245: 573–583.

CHAPTER 11

Microbiological examination and investigation

LARRY BENJAMIN

Introduction

The internal ocular environment, unlike the external one, is normally sterile. Conjunctiva and lid skin harbour commensal organisms which may themselves cause intraocular infection if introduced into the eye at surgery.

This chapter will describe the examination and investigation of common eye infections starting from the lids and working inwards to the retina.

The broad principles of managing microbiological disease in the eye are to:

- establish a cause (history, examination, investigations)
- treat appropriately
- limit inflammation and scarring where it may cause visual deficit.

Some infections are self-limiting and do not have serious visual consequences while others can progress rapidly without appropriate intervention and cause blindness.

General symptoms of external eye infections

Bacterial

Conjunctival inflammation causes excess discharge and the nature of this discharge can give valuable clues to the cause of the conjunctivitis. Generally, bacterial infections cause a sticky mucoid or muco-purulent discharge which causes matting of the eyelids and lashes overnight. The eyes feel gritty, with the sensation that the grit is moving around under the lids.

A bacterial corneal ulcer (Fig. 11.1) causes pain, photophobia and often reduced vision. There is often a history of trauma or contact lens wear. Infective

ulcers are also seen in patients with other corneal disease.

Viral

A typical history of an adenoviral infection is of an upper respiratory tract infection or sore throat followed a week or two later by red eyes with a watery discharge with little mucoid content. Photophobia may also be a problem, particularly if the cornea is affected. Vision may be affected with corneal involvement.

Severe photophobia may also be found in patients with a herpetic dendritic ulcer which can also affect the vision if it is in the visual axis.

Severe itching and eye-rubbing are likely to be caused by viral shedding from a molluscum conta-giosum lesion which is usually obvious clinically. This is a common poxvirus infection, particularly in childhood (Fig. 11.2).

Chlamydia

A chronic conjunctivitis with intermittent discomfort should raise the possibility of chlamydial infection, especially if associated with a partial ptosis.

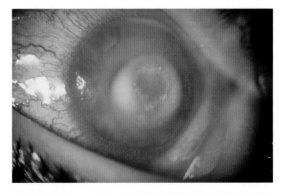

Fig. 11.1 A bacterial corneal ulcer.

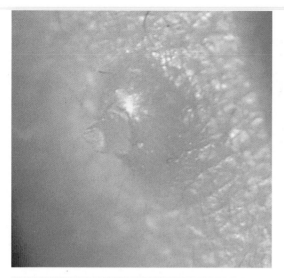

Fig. 11.2 A molluscum contagiosum lesion with cheesy material extruding from the umbilicated centre.

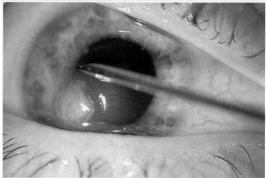

Fig. 11.3 Sterile needle being used to debride a corneal ulcer.

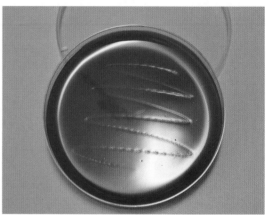

Fig. 11.4 Plating out on to blood agar. Avoid deep inoculation into the jelly.

Acanthamoeba

This organism is ubiquitous and resides in cold-water storage tanks, which are common in the UK as a source of cold-water supply in houses. Infections with this organism are most often associated with contact lens wear. The initial presenting picture can look very similar to herpes simplex keratitis, but quite often the pain of the condition is in excess of the clinical signs present. There is little discharge.

Examination

Bacterial infections

In conjunctivitis examination of the tarsal conjunctiva with the slit lamp reveals a papillary conjunctival reaction due to inflammatory cell accumulation around the conjunctival arterioles. The vessels of the bulbar conjunctiva are also dilated and engorged. The diagnosis is usually easily made and does not require swabs to be sent.

Examination of the patient with a corneal ulcer reveals an epithelial defect and surrounding stromal infiltrate. There may be anterior-chamber activity, including an hypopyon. If a corneal ulcer is present then samples should be taken from the bed of the ulcer. These can be taken from the cornea with a sterile hypodermic needle (Fig. 11.3). A gentle debriding motion at the base of the ulcer is required. There is little point in sampling the mucoid material that often accumulates in the ulcer crater. The sharp edge of the needle is then placed directly on to the culture media and spread with a sterile cotton bud (Fig. 11.4). The specimen should be gently wiped across the surface in a zig-zag pattern and not buried below the surface of the agar.

A Gram stain should always be performed, as early clues to the type of organism can be very helpful in treatment. Figure 11.5 shows the equipment that is necessary for a Gram stain and culture. The Gram stain sample may be minute and so glass slides with a small central well are used. This ensures that the

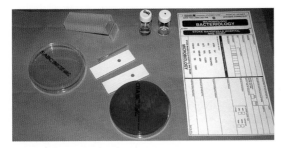

Fig. 11.5 The collection of apparatus and culture media needed when taking a corneal scrape. Included are blood agar and Sabouraud's agar and glass slides for Gram staining. A special transport case for the slides ensures that it is not damaged en route to the lab. The enrichment media used will depend on the protocols of local laboratories. It is important that everything is correctly labelled.

microbiology technician knows where to look for the specimen. Alternatively the site of the sample must be marked on the slide.

Table 11.1 lists the various culture media and the organisms that they support. These should be stocked routinely in eye departments. It is important that they are kept in date by regularly changing the stocks in conjunction with the microbiology department.

If contact lenses are associated with the infection they should be retained and, along with the contact lens cases and if possible solutions, should be sent for culture and sensitivities. Patients should be warned that they will not get the lenses back.

Failure to respond to treatment should alert the clinician to the possibility of resistance to treatment, incorrect choice of antibiotics, or possibly a fungal infection, although hopefully this would have been picked up at an early stage with the use of Gram stain and the relevant cultures. In these circumstances after 48–72 h antibiotics should be stopped for 24 h and the cornea rescraped.

Viral infections
Adenovirus
On examination at the slit lamp a follicular tarsal reaction due to lymphocytes aggregating into small nodules (follicles) is seen on the lower tarsal conjunctiva. There is little stickiness because of the lack of excess mucus. With some strains of adenovirus, conjunctival pseudomembranes are formed, and may cause bleeding if removed. A preauricular lymphadenopathy, which may be tender, should be looked for.

A swab can be taken if there is doubt about the diagnosis, with a cotton applicator wiped around the fornices (Fig. 11.6). This is transported to the laboratory in viral culture medium. Cell cultures are used in the laboratory and examined at the appropriate interval for a cytopathic effect of the virus on the cultured cells. Different cell lines are used for different viruses. Polymerase chain reaction (PCR) techniques are also used to detect viruses (see later).

The infection is very contagious and great care must be taken by family members to avoid cross-infection. Examining doctors are also at risk and hand-washing and equipment-sterilizing are important to prevent contamination. The slit-lamp switch may act as a reservoir for infection as it tends to be switched off between patients and before hand-washing occurs and then switched back on after

Table 11.1	Culture media and the organisms that they support
Clean glass slides for Gram stain	Gram stain
Blood agar	Most corneal bacterial pathogens
Chocolate agar	*Moraxella, Neisseria* and *Haemophilus* species
Sabouraud's agar	Fungi
Thioglycolate broth	Anaerobic and microaerophilic bacteria
Brain/heart infusion broth	Fastidious bacteria and fungi. Particularly useful if the patient has been treated with antibiotics prior to sampling

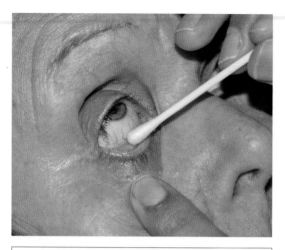

Fig. 11.6 A moistened sterile cotton applicator being used to swab the conjunctival fornices. A drop of local anaesthetic can be helpful in the recovery of material by making the procedure much more bearable.

hand-washing and just before examining the next patient.

Herpes simplex

Antibody studies show that approximately 90% of humans have been exposed to herpes simplex virus at some time in their life. The virus tends to live in a ganglion, close to the initial site of infection, and may break out on the dermatome served by that ganglion years later as either a cold sore, or, in the case of the cornea, a dendritic ulcer. On examination at the slit lamp a follicular conjunctival reaction is commonly seen. Staining the cornea with fluorescein and/or rose Bengal shows up a typical branching ulcer in the epithelium. If the diagnosis is in doubt it is worth taking a swab from the ulcer itself with a moistened sterile cotton applicator and sending it to the laboratory in viral culture medium to prove the diagnosis. A negative culture does not exclude the disease, however. Other conditions, such as acanthamoeba, can mimic herpetic keratitis; furthermore herpetic eye disease can smoulder on for many years and it is useful to have a definitive diagnosis in the notes upon which to base future treatment.

Stromal disease may ensue some weeks later, with the typical disciform appearance of corneal stromal oedema and keratic precipitates clustered around the original site of the epithelial disease. This is an immunological reaction to viral proteins in the stroma.

Chlamydia

Chlamydia trachomatis (serotypes D–K) is the cause of conjunctivitis associated with genital disease. Other serotypes are associated with trachoma, a major cause of world blindness. Examination of patients with conjunctivitis associated with genital disease reveals a follicular conjunctival reaction. The genital association of the disease must be borne in mind once the diagnosis is made. Patients should be referred to specialist genitourinary clinics for contact tracing and treatment of their systemic disease, rather than just treating the eye disease alone. Failure to do this can result in pelvic inflammatory disease in females and urethral strictures and other problems in males. This should be done before starting treatment.

Conjunctival swabs for chlamydia should always be taken and it may be advisable to look for adenovirus and herpes simplex as well with any follicular conjunctivitis. An enzyme-linked immunosorbent assay (ELISA) test is performed to identify the chlamydial organism. The results of this are usually available in 24 h. This test detects the binding of antibodies in the test serum to solid-phase antigen from the swab by the binding of a labelled secondary agent, often an enzyme, which can be detected by a colour reaction.

Fungi

Fungal external eye infections should be considered in:

- chronic infection which fails to resolve
- immunocompromised patients
- patients using steroids

These tend to present as indolent ulcers that fail to respond to antibiotic therapy. They are more common in tropical and subtropical climates. Any corneal ulcer failing to respond to broad-spectrum antibiotic therapy should be rescraped for fungi and plated on to a Sabouraud's agar plate. *Aspergillus* and *Fusarium* species ulcers often have a greyish appearance with deep stromal infiltration and filamentous extensions. They are commonly associated with agricultural trauma. *Candida* are more commonly suppurative and associated with an immune-compromised patient or one who has been treated with topical steroids.

Molluscum contagiosum

Examination reveals a chronic follicular conjunctivitis. The lids should be closely inspected on the slit lamp for a classic molluscum lesion which has an umbilicated centre with cheesy material exuding from the middle. The virus particles are in this material and are often shed into the conjunctival sac, resulting in the follicular conjunctival reaction. Multiple lesions can occur around one or both eyes and sometimes the rest of the face. Culture is not necessary. They can disappear spontaneously but if the child is symptomatic they can be shaved flat with a scalpel blade and the base cauterised to kill the virus. The diagnosis can be confirmed on histology.

Acanthamoeba

Examination, as well as revealing a corneal ulcer, infiltrates or epithelial defects, may also show perineural infiltrates which are probably pathognomonic for this condition. There is usually marked conjunctival injection; there may be an anterior uveitis or scleritis. After a week or 10 days of infection a typical ring ulcer appears which should immediately alert a physician to the diagnosis (Fig. 11.7). Patients using bathroom tap water to clean out their contact lens cases are at increased risk of infection. In suspected cases samples should be taken from the corneal epithelium and contact lens cases and if possible solutions used with the contact lenses. Samples are plated in the microbiology laboratory

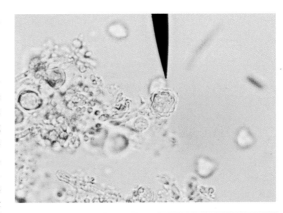

Fig. 11.8 Acanthamoeba cysts recovered from a contact lens case.

on to agar freshly seeded with *Escherichia coli* organisms upon which the acanthoemeba feed. Again it is important to culture the contact lenses themselves and the case in which they are kept (Fig. 11.8).

Intraocular infection

Endophthalmitis

Endophthalmitis is an inflammation of both the anterior and posterior chambers and the vitreous gel of the eye. When resulting from infection it can result in disastrous visual loss. Infectious endophthalmitis is often classified according to its source, for example, postoperative endophthalmitis follows surgery, traumatic endophthalmitis following injury and endogenous endophthalmitis is often seen in immunocompromised patients or intravenous drug abusers. Postoperative endophthalmitis has as its hallmark increasing severe ocular pain and decreased vision. It usually comes on in the first week after surgery and may result in an hypopyon and/or severe fibrinous reaction in the anterior chamber, with a reduction in the red reflex and severe vitritis (Cooper, 2003).

Any patient complaining of increasing pain or decreasing vision, or both, following eye surgery should be assessed very rapidly and carefully. If infection is suspected samples should be obtained from the anterior chamber by aspiration and from the posterior segment by way of a vitreous tap (Fig. 11.9). Specimens are sent for microscopy

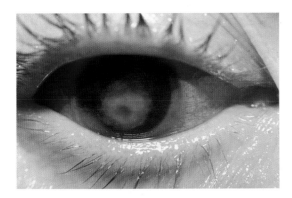

Fig. 11.7 A ring ulcer typical of late acanthamoeba keratitis.

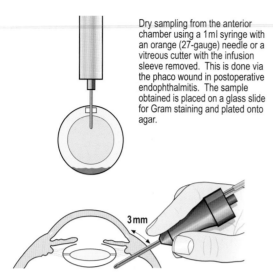

Dry sampling from the anterior chamber using a 1ml syringe with an orange (27-gauge) needle or a vitreous cutter with the infusion sleeve removed. This is done via the phaco wound in postoperative endophthalmitis. The sample obtained is placed on a glass slide for Gram staining and plated onto agar.

3mm

Dry vitrectomy sampling, using a sleeveless vitreous cutter placed through a wound 3mm to 3.5mm from the corneoscleral limbus in a pseudo-phakic eye. As infected fluid is drawn into the tubing, the cutter is removed and the tubing cut. The entire handpiece and short piece of tubing are sent to the laboratory and the vitreous sample extracted for Gram staining, culture and sensitivities. Intravitreal antibiotics are injected through the same wound.

Fig. 11.9 Sampling the anterior and posterior segments in post-operative endophthalmitis. If a full vitrectomy is performed (as recommended in patients with vision of perception of light), the entire cassette and contents can be sent after the procedure.

culture and sensitivities, as well as Gram staining, and intraocular antibiotics are introduced at the time of tissue sampling.

Retinitis

A good history is important in determining the cause of retinitis. For example, in immunocompromised patients cytomegalovirus (CMV) retinitis is much more common while in otherwise healthy patients herpetic retinitis with acute retinal necrosis is more likely. CMV has a fairly typical clinical picture with venous sheathing, exudation and retinal haemorrhages and is more common in acquired immunodeficiency syndrome (AIDS) patients. Suspected herpetic retinitis (zoster or simplex) must be confirmed rapidly with PCR tests on intraocular fluids as it needs aggressive treatment to prevent a poor visual outcome (Fig. 11.10). The acute picture is of a peripheral retinitis which rapidly spreads centrally and causes acute retinal necrosis.

Toxoplasmosis is another cause of retinitis or retinochoroiditis. The organism is contracted by eating undercooked meat, by accidental ingestion of the sporocyst form from cat litter or by transplacental spread during acute toxoplasmosis in a pregnant woman. The majority of cases presenting to an eye department are from congenital retinal disease that has reactivated. The acute ocular disease is a retinitis with secondary choroidal involvement, possibly via an immune response. A typical *Toxoplasma* lesion will often help to confirm the diagnosis (Fig. 11.11).

Laboratory tests include:

- A latex test, often used for screening patients to detect antibody prior to performing other tests. Antigen coupled to latex particles detects the presence of serum antibody in the sample
- ELISA tests against antibodies in the patient's serum or, more sensitively, in aqueous
- Haemagglutination tests can also be used. This utilises red blood cells coated with the lysed organism which are then exposed to the patient's serum. Positive sera cause the red cells to agglutinate
- Toxoplasma antibody levels (immunoglobulin A (IgA) and IgM).

Toxocariasis is caused by ingestion of ova from the roundworm *Toxocara canis*, shed in dog faeces. The ocular manifestations are peripheral or central (posterior pole) granulomata or a chronic inflammatory picture. The patient is usually a young child and presents with leukocoria, strabismus as a consequence of poor vision or unilateral visual loss.

Diagnosis is made clinically but with dense posterior uveitis and vitritis care must be taken to exclude a retinoblastoma. Peripheral granulomata may be compatible with good vision but posterior pole lesions are often associated with a poor visual prognosis. Ultrasound scans may demonstrate a traction retinal detachment.

Summary

Infections on and in the eye need rapid assessment and treatment in order to limit sight-threatening inflammation and fibrosis. It is important to take samples correctly and to discuss the patient with the microbiology department if any doubt exists about the correct culture media to use.

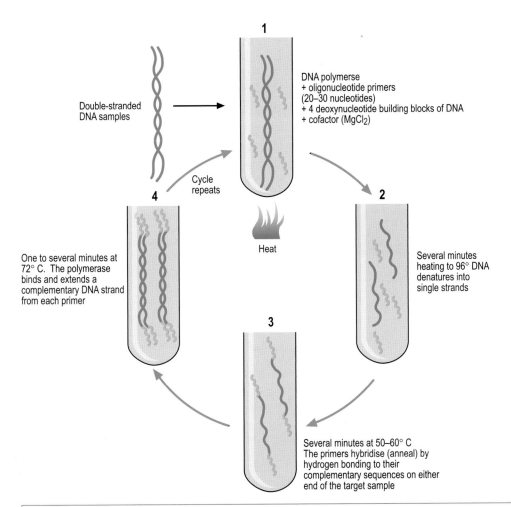

1

Double-stranded
DNA samples

DNA polymerse
+ oligonucleotide primers
(20–30 nucleotides)
+ 4 deoxynucleotide building blocks of DNA
+ cofactor (MgCl₂)

Cycle
repeats

4

Heat

2

One to several minutes at
72° C. The polymerase
binds and extends a
complementary DNA strand
from each primer

Several minutes
heating to 96° DNA
denatures into
single strands

3

Several minutes at 50–60° C
The primers hybridise (anneal) by
hydrogen bonding to their
complementary sequences on either
end of the target sample

Fig. 11.10 Polymerase chain reaction (PCR) explained. PCR is a molecular biological technique that enables extremely small samples of DNA to be amplified and then analysed to aid in diagnosis. The sample tissue may contain as few as 10 copies of the sequence of interest as it multiplies them exponentially. It is particularly useful for detecting viruses, which can often be diagnosed from their unique DNA or RNA sequences. The first stage of this figure shows a test tube with the ingredients for the PCR. These are heated to 96°C to denature the DNA into single strands. By keeping the mixture at 50–65°C for several minutes, the oligonucleotide primers bind to complementary sequences at the extremes of the sample DNA strands and then by heating to 72°C the DNA polymerase extends a complementary strand from each length of DNA. This cycle is repeated many times to multiply the original DNA sequence millions of times. The DNA sequence is then analysed.

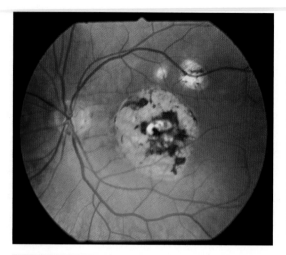

Fig. 11.11 A typical congenital chorioretinal scar from toxoplasmosis, in this case affecting the macula and causing severe central visual loss.

- Commensal organisms from the ocular environment are a not uncommon cause of intraocular infection
- Accurate history-taking is essential to differentiate different types of infectious eye agents
- Eye infections may be mild and self-limiting but with some organisms may progress rapidly, to destroy sight and possibly the eye itself
- Modern techniques such as polymerase chain reaction are helpful but still require an educated guess as to the possible causative organisms so that appropriate investigative techniques are employed

Reference

Cooper BA, Holekamp NM, Bohigian G, et al. Case control of endophthalmitis after cataract surgery comparing scleral tunnel and clear corneal wounds. AM J Ophthalmol 2003; 136: 300–305

Ultrasound techniques in ophthalmology

CARLOS EDUARDO SOLARTE and ASIFA SHAIKH

Introduction

Ultrasound examination techniques have evolved rapidly in the past decade. Improvements in computers and electronics have increased the resolution of ultrasound equipment, but the principles and the techniques remain unchanged. It is easy to perform, non-invasive, with little morbidity. This chapter outlines the principles and practical technique of ophthalmic ultrasound.

Mundt and Hughes described the first application of ultrasound in the USA in 1956. Several groups (for example, those of Oksala in Finland and Baum in the USA) worked very actively in the development of new equipment. In the 1960s Ossoinig, an Austrian ophthalmologist, emphasised the importance of standardising instrumentation and techniques, so that sonographers could rely on the results of fellow investigators. This standard is used by most ultrasound specialists around the world and its principles remain intact today. In the 1990s new applications, including the use of Doppler ultrasound, new high-frequency probes and software for anterior segment evaluation, have further increased the value of the technique. Three-dimensional imaging is part of the continuing evolution of ophthalmic ultrasound.

Indications for ophthalmic ultrasound (Box 12.1) include the study of the posterior segment and the anterior segment (ultrasound biomicroscopy, UBM), vascular evaluation and, of course, biometry (see Ch. 13).

Basic principles

Physics and instrumentation

Ultrasound is a high-frequency acoustic wave using frequencies outside the normal hearing range (20 Hz to 20 kHz). Most ophthalmic equipment is set at 8 MHz (8 million/cycles per second) or higher. This contrasts with ultrasound equipment used for general surgery or obstetrics that works at 5–6 MHz, allowing a greater depth of tissue penetration but reduced resolution. Probes generating frequencies up to 20 MHz and, in the case of UBM, up to 50 MHz, are now also used in ophthalmology. These allow resolution of very small structures. The probe contains quartz or ceramic crystals (usually lead zirconate titanate) that vibrate when a voltage is applied, generating a sound wave of constant frequency and amplitude. This is known as the piezoelectric effect.

The application and principles of the physics of sound apply. Ultrasound is propagated as longitudinal

---

Box 12.1

Indications for ultrasound evaluation of the eye

Opaque ocular media
- Corneal opacification
- Hyphaema
- Small pupil
- Cataract
- Vitreous haemorrhage or inflammation

Clear ocular media
- Iris lesions
- Ciliary body lesions
- Tumours
- Retinal detachment
- Optic nerve abnormalities
- Evaluation of extraocular muscles and the orbit
- Intraocular foreign-body detection and trauma evaluation
- Evaluation of the iridocorneal angle
- Biometry

Table 12.1	Sound wave velocities in different media
Medium	**Wave velocity (m/s)**
Silicone oil	980
Water	1480
Aqueous/vitreous	1532
Soft tissue	1550
Crystalline lens	1641
Bone	3500

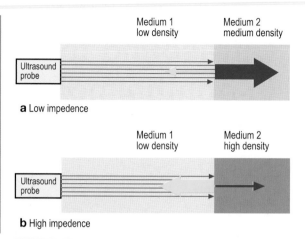

a Low impedence

b High impedence

Fig. 12.1 The effect of an interface between media of different densities on echo generation. **(a)** The difference in density is slight, with only little reflection. **(b)** There is a greater difference and the reflection is increased.

waves that change in velocity as they pass through tissues of different density. The higher the frequency, the shallower is the depth of tissue penetration. Increasing the energy of the wave will increase penetration but will increase heat generation. Ultrasound waves travel faster in solids and slower in liquids (Table 12.1). This is important in the use of ultrasound for measurement (biometry). Ultrasound waves can be reflected and refracted and waves reflected back towards the ultrasound source are known as echoes. These can be analysed and processed to form images.

Reflections (echoes) are produced at the junction of tissues with different densities or impedance to sound (impedance = sound velocity × density). The greater the difference in density between the two tissues, the stronger is the reflection or echo (Fig. 12.1). The returning echoes themselves can be influenced by many factors, including absorption, refraction and, importantly, the angle of incidence of the ultrasound wave. The ultrasound wave emitted by the probe is constant, while the reflected echoes will vary in amplitude and frequency. Echoes generate a current in the quartz crystal through the piezoelectric effect and this is computed into a display by the ultrasound machine. The most efficient system would have all the sound reflected towards the source (the probe). This only occurs if the probe is placed perpendicular to the structure being analysed. If it is placed in an oblique position, more sound will be scattered and the returning echo to the probe will be weaker. Amplification will be needed (Fig. 12.2a–c). This amplification is known as gain, and it is measured in decibels (dB). The echo will

also be reduced if the ultrasound wave is reflected from an irregular surface (Fig. 12.2d).

Ultrasound waves can also be refracted (bent). Refraction occurs when a sound wave is directed obliquely at an interface between media of different densities. No refraction occurs when a sound wave is directed perpendicularly or the interface is between two media of the same density.

As the ultrasound waves and echoes pass through the tissue a very small amount of energy is absorbed and is converted into heat. This is not known to result in tissue damage. Assessing the amount of absorption is useful in evaluating solid lesions that absorb more ultrasound energy.

The echoes from a single longitudinal sound wave focused through the eye is called an A-scan (see Ch. 13). It is used to measure the length of the eye and analyse the sound characteristics of sections on the B-scan (Fig. 12.3a). A B-scan uses a probe to send multiple sound waves simultaneously at slightly different angles (each one corresponding to an A-scan). Merging the echo from each scan creates a composite picture, a two-dimensional slice of tissue (Fig. 12.3b).

Technique

Ultrasound is a dynamic test; the results are most easily interpreted from the moving images on the

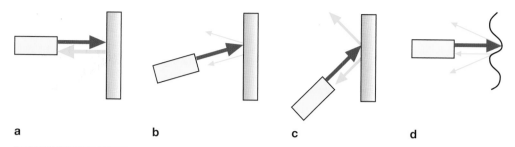

Fig. 12.2 (a–c) The effect of probe positioning on the return of the echo. The greater the obliquity of the probe, the less echo returns. **(d)** The effect of an irregular interface on the echo. Again, the strength of echo returning to the probe is reduced.

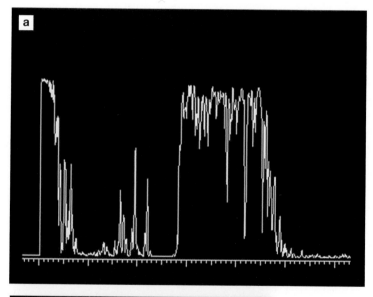

Fig. 12.3 (a) A typical A-scan. **(b)** A typical B-scan.

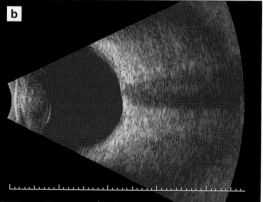

screen during the course of the examination rather than from still pictures.

The patient needs to be sitting comfortably on a reclining chair. The ultrasound machine is positioned so that the examiner can see both the screen and the probe. A foot pedal or switch on the machine allows the examiner to freeze the image on the screen. On modern machines an additional pedal allows the frozen picture and video clips of a dynamic scan to be saved on a computer. An explanation of the test needs to be given to the patient, emphasising that it is painless.

The examination includes:

- topographic examination, to assess the shape and location of any abnormality
- quantitative assessment, to assess reflectivity, attenuation and structure of any abnormality within the eye or orbit: this usually also requires an A-scan
- kinetic evaluation, to assess the mobility of normal and abnormal structures within the eye

Each of these is important and plays a part in reaching a diagnosis. Many lesions may initially appear similar on simple topographic examination. A B-scan is also useful in localising lesions, in assessing extension through ocular tissue and in examining shape.

The B-scan probe has a distinct mark, usually a white line or dot at its head (Fig. 12.4). This indicates to the examiner which part of the eye will appear in the upper part of the screen. The probe, covered with a protecting cap, can be applied directly on the surface of the anaesthetised eye. The scan can also be

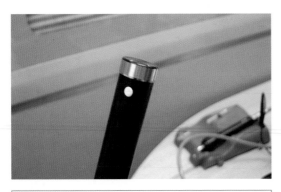

Fig. 12.4 The B-scan ultrasound probe. Note the white dot marker.

performed through the eyelids using no anaesthetic but a coupling jelly is required.

A grey-scale image is displayed on the screen. This represents the reflectivity of the structure being examined: high reflectivity is white, low reflectivity is black. When low-reflectivity lesions are imaged, for example, lesions in the vitreous, the gain may have to be increased. The gain is reduced when high-reflectivity lesions are to be imaged to create a clear image. The brightness and contrast of the screen can also be adjusted. A zoom control allows the image to be magnified. On some machines the energy of the ultrasound wave can be adjusted; this increases the depth of tissue visualised with higher-frequency probes. Some machines also permit the duration of the ultrasound pulse to be varied. A shorter pulse increases resolution but depth of field is reduced. Longer pulse duration is helpful in looking at the vitreous or eyes filled with silicone oil.

Probe orientation is important in the performance of a B-scan. The probe scans from side to side; axial, transverse and longitudinal scans can be performed (Fig. 12.5). Axial views scan through the lens of the eye; longitudinal and transverse scans are made eccentric to the lens scanning through the sclera. To try and maintain a perpendicular scan with respect to the retina and choroid the patient is asked to look away from the probe.

Scanning sequence

It is important to scan the eye in a systematic manner. Initially a high gain is used, particularly to visualise the vitreous. Subsequently a lower gain is used to look at the retina, choroid and any solid lesions.

An axial transverse scan is first performed (Fig. 12.5a); the probe is positioned between 3 and 9 o'clock with the white mark pointing to the nose so that the nasal part of the retina appears superiorly on the screen. The optic nerve acts as a reference in the middle of the picture (Fig. 12.6).

Transverse scans are then made (Fig. 12.5b). The probe is positioned inferiorly, the white mark points towards the nose and the patient is asked to look upward. The probe is gently rotated to examine the superior quadrants of the eye. It is then placed superiorly, the white mark points to the nose and the patient is asked to look downwards to enable the inferior quadrants to be seen. Examination of the temporal and nasal retina requires the probe to be placed nasally and temporally respectively. The eye

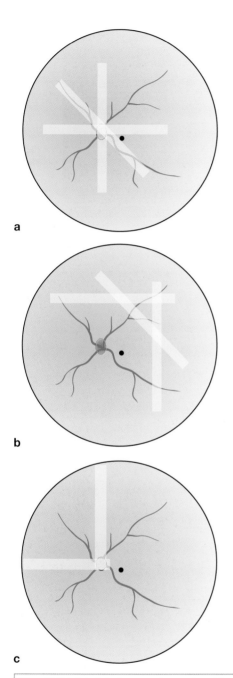

a

b

c

Fig. 12.5 (a) Axial ultrasound scanning. The optic nerve appears in the centre of the screen. The probe can be rotated through 360° to examine any part of the posterior pole. **(b)** Transverse scanning. The probe is placed opposite the part of the eye to be studied. The scan passes through the sclera and not the lens. The optic nerve is not visualised. **(c)** Longitudinal scanning. This allows the peripheral retina to be viewed. The optic nerve appears at the bottom of the scan.

again looks away from the probe but the white mark now points upwards. Oblique scans can be performed in a similar manner. This allows the topographic localisation and extent of any abnormality to be determined. Carefully performed, it can also help to localise an intraocular foreign body.

The anterior extension of a lesion can be determined from a longitudinal scan (Fig. 12.5c). The probe is placed with the white mark pointing towards the centre of the cornea or the limbus. The patient again looks away from the probe. This displays the optic nerve at the bottom of the screen and the anterior retina and sometimes the pars plana in the upper part of the screen. This view is also useful to look for anterior retinal pathology such as breaks or tears (Fig. 12.7). If the anterior vitreous is to be examined, a higher-frequency (20 MHz) probe can be placed on the cornea to produce an axial projection.

B-scan evaluation also produces a dynamic picture of the eye. The patient moves the eye while the probe remains still. This is particularly useful in studying the detached vitreous gel and retinal detachment. After-movement of the vitreous, when the eye has stopped moving, is a helpful sign in differentiating a posterior vitreous and retinal detachment.

If the B-scan reveals an abnormality, a complete A-scan should also be performed. Some machines will effectively perform both scans automatically and allow the orientation of the A-scan to be changed on the frozen or stored B-scan image to aid analysis. Remember that a transcleral (non-axial scan) will show only one initial spike (sclera) while an axial scan will show two. The A-scan should be as perpendicular as possible to the abnormality. It is displayed as a single line on an x–y axis, where x is distance and y height. The height indicates the amount of reflectance (Fig. 12.8). The A-scan also helps when measuring objects on the ultrasound picture. Two markers can be independently moved on the screen and the distance between them calculated. Using the peaks on the A-scan helps to locate these markers accurately on the abnormal region of the B-scan.

Scanning an eye following penetrating trauma requires great care. It is probably best left until a primary repair has been undertaken to avoid pressure on the eye causing further damage.

The combined use of standardised A-scan and contact B-scan is referred to as standardised echography. An optimal echographic examination results

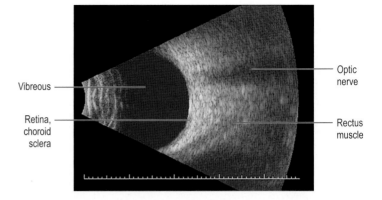

Fig. 12.6 A transverse scan. The optic nerve appears in the centre of the picture.

Vibreous

Retina, choroid sclera

Optic nerve

Rectus muscle

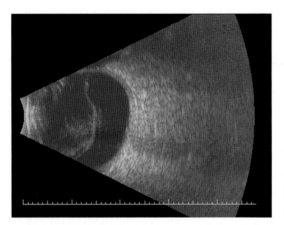

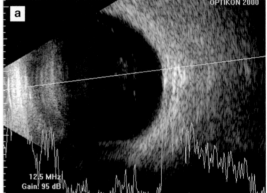

Fig. 12.7 A longitudinal scan. The patient has a posterior vitreous detachment. The optic nerve appears towards the bottom of the scan. Superiorly the attachment of the vitreous can be seen.

from the appropriate combination of both A- and B-scans.

Clinical application of ultrasound

Vitreous and retina

Suspected abnormalities of the vitreous and retina are a very common indication for ultrasound examination. It is particularly useful in assessing the vitreous and posterior segment when the media is opaque. The sound characteristics of the *normal* vitreous include the following:

- no reflection
- the need for high gain settings to see small condensations

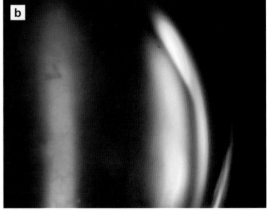

Fig. 12.8 (a) A combined A- and B-scan showing a vitreous opacity. The axis of the A-scan is shown by the line on the B-scan. The A-scan is displayed at the bottom of the picture. Note the high reflectance (the peak on the *y*-axis) corresponding to the opacity seen on the B-scan. **(b)** The clinical appearance of the vitreous floater.

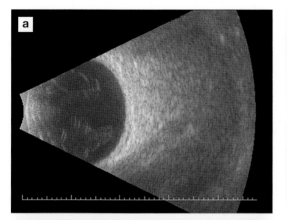

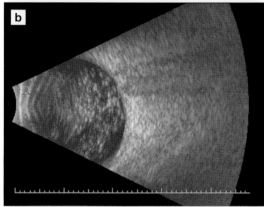

Fig. 12.9 The ultrasound appearance of a vitreous haemorrhage in the early **(a)** and late **(b)** stages.

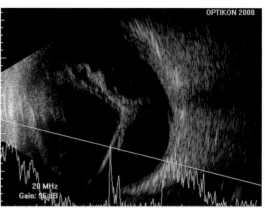

Fig. 12.10 A funnel-shaped detachment. The retina remains attached at the disc. Note that on the A-scan the retinal peak has a similar reflectivity to the sclera.

• little movement on dynamic testing in the absence of a posterior vitreous detachment (PVD).

Vitreous haemorrhage, endophthalmitis, asteroid hyalosis, clumps of inflammatory cells and any other condition that creates vitreous condensations cause reflectivity to be increased. The gain is decreased to assess the pathology. Vitreous haemorrhage varies from medium to high density initially; once the coagulation cascade starts with fibrin formation, reflectivity increases further. This high reflectivity is very characteristic of a haemorrhage (Fig. 12.9).

The retina shows a similar reflectivity as sclera under normal conditions. When assessing the retina it should always be compared to the reflectivity of the underlying sclera using the A-scan (Fig. 12.10).

This is particularly useful when trying to differentiate a vitreous membrane from the retina.

The echographic features of a rhegmatogenous retinal detachment are thus quite typical (Figs 12.10, 12.11):

• a bright, continuous smooth or folded membrane on B-scan
• a highly reflective spike on A-scan similar to the sclera.

A complete examination will also provide topographic information and an assessment of retinal mobility. This may be reduced in proliferative vitreous retinopathy (PVR). Associated findings such as membranes, intraocular foreign bodies and tumours may also be present.

It is important to differentiate a retinal detachment from a PVD or PVR. Superficially they may appear to have similar patterns. The clinical history aids a detailed evaluation with the B-scan. A PVD usually produces weaker reflectivity than a detached retina. Associated findings on ultrasound may also help with the diagnosis; for example, breaks or tears in the peripheral retina, membranes or PVR suggest a retinal detachment. As a retinal detachment advances it becomes funnel-shaped, reflectivity increases and less movement occurs (Fig. 12.10). However, care must be taken in assessing what appears to be a funnel-shaped detachment anchored at the optic nerve head, a PVD can also appear like this. The dynamic scan will help. A PVD tends to

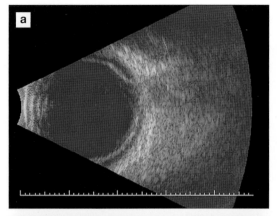

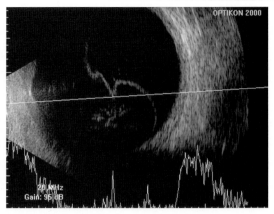

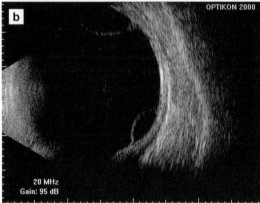

Fig. 12.12 This patient has had a vitreous haemorrhage associated with a posterior vitreous detachment. There is blood on the posterior vitreous face, an ochre membrane. Note the folded appearance of the posterior vitreous face. Even with the deposition of blood, the peak on the A-scan is not as great as that of the sclera.

Fig. 12.11 (a) A rhegmatogenous retinal detachment. **(b)** Retinoschisis.

flow as the eye moves from side to side, causing significant after-movement when the eye comes to rest. A retinal detachment appears less mobile with less after-movement (Fig. 12.12).

Traction retinal detachments may produce a tent-like configuration of the retina, with one or more points of traction and contraction. Topographic evaluation is important, particularly if a clear view of the retina is not possible (Fig. 12.13).

Although the diagnosis of retinal detachment is generally easy to make, it can be mimicked by a number of other pathologies (Box 12.2).

The choroid

Under normal conditions ultrasound is unable to differentiate the thin layer of choroid from the over-

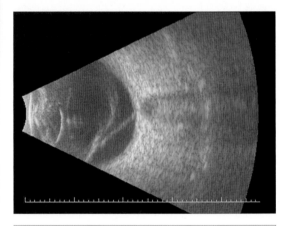

Fig. 12.13 A traction retinal detachment inferiorly. The retina appeared immobile on kinetic testing.

lying retina and underlying sclera. This complex is usually seen on a B-scan as a bright band and as a layer of multiple echoes on A-scan. However, fluid or infiltrative lesions may result in separation of the layers.

Choroidal thickening and/or detachment may be seen in inflammatory disease, hypotony, trauma,

Differential diagnosis of a retinal detachment on ultrasound

- posterior vitreous detachment with attachment to optic nerve
- Vitreous haemorrhage
- Bridging vitreous membrane
- Vitreous track from a penetrating injury
- 360° peripheral choroidal detachment
- Kissing choroidal detachment

following intraocular surgery and with tumours. All of these conditions may share common findings but the clinical history usually helps pinpoint the diagnosis.

A choroidal detachment typically shows a smooth, thick, dome-shaped membrane, with no movement on B-scan and a double-peaked spike on A-scan with 100% reflection (Fig. 12.14). Between the anterior spike (retina and choroid) and the posterior spike (sclera) there is no reflectivity at all from the intervening clear fluid. If haemorrhage or other material is present in the choroidal space, spikes of variable reflectivity appear. Sometimes choroidal detachments can approach from nasal and temporal sides touching centrally. These are known as kissing choroidals.

Intraocular tumours

Ultrasound examination is of great importance in the diagnosis and investigation of intraocular tumours, even if the medium is clear. An assessment of location, size, reflectivity and sound absorption may help arrive at a diagnosis. The major tumours will be covered below.

Retinoblastoma

Ultrasound is very useful in the differential diagnosis of leukocoria and retinoblastoma in infancy. Retinoblastoma can be focal or multifocal, unilateral or bilateral. It may grow towards the vitreous (endophytic) or the choroid (exophytic). Clinically it has a creamy-yellow appearance. Internally calcium deposits are characteristic. These can be very small and focal or large, occupying much of the tumour. Ultrasonically they can present as mildly elevated, diffuse lesions at the level of the retina, with a bumpy irregular contour. The presence of calcium is extremely important in diagnosing the tumour. In advanced cases, the calcium reflects all the sound, producing a complete shadow posteriorly. On the A-scan there is variable absorption and reflection of sound. A high initial spike with very variable intermediate spikes from calcium and dense tissue and a final spike of high reflectivity that corresponds to sclera are typical. There may be associated changes in the vitreous and indeed the orbit. Due to the high risk of metastasis, very careful evaluation of the choroid is important (Fig. 12.15).

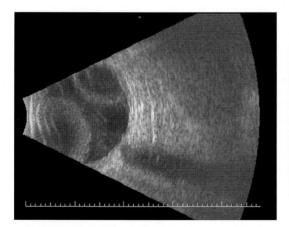

Fig. 12.14 A choroidal detachment.

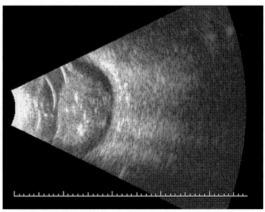

Fig. 12.15 A retinoblastoma.

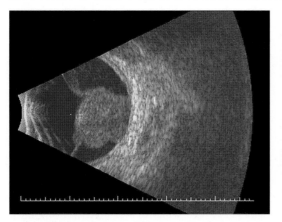

Fig. 12.16 The mushroom configuration of a melanoma.

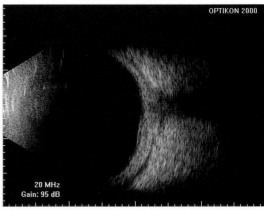

Fig. 12.17 Posterior scleritis. This has caused fluid to form in Tenon's layer. In this case the optic nerve sheath is also involved, producing a T-sign.

Melanoma and haemangioma

Both these tumours have a similar appearance in the posterior segment on B-scan, particularly in the early stages, when both may appear dome-shaped. At a later stage a melanoma may take the typical mushroom configuration. A melanoma may rupture Bruch's membrane. It is very important to locate the tumour accurately with very detailed topographic evaluation and to look for extension to neighbouring structures (Fig. 12.16).

The difference in ultrasound appearance between these lesions is best appreciated with an A-scan examination of the internal structure. A melanoma is a very solid and compact tumour, with low flow of blood and high absorption of sound, producing low reflectivity. Reflectivity increases following radiotherapy treatment. Conversely a haemangioma has a very high flow of blood with no absorption of sound, resulting in high reflectivity, making a very clear difference between the two.

Choroidal metastases may appear similar to melanomas on ultrasound. They are associated with retinal detachment at an earlier stage than melanomas. They tend to have more reflectivity than melanomas.

The sclera

Ultrasound can be helpful in diagnosing posterior scleritis. Fluid with low reflectivity accumulates between Tenon's layer and the orbital fat. With involvement of the optic nerve this fluid tracks along the sheath, giving rise to the appearance of a horizontal T (the T-sign). The sclera may also appear thickened (Fig. 12.17).

The optic nerve orbit and extraocular muscles

Although magnetic resonance imaging and computed tomography scans are commonly used to examine the orbit and extraocular muscles, ultrasound also has a role. It helps to differentiate between solid and cystic masses. The optic nerve can be evaluated and the extraocular muscles imaged. It is not possible to image the posterior quarter of the orbit.

Ultrasound examination of the optic nerve is particularly useful in the diagnosis of optic nerve head drusen (Fig. 12.18). These have a high reflectivity due to their calcium content and are readily demonstrated on axial scanning.

Fluid and solid distension of the anterior optic nerve can also be demonstrated.

A B-scan is also performed to look for signs of high reflectivity and masses in the orbit. In Graves disease the muscles gain width, which can be measured with the A-scan and recorded for further follow-up. The probe is placed on the opposite side to the muscle to be assessed. The fascia produces a very distinct double peak on the A-scan marking the limits of the muscle. In between the muscle itself usually shows low reflectivity. Infiltrative lesions show high reflectivity.

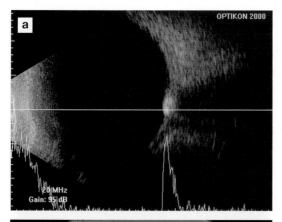

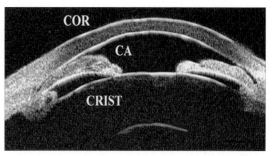

Fig. 12.19 An ultrasound biomicroscopy picture of the anterior segment. COR, cornea; CA, anterior chamber; CRIST, crystalline lens. (Courtesy of Dr Mario de la Torre, Peru.)

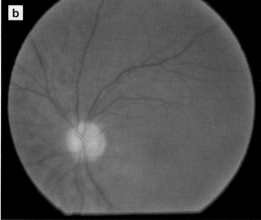

Fig. 12.18 (a) The appearance of optic nerve head drusen on ultrasound. **(b)** The clinical appearance of the nerve head.

The superior rectus appears to share the anterior portion with the levator muscle of the lid, which makes it seem larger.

Anterior-segment ultrasound biomicroscopy

This ultrasound technique requires immersion using a special cup placed directly over the cornea to provide an interface between the probe and the anterior segment. The images show the anterior segment very clearly, particularly the cornea, iridocorneal angle and the relation between the iris and the lens (Fig. 12.19). The probe uses frequencies of 35 and 50 MHz, giving great resolution but low tissue penetration.

The UBM is useful in the evaluation of anterior-segment angle anomalies such as plateau iris, tumours and elevated lesions. As with posterior-segment tumours, topographic localisation and measurement of the tumour are possible.

Colour Doppler imaging

Introduction

The depiction of blood flow information on a real-time grey-scale B-mode background is termed colour Doppler imaging (CDI). It uses a combination of B-scan and Doppler images (duplex scanning). Originally described in 1979, it became a major advance in cardiological investigation. It has gained increasing clinical use since then, for example in the assessment of peripheral vascular disease. In ophthalmology it has been used extensively in research, and is increasing in clinical use, particularly in the investigation of orbital disease. A brief overview of the technique is given here.

The Doppler phenomenon

To understand how CDI works it is first necessary to understand the Doppler phenomenon. If an ultrasound wave generated by a fixed source is reflected from a moving object the frequency of the reflected wave changes (Fig. 12.20). It is higher than the incident wave when the object is moving towards the ultrasound probe and lower when it is moving away. The velocity at which the object moves towards the probe will also affect the frequency of the reflected wave. This change in frequency is

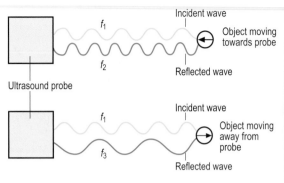

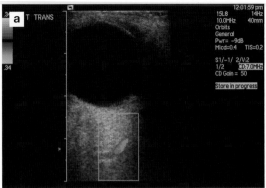

Doppler shift frequency = $f_1 - f_2$ and $f_1 - f_3$

Fig. 12.20 The Doppler phenomenon. Note the difference in the frequency of the reflected wave when the object is moving towards and away from the probe.

known as the Doppler shift. Mathematically it can be represented by the following equation:

$$D f = \frac{2FV \cos\theta}{c}$$

where:

- $D f$ is the measured frequency shift
- F is the frequency of ultrasound waves emitted from the transducer
- V is the blood flow velocity
- θ (A) is the angle of incidence of the sound beam to the direction of blood flow
- c is the velocity of ultrasound in tissue.

It is apparent from this formula that the angle at which the ultrasound wave impacts the moving object is important. The maximum Doppler shift is when the angle is 0°, that is, the probe is parallel to the moving object, in comparison to B-scan ultrasound where the maximum echo occurs when the probe is at a right angle to the interface. An angle greater than 45° will result in a significant error in analysing the Doppler shift from blood flowing in a vessel. This has practical implications in the measurement of CDI.

Colour Doppler imaging

Information regarding blood flow is superimposed on the conventional B-scan grey-scale image. Analysis of the Doppler shift of the ultrasound wave provides information on movement in tissue. Usually

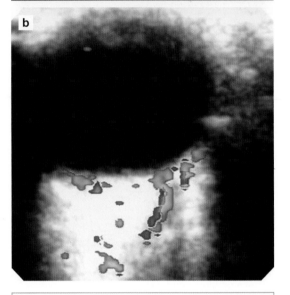

Fig. 12.21 (a) Colour flow map showing the normal ophthalmic artery (red). (Courtesy of Marie Restori, Moorfields Eye Hospital, London.) **(b)** Colour flow map showing normal ciliary and retinal blood vessels. (Courtesy of Tom Williamson, St Thomas' Hospital, London.)

this movement represents the flow of blood in the vessels (Fig. 12.21). The relative Doppler shift frequency is colour-coded on the greyscale of the B-scan, providing a velocity map of the blood flow in the tissue or vessel being studied. Flow towards the probe is designated red and flow away from the probe is blue. In arterial vessels the velocity of the blood will change throughout the cardiac cycle. In turn this will result in a change in the Doppler frequency shift throughout the cycle. Analysis of this change enables a continuous measure of blood velocity in the vessel to be made. As the change in frequency is within the audible range it can also be heard. The ultrasound transducer switches between pulses recording the B-scan and pulses recording the Doppler shift (these are usually longer than the pulses used to record the B-scan).

The operator adjusts the area of tissue being sampled for Doppler measurements to localise the vessel to be studied. Analysis of the Doppler frequency (spectral analysis) enables the velocity of blood in the vessel under investigation to be calculated, for example the peak and trough velocity values to give the peak systolic and end-diastolic velocities. Additionally an assessment of vascular resistance (pulsatility) can be made.

Clinical applications

A number of studies have demonstrated abnormal CDI in ophthalmic conditions. Reduced flow in the central retinal artery and vein has been found in patients with a central retinal artery occlusion. The short posterior ciliary arteries, although sometimes difficult to identify, have a reduced flow in anterior ischaemic optic neuropathy, particularly when associated with giant cell arteritis. There has also been much interest in these vessels in glaucoma research. The venous flow may be pulsatile and blood flow velocity increased in carotid-cavernous sinus fistula. CDI also allows the vascularity of orbital lesions, tumours or varices to be assessed.

Box 12.3

The major parts of an ultrasound examination

Topographic
- Localisation
- Extension
- Shape

Quantitative
- Reflectivity
- Internal structure

Kinetic
- After-movement
- Vascularity

Summary

Ultrasound examination of the eye is useful in diagnosis, particularly when media opacity prevents a view of the posterior segment. The echo pattern may help confirm a diagnosis in an eye with clear media. Measuring the size of a lesion is helpful in following patients with tumours and in judging the success of treatment.

The component parts of an ultrasound examination are summarised in Box 12.3.

- Technological advances allow examination with higher resolution of ocular structures by utilising higher frequencies of ultrasound (up to 50 MHz)
- Examination by ultrasound is relatively easy to perform, with little morbidity
- Ultrasonographic examination is a dynamic technique, with much interpretation of the scans taking place during the examination. Still pictures are a useful record but should not be the only source of information diagnostically

References and further reading

Aburn NS, Sergott RC. Orbital colour Doppler imaging. Eye 1993; 7: 639–647.

Atta HR. Ophthalmic ultrasound: a practical guide. Edinburgh: Churchill Livingstone; 1996.

Baum G, Greenwood I. The application of ultrasonic locating techniques to ophthalmology: theoretic considerations and acoustic properties of ocular media: Part I. Reflective properties. Am J Ophthalmol 1958; 46: 319–329.

Mundt GH, Hughes WE. Ultrasonics in ocular diagnosis. Am J Ophthalmol 1956; 41: 488–498.

Oksala A, Lehtinen A. Diagnostic value of ultrasonics in ophthalmology. Ophthalmologica 1957; 134: 387–394.

Ossoinig KC. Standardized echography: basic principles, clinical applications and results. Int Ophthalmol Clin 1979; 19: 127–210.

White DN. Johann Christian Doppler and his effect: a brief history. Ultrasound Med Biol 1982; 8: 583–591.

13

Biometry

DAVID SCULFOR

Introduction

Biometry is the measurement of living tissue. It is an essential part of preoperative assessment for cataract surgery. Calculating the power of the intraocular lens (IOL) to be implanted requires at least the measurement of corneal curvature and axial length of the eye.

Accuracy in biometry is vital because cataract surgery alters patients' refractive error. Their postoperative refractive error is one of the key 'take-home' outcomes for patients, and the one they will be reminded of every time they have to put their glasses on to see. However careful the surgery, however good the nursing care and hospital food, if patients cannot comfortably wear glasses for the rest of their life, they will never forgive those involved. IOL exchange or the implanting of a

second 'piggy-back' lens may be possible, but it is technically difficult and exposes patients to further, often avoidable risk.

Calculation of IOL power is not an exact science. The components of the eye that influence the final outcome are normally distributed, so it is reasonable to assume that the outcome will also be normally distributed. All the clinician can do is to minimise the mean error and standard deviation so that most patients are clustered around the intended outcome. However, there will always be those who are at the extreme ends of the tails of the distribution. It is recommended that the clinician spends some time explaining to patients and carers about the limitations of the technique (Box 13.1).

However, there are three things that can and must be done to minimise errors:

1. accurately assess the patient's post-surgery requirements and expectations
2. optimise the biometry
3. check the quality of the biometry prior to surgery. This is the surgeon's responsibility, regardless of who performed the biometry.

Principles

The refractive error of an eye is determined by three elements: (1) the length of the eye; (2) the power of the cornea; and (3) the effective power of the crystalline lens (in a phakic eye) or IOL (pseudophakic eye). Various formulae have been developed whereby, for a given refractive error, if any two of these elements are known, the third can be calculated. The original Sanders, Retzlaff and Kraff (SRK) formula, although long obsolete, indicates the relationship between these elements:

For zero refractive error, IOL power = A-constant − (2.5 × axial length in millimetres) − (0.9 × keratometry in dioptres).

Box 13.1

Suggested advice to patients

We are going to measure the length and curvature of your eyes so that we can calculate the strength of the plastic lens that goes inside the eye in place of your cataract. Although we will take great care to get the measurements as accurate as possible, it is not an exact science. The problem is that in doing the calculations, the equipment has to assume that your eyes are average. Most eyes will be close to that average, but there are some that are not, and there is no way of knowing which they are. The result is that you might end up a little more long- or short-sighted than intended, and that would have to be corrected with glasses after the operation, whether for distance, close work or both

---

Keratometry

Keratometry is the measurement of the curvature of the cornea and is performed with an instrument called a keratometer (see Ch. 6). From the formula for the refractive power of a surface in air:

$$F = \frac{n - 1(1000)}{r}$$

if n is the assumed refractive index of the cornea and r is the radius of curvature of the cornea in millimetres, then F is the refractive power of the cornea in dioptres. Most keratometers have scales marked with the corneal power in dioptres, and the radius of curvature in millimetres, and will show, either on the instrument itself or in the handbook, what refractive index is assumed for the cornea. Commonly it is 1.336, but different manufacturers use values from 1.332 to 1.338. For a typical cornea of radius 7.70 mm, that gives a dioptric value ranging from 43.12 to 43.90. The refractive index used is less important than ensuring that the same value is used consistently in a department, regardless of the instrument used to record the measurement.

The cornea is a very powerful optical surface, and accounts for some two-thirds of the refractive power of the eye. As such, small errors in measuring the radius of curvature can give large errors in the choice of IOL power. Unfortunately there are a number of sources of error in keratometry, some of which can be controlled, and some that cannot.

Studies have shown that the refractive index of the cornea varies not only between subjects, but also within subjects during the day as the hydration of the cornea changes. The assumed value used in the calculation is an average, and, as pointed out earlier, some corneas will deviate significantly from this. It is not feasible to measure a true refractive index for each patient, so a non-standard corneal refractive index cannot be controlled for.

For practical purposes, another non-controllable source of error derives from the fact that the cornea is not a sphere. The common profile is a prolate ellipse, so that the cornea flattens from centre to edge, but that rate of flattening varies between eyes. Most keratometers measure only the central 3 mm of the cornea, so, given an average total corneal diameter of some 11 mm, the limitations are obvious. Equally obvious is that the patient must be viewing the central fixation target in the instrument when the reading is taken. The corneal apex will be found

to be slightly nasally displaced, and if performing keratometry on a patient under anaesthetic, that is where the central fixation point should be placed.

Keratometers, whether manual or automatic, work by projecting lights of known separation on to the corneal surface, and then measuring the separation of the reflected image (see Ch. 6). By trigonometry, the corneal radius of curvature is calculated. For this to be valid, the instrument must be a certain distance from the eye. All instruments require the images to be accurately focused by the operator, but some also require the eyepiece to be adjusted for the user, in particular the Haag–Streit type found in most ophthalmology departments. To do this, look through the eyepiece. There will be a black line running across the middle. Wind the eyepiece anticlockwise until the line is blurred, then slowly turn it clockwise until the line *first* becomes clearly focused. Further movement clockwise will result in the operator accommodating and give a false result. This adjustment need only be done once for each user, who should then remember his or her own setting for that particular instrument.

Difficult keratometry
Corneal disease

A poor corneal surface will give rise to irregular reflections from the tear film, resulting in variable readings, if they can be obtained at all. Typical causes include dry-eye problems or corneal scarring from trauma. A drop of saline or hypromellose may permit measurements to be taken, but in extreme cases, it may be necessary to use readings taken from the other eye. Since most pairs of eyes show reasonable symmetry, this technique is valid, but its use should be recorded, and the reason explained to the patient.

Previous refractive surgery

Corneal refractive surgery of whatever type alters the rate of flattening of the cornea, and in some cases, the curvature of the posterior corneal surface and the refractive index. Keratometry readings taken from such eyes, whether by manual, automatic or corneal mapping instruments, invariably give large hypermetropic errors and must not be used in IOL calculations.

Various methods have been proposed to overcome this difficulty, but none is accurate. In order of least inaccuracy, the two commonest are the prior data and contact lens methods.

The prior data method requires knowledge of:

- pre-refractive surgery refraction and keratometry
- post-refractive surgery refraction, which must have been obtained once the result had stabilised, but prior to the onset of any index myopia due to cataract.

An example is shown below:

> Pre-photorefractive keratectomy (PRK) refraction at cornea = −6.00 D
>
> Pre-PRK keratometry = 44 × 46 D (mean value = 45 D)
>
> Post-PRK refraction at cornea prior to myopic shift = −1.00
>
> Change in refraction = −5.00 D
>
> Mean keratometry to use in IOL calculation = 45 − 5 = 40 D

Where prior data cannot be obtained, the contact lens method may be used. The patient is refracted with and without a plano-powered contact lens (CL) of known back-surface power. The corrected keratometry value is given by:

$$CL_{\text{back-surface power}} + \text{refraction}_{\text{over CL}} - \text{refraction}_{\text{without CL}}$$

The refraction is corrected for back vertex distance, i.e. at the cornea.

> An example is given below:
>
> Post-PRK mean keratometry = 34.75 D
>
> Choose a plano contact lens with a base curve 0.95 × 34.75 = 33 D
>
> Refraction with this contact lens in place = −2.75 D at cornea
>
> Refraction without the contact lens = −0.50 D at cornea
>
> Keratometry to use in IOL calculation = 33 + (−2.75) − (−0.50) = 30.75 D

Whichever method is used, it is essential to advise such patients that the outcome is highly unpredictable, and that further surgery to correct refractive error may well be necessary. That advice must be recorded in the notes.

It is not unusual for elderly patients to require both cataract surgery and penetrating corneal keratoplasty (corneal grafting) (PKP). The dilemma for the surgeon is that the preoperative keratometry used in the IOL power calculation will bear little relation to that following PKP. Ideally, the PKP should be performed first, and, following removal of sutures, keratometry can be repeated prior to performing cataract surgery as a secondary procedure. The refractive benefits must be weighed against the risks involved in two lots of surgery, and the delay before full visual potential is realised.

Axial length measurement

There are two ways to measure the axial length of the eye. Ultrasound is a long-established method, but it has now been superseded by partial coherence interferometry, although that technique has its limitations, as will be discussed later.

A-scan ultrasound biometry

Ultrasound is defined as sound above the frequency of normal human hearing, that is, above 20 kHz. The frequency used for ultrasound biometry is 10 MHz, chosen as a compromise between resolution and penetration of the tissues. Lower frequencies have greater penetration of tissue, whereas higher frequencies have better resolution. Obstetric ultrasound has to penetrate to a much greater depth, so a frequency of 3.5–7 MHz is used, compared with 35 MHz for high-resolution ultrasound biomicroscopy of the eye's anterior segment.

The sound is both generated and received by a piezoelectric probe called a transducer. Piezoelectric materials have the useful property of producing an electrical charge when stressed, and the inverse effect of flexing when an electrical potential is applied, allowing the crystal to act as both transmitter and receiver.

An electrical potential is applied to the piezo crystal in the transducer, causing it to flex, and produce a sound wave that travels towards the tissue being investigated (Fig. 13.1). A simultaneous trigger pulse initiates detection. At any interface between materials of different sonic density, some sound is

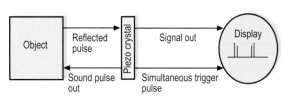

Fig. 13.1 Schematic principle of ultrasound.

reflected, and the rest transmitted. Reflected sound travels back to the transducer, causing the piezo crystal to flex and produce an electrical signal which is detected and displayed. The two parameters of interest are the amplitude of the signal reflected at each interface (the 'A' in A-scan is amplitude), and the calculated distance of the interface from the probe.

The tissue type and the perpendicularity of the beam of sound to the interface determine the amplitude. A high proportion of the sound will be reflected from an interface with a smooth surface and large difference in density. If the beam strikes the interface perpendicular to the surface, again most of the sound will be returned to the transducer. Conversely, if the incidence is not perpendicular, some of the sound will be reflected away from the transducer, and the displayed amplitude will be lower. An understanding of this principle will help explain an important source of error in A-scan ultrasound (Fig. 13.2).

The instrument uses the short time delay (typically 100 ns) between the sound pulse being produced and the reflected sound being received by the transducer in a time–velocity calculation to give the distance from the transducer to the interface.

$$\text{Distance} = \text{time} \times \text{assumed velocity}$$

This brings us to a limitation of the technique. The velocity of sound varies with the density of the medium through which it is passing. For example,

the average velocity of sound through the cornea and the lens is 1641 m/s, whereas the velocity through the aqueous and vitreous is 1532 m/s. As with corneal refractive index, these figures are averages, and will vary between subjects. In particular, the density and velocity of sound in the crystalline lens will increase with age. Most A-scan instruments allow the user to adjust the figure used for velocity, although this is not common practice. However, later instruments incorporate an age correction which makes this adjustment automatically.

Performing an A-scan

There are two methods of performing ultrasound biometry: the immersion technique or the more commonly used contact method. A hand-held probe or, better, one mounted on a holder at the slit lamp (often the Goldmann tonometer with the prism removed and the pressure set to 10 mmHg) is used with the contact method. The eye is anaesthetised (proxymetacaine) and the probe advanced like a tonometer to touch the eye gently. In immersion A-scanning, a shell containing saline is placed over the eye. The probe does not touch the cornea. With the contact method, the tip of the probe touches and partially flattens the cornea (Fig. 13.3).

The immersion technique is possibly more difficult to acquire, can be messy and may be intimidating for the patient. It is not available on all instruments. However, it is more accurate than the contact method because it is easier to recognise when the probe is not correctly aligned, and because the probe does not compress the cornea. Corneal compression in contact A-scan reduces the measured axial length by 0.1–0.3 mm, even for a careful user.

Sources of error in A-scan

There are a number of sources of error in A-scan biometry, but fortunately good technique can eliminate or reduce their effect. A typical good A-scan is shown in Figure 13.4, in this case for an immersion scan. For a phakic eye, there should be five clearly identifiable peaks (six for the immersion method): (1) the anterior corneal surface (immersion only); (2) the posterior corneal surface; (3 and 4) the anterior and posterior surface of the crystalline lens; (5) the retina; and (6) the sclera. The lens peaks should be around 90% of the maximum, with the second peak just slightly shorter than the first. Of particular importance is a sharp retinal peak, rising

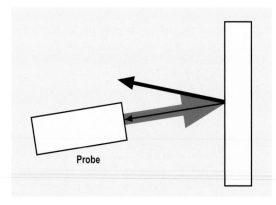

Fig. 13.2 Oblique scan. If the sound strikes the interface at an oblique angle, only a proportion of the beam will be reflected back to the transducer.

Probe

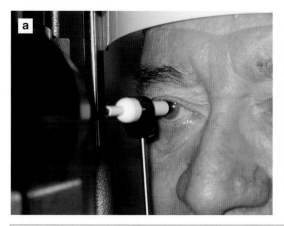 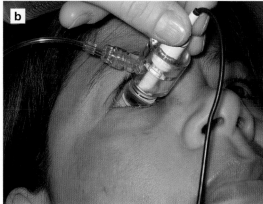

Fig. 13.3 (a) Contact and **(b)** immersion A-scans.

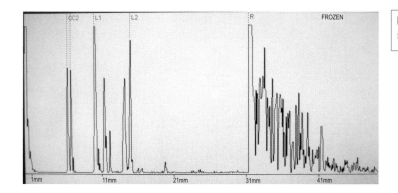

Fig. 13.4 Example of a good immersion A-scan.

quickly from the baseline. The scleral return usually comprises multiple peaks. The dotted lines, called gates, show where the instrument is taking the measurements from. Their appearance differs between manufacturers: the examples in Figure 13.4 are from the Alcon OcuScan RxP.

The software looks for a peak occurring within a predetermined measurement, and will, for example, assign the retinal gate to the first significant peak after the posterior lens marker. It is vital therefore to make sure that the gates have been correctly placed, because the instrument uses a different velocity to calculate the distance between the gates depending on where they lie. The first gate is set at the anterior cornea, and the second at the anterior lens surface. The instrument places the next gate at the posterior lens surface, with the final gate marking the inner limiting membrane of the retina. The velocity between the first two gates delimiting the anterior chamber is usually taken as 1532 m/s. The corneal velocity is ignored because the cornea is thin, and thus makes very little difference. A velocity of 1641 m/s is assumed between the next two gates which represent the lens, and finally 1532 m/s is again used for the posterior chamber. An individual distance calculation is made for each of these three sections, and their sum is displayed as the axial length. If a gate is incorrectly placed, most instruments allow you to adjust them manually, otherwise the scan must be deleted.

The commonest A-scan error occurs when the beam of sound is not aimed along the visual axis. As a result, the instrument measures a chord drawn across the eye, rather than the full diameter, giving a falsely short reading. The clue that this has happened is that the second lens peak is significantly longer or shorter than the first. Figure 13.5 shows why this occurs. The sound is incident on the anterior

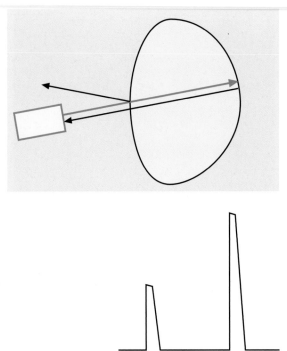

Fig. 13.5 An oblique lens scan produces uneven peaks.

If tonometer-mounted, the tonometer should be set to no more than 10 mmHg, and care taken to stop forward movement as soon as adequate contact is achieved. Another advantage of having the probe mounted rather than hand-held is that it is much easier to make small adjustments to the alignment, for example, moving the probe slightly up or down without altering the horizontal angle. Vertical alignment is aided by having the patient fixate a high-contrast target fixed to a wall behind the operator, with the fellow eye. The target should be positioned at the patient's eye height when the patient's head is on the headrest.

A falsely short measurement will result in a higher then necessary IOL power being indicated. The patient is likely to be myopic as a result, but may at least have some useful unaided near vision. A far worse error is to record an eye as being incorrectly long, because the IOL power will be too low. As a consequence the patient will be left hypermetropic,

lens surface at an oblique angle, and consequently much of the reflected signal does not reach the probe. At the second surface, although the beam is off-centre, it is more perpendicular, and consequently the returned amplitude is higher.

Using the contact technique, it is possible to compress the cornea significantly, particularly if the probe is hand-held. This source of error is the main cause of interoperator variability. It too will result in a short measurement, and may be detected by inspecting the measured anterior-chamber depth. Most instruments show this as a separate measurement specifically for this purpose. Any readings where the anterior-chamber depth is shorter than the rest should be discarded. The continuous bleep emitted by many instruments during measurement indicates that the probe has adequate contact on the cornea, and once achieved, no further forward pressure should be applied.

Corneal compression and failure to align the probe along the visual axis can be avoided by using the probe in a tonometer at a slit lamp, or using the spring-loaded mount supplied with some instruments.

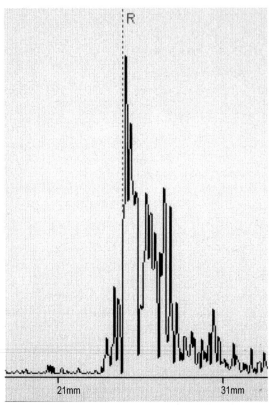

Fig. 13.6 A small retinal peak will be ignored by the instrument.

and will be very unhappy, having blurred unaided vision at all distances. The commonest cause for this is a failure of the instrument to identify the retinal peak correctly. If the return from the retina is very small or entirely missing, the retinal gate will be erroneously placed at the sclera, giving an error of up to 1 mm (Fig. 13.6).

This is a particular problem with dense cataracts because much of the sound energy is absorbed by the lens, and in myopic eyes, where the retina is thinner than normal. A falsely long measurement will also result if the rising face of the retinal peak is sloping rather than perpendicular. Poor alignment is again the chief cause (Fig. 13.7).

If the retinal peaks are consistently short, the gain of the instrument may be increased. This will increase the height of the returns, but care should be taken not to introduce clipping. This is where all the peaks reach the top of the display, which cuts off (clips) the top of the spike. It is then impossible to separate the retinal from the scleral peak, or to say whether the lens peaks are the correct height.

It is common practice to take several scans and use the mean axial length in calculations. This is perfectly valid; however, averaging several poor scans does not make them any more reliable. All the averaged scans should be within 0.2 mm of each other, and any outliers carefully assessed, and discarded and rescanned if necessary. The following checks should be applied (Box 13.2).

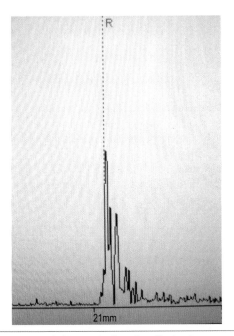

Fig. 13.7 A sloping retinal peak will give incorrect placement of the retinal gate.

Box 13.2

A step-by-step guide to contact ultrasound biometry

Before the patient comes in:
- Know the machine: practise with the software and on fellow staff
- Carry out calibration (more detail later)
- Read the notes to determine:
  - Which eye? Right/left/both?
  - Previous surgery
  - Preoperative refractive error
  - Intended (target) refraction
- Position the machine so you can see the screen while measuring
- Clean probe, following local infection control guidelines
- Enter patient details
- Check machine settings:
  - Right/left eye
  - Select eye type: phakic/aphakic/pseudophakic
  - Check contact/immersion setting
  - Auto/manual
- Do keratometry *before* contact ultrasound
- Sit the patient comfortably at the slit lamp
- Attach a bright, high-contrast, movable fixation target at the patient's eye level on far wall
- With the probe 2 cm away from the eye, ask the patient to fixate the light-emitting diode in the end of the probe and note the corneal reflex position
- Have the patient fixate the distant target
- Move the probe forward until contact is achieved, then stop!
- Watch the display and adjust probe alignment in small steps, one axis at a time
- Review and edit results
- Print out a representative scan for the patient records
- There should be five (six) clearly identifiable peaks
- The lens peaks should be around 90% of the scale maximum, and approximately equal height
- The retinal peak should be 70% of the scale maximum with a steeply rising face, and be clearly distinguishable from the scleral peak
- The gates should be where expected.

A majority of patients will have right and left axial lengths within 0.3 mm of each other. Some 96% of eyes have an axial length between 21 and 25.5 mm, and 60% fall between 22.5 and 24.5 mm. Axial lengths outside this range, or showing a difference of more than 0.3 mm, should be viewed with suspicion, and corroborating evidence sought. For example, with due allowance for index myopia in nuclear sclerotic cataract, if the refractive errors and keratometry are similar in the two eyes, then the axial lengths should also be similar. An eye that is 29 mm axial length should be highly myopic. An old, pre-cataract, spectacle prescription can be useful. Patients are usually quite willing to obtain this evidence from their optometrist if requested.

Partial Coherence Interferometry – the Zeiss IOL Master

The introduction of the Zeiss IOL Master in the late 1990s was a major step forward in improving the accuracy of biometry for cataract surgery (Fig. 13.8).

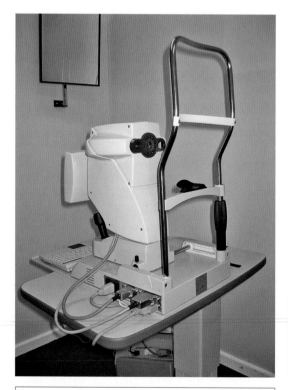

Fig. 13.8 Zeiss IOL Master.

For the first time, reliable measurements could be taken with a minimal amount of training, although some limitations of the equipment soon became apparent.

The IOL Master was developed as an offshoot of the technology used in Zeiss' ocular coherence tomography (OCT) instrument (Ch. 17). This uses a technique analogous to B-scan ultrasonography, but using light. It has 10 times the resolution of ultrasound, but the time delay is very short at 30 fs (30×10^{-15}). Both instruments therefore use the principle of partial coherence interferometry to determine the depth of living tissue. Interferometry compares the length of one beam of light with a reference beam.

The classic interference experiment, Young's slits, demonstrates the principle of interference. A beam of monochromatic light is incident on two slits in a plate. The slits then act as two new sources of coherent light beams (i.e. in phase and having the same wavelength) which then fall on a screen. Where the light arrives at the screen such that the difference in distance travelled by each beam is a whole number of wavelengths $(n\lambda)$, the light waves arrive in phase and interact to produce constructive interference, forming a light band on the screen. Conversely, if the path difference of the two beams is a multiple of a half-wavelength $(n\lambda/2)$, the waves arrive out of phase, cancelling each other out by destructive interference, and a dark band appears (Fig. 13.9).

The IOL Master uses low-coherence near-infrared light at 820 nm. The reason for this is that, with low coherence light, constructive interference only occurs when the two path lengths are identical. It thus gives a very accurate way of comparing the path length of two beams. The schematic shows how this is done (Fig. 13.10).

Light is incident on a semi-silvered mirror. Half is reflected to the movable reference mirror, and thence to the detector as shown. The other half is

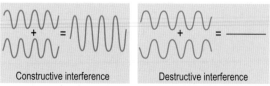

Constructive interference   Destructive interference

Fig. 13.9 Constructive and destructive interference.

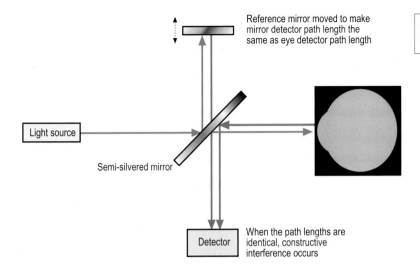

Reference mirror moved to make mirror detector path length the same as eye detector path length

Light source

Semi-silvered mirror

Detector

When the path lengths are identical, constructive interference occurs

Fig. 13.10 Schematic of interferometer.

transmitted to the eye, where it is reflected to the semi-silvered mirror, and then to the detector. The reference mirror is moved until the length from the reference mirror to the detector path is the same as the distance from the eye to detector. Only when this condition is met does constructive interference occur, resulting in a maximum intensity recorded by the detector. Users of the IOL Master will be familiar with the whirring sound as the measurement is taken, and that sound is the motor moving the reference mirror.

Although the IOL Master is straightforward to use, the operator and surgeon must know how to assess the scan quality, just as they must when using ultrasound.

The main features of the print-out are shown in Figure 13.11.

1. Axial length and signal-to-noise ratio (SNR) for each scan. The SNR indicates the height of the highest peak above the baseline, and as such is a measure of scan quality

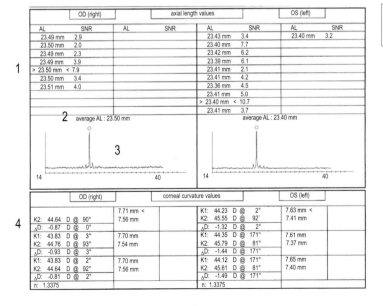

Fig. 13.11 IOL Master print-out with key features indicated.

2. Mean axial length. If any one axial length differs by more than 0.2 mm, the mean will not be calculated, and an 'Evaluation' error message appears instead. IOL calculations cannot be performed until this is corrected

3. The scan with the highest SNR is arrowed, and the actual display obtained appears at the bottom of the list so that its quality can be assessed

4. Keratometry readings. The arrowed measurement will be used in the IOL calculation. The instrument calculates an average value of R1 and R2 for each reading, and if the difference between the highest and lowest is greater than 0.50 D, an 'Evaluation' error message appears.

An ideal axial length scan is shown in Figure 13.12, the key features being a centralised peak and an even baseline. The SNR will typically be over 5.0. Note the appearance of secondary and tertiary maxima at around 0.8 mm from the central peak. An example

of a good scan is shown in Figure 13.13. It will have an SNR > 2.0. Scans with an SNR between 1.6 and 2.0 will be marked 'Borderline', and will have an exclamation mark next to them (Fig. 13.14).

Provided the main peak is clearly distinguishable from the baseline, and four or more repeatable scans are obtained, they may be used. If there is any doubt, then an ultrasound scan should be used to verify the result, remembering that the ultrasound result will be up to 0.3 mm shorter if contact ultrasound is performed, due to corneal compression.

Where the SNR is less than 1.6, the main peak will be virtually indistinguishable from the baseline, and an 'Error' message will appear in the average table (Fig. 13.15). These results cannot be used in the IOL calculation, but they may be usefully compared with the result of a subsequent ultrasound scan.

Although the instrument is set to reject any measurements which differ from the others by more than 0.2 mm, in practice a spread of no more than

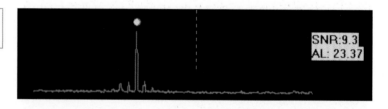

Fig. 13.12 Example of ideal IOL Master scan.

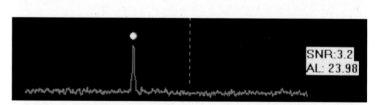

Fig. 13.13 Example of a good IOL Master scan.

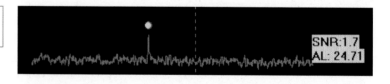

Fig. 13.14 Example of a borderline IOL Master scan.

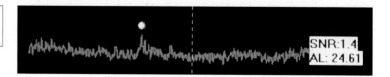

Fig. 13.15 Example of an unacceptable IOL Master scan.

0.05 mm is readily obtainable. Close inspection of each scan, with subsequent editing of the results, is essential. Commonly, instead of a sharp central peak, fine retinal structures may result in a double-tipped peak (Fig. 13.16). The resultant error is small, but careful editing can eliminate even these small differences. By left-mouse-clicking on the peak, the display will zoom in, and the separate peaks can be identified. The commonest cause of a double peak is light reflected from the inner limiting membrane of the retina, represented by the left-hand peak, in addition to the retinal pigment epithelium, which is the right-hand peak. The two peaks will be separated by less than 0.35 mm, and are thus distinguishable from secondary maxima which lie at 0.8 mm either side of the central maximum peak. Provided the marker has stopped at the second, retinal pigment epithelial peak, the scan is acceptable. It is possible to move the marker manually, and the resultant axial length will be highlighted with an asterisk. This should be used with caution, and care taken always to place the marker over the *right-hand* peak.

Tips on using the IOL Master

To limit a patient's exposure to the laser, the IOL Master allows up to 20 axial length measurements per eye per day for an individual patient. It is not necessary to use all 20, but at least four acceptable, repeatable scans should remain after editing.

To begin with, the reflection of the fixation light should be sharply focused and central. If good SNR results are obtained in this position, no further scans need to be taken. If the results are poor or variable, further readings should be taken at 12, 3, 6 and 9 o'clock with the reflection positioned at the inner edge of the circle, and note taken of the position giving the best SNR. In addition, focus in and out so that the reflection fills the circle, and take further readings. Provided the SNR is acceptable, and the results are repeatable, the axial length readings will be valid.

A poor tear film will result in a low SNR, and a drop of artificial tears will be helpful in improving the readings. A restless patient who moves or has poor fixation will give an unstable baseline. Patients may wear their glasses if it aids fixation, but contact lenses must not be worn.

Artificial tears are also useful when taking keratometry readings. All six of the outside dots must be sharply focused. Note that the central dot is used for centration only, and need not be in focus. The instrument will remind the operator to instruct the patient to blink once, and then open the eyes wide. Any obscured dots will result in an error message and will be highlighted with a cross on the print-out (Fig. 13.17).

As stated earlier, the instrument will reject any readings falling outside a given limit. However, the operator should seek to obtain three readings where the spread between the highest and lowest K1 readings is less than 0.3 D, and similarly all the K2 readings are within 0.3 D of each other.

Calculation of IOL power and the A-constant

Since the 1970s various formulae have been used to calculate the IOL power required for a given refractive outcome. A detailed discussion of lens formulae is beyond the scope of this book, but it is important to have an understanding of the elements involved, and the limitations of the formulae.

In 1980, Sanders, Retzlaff and Kraff used regression analysis to examine the refractive outcomes of cataract surgery they had performed. The basic formula they developed using this method is shown below:

For zero refractive error, IOL power =
A-constant − (2.5 × axial length in mm) −
(0.9 × keratometry in dioptres)

While this formula represented a considerable step forward, it is now obsolete. However, it introduced an important concept still used in modern lens formulae – the A-constant.

This figure will be found on the packaging of all IOLs, and is individual for that lens type. The manufacturer's figure should be regarded as a starting point, and refined as soon as results are available. It is often suggested that the A-constant should be adjusted for an individual surgeon, and while this may be possible for a small practice, it is more common to have a 'departmental' A-constant. This approach is valid, since intersurgeon differences are usually small. Some biometry instruments, including the IOL Master, incorporate a program for refining the A-constant using actual results. It is important to be aware of the limitations of this technique. Figure 13.18 shows a typical plot of deviation

Fig. 13.16 (a) Scan showing a double peak. **(b)** Zooming in shows that the cursor has picked up the return from the inner limiting membrane rather than the retinal pigment epithelium. **(c)** Note the change in axial length when it is repositioned by hand.

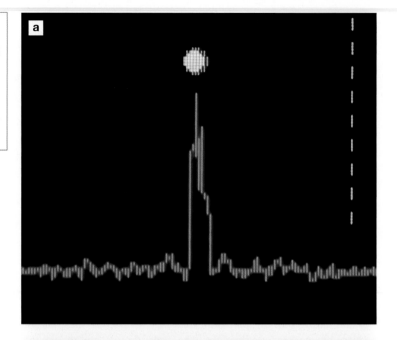

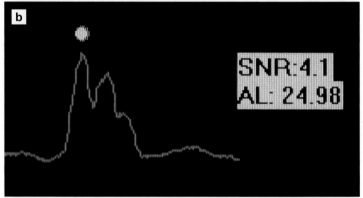

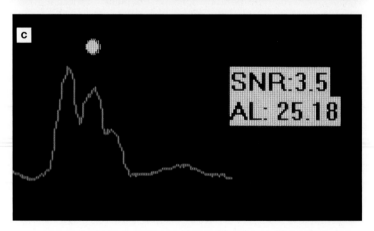

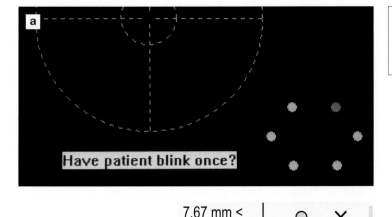

Fig. 13.17 (a) Error message and **(b)** print-out highlighting an obscured point from the IOL Master keratometer reading.

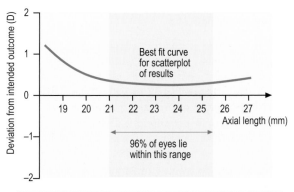

Fig. 13.18 Example plot of refractive error versus axial length.

The manufacturer's figure is usually for contact ultrasound biometry. If immersion biometry is performed, the A-constant must be adjusted, and will generally be around 0.3 higher. This is because the measured axial length will be consistently longer due to the absence of corneal compression.

The A-constants used with the IOL Master also require adjustment from the stated figure, as it too measures consistently longer than contact ultrasound. This is often wrongly assumed to be because the optical path length is measured to the retinal pigment epithelium, rather than the inner limiting membrane used in ultrasound. The correct reason is that the IOL Master was originally calibrated against a high-frequency immersion ultrasound instrument. It does not directly calculate axial length, but instead, once the optical path length is found, it goes to a 'look-up' table to find the corresponding axial length. As might be expected, the A-constant for the IOL Master is also higher, being typically around 0.4.

Later generations of IOL formulae aim to improve the predicted effective lens position, i.e. the distance from the cornea to the IOL. If the lens sits forward of the predicted position, the patient will be left myopic. These formulae require measurement of the anterior-chamber depth, or the corneal diameter (known as the 'white-to-white' measurement). They are thus slightly more complicated to use, but have

from the intended refractive error against axial length for a surgeon using the SRK-T (theoretic) formula. The curve is representative, as the formulae are generally less accurate for very long, and in particular, for very short eyes. Adjusting the A-constant of a given IOL will simply move the entire curve up or down, but will not flatten the extreme ends. Therefore, while it is valid to alter the A-constant to reduce the mean error in the central flatter portion of the graph, outliers should not be allowed to influence that adjustment unduly.

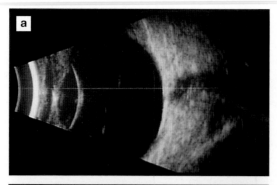

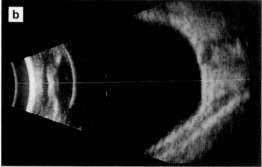

Fig. 13.19 Ultrasound B-scans showing **(a)** a normal eye and **(b)** an eye with a staphyloma.

the major advantage of being more accurate for eyes that are shorter or longer than average.

Difficult biometry

Where a patient is unable to cooperate with biometry, it can be performed under anaesthetic. However, the characteristics of some eyes make accurate biometry difficult, or in some cases, impossible.

A highly myopic eye presents two difficulties: (1) the retina may be very thin, making it difficult to obtain a good retinal peak; or (2) it may be an irregular shape due to a thinning and bulging of the sclera, known as a staphyloma (Fig. 13.19). Increasing the gain will give a stronger retinal return, but careful inspection of the gate position is required. A staphyloma may be suspected in highly myopic eyes where seemingly adequate scans show a wide variation in axial length. If the fovea lies on the sloping part of the staphyloma, a small change in scan direction gives a large difference in measurement. A B-scan will help to diagnose the condition,

but it may still be difficult to identify the position of the fovea to allow placement of the callipers. Where available, the IOL Master should be used instead. Provided the patient has good fixation, the axial length will always be measured along the visual axis.

Myopic eyes are also prone to retinal detachment, and cataract is a common sequel where vitrectomy and silicone oil are used in detachment surgery. The velocity of sound in silicone oil is much slower than that of vitreous, and so ultrasound greatly overestimates the axial length. Again, the IOL Master with its silicone oil setting will overcome this problem. It is advisable to perform biometry soon after detachment surgery in anticipation of cataract formation.

If biometry proves impossible, then, just as for keratometry, a reasonable estimate may be obtained by measuring the fellow eye. Intelligent inspection of a preoperative refraction will indicate whether the two eyes are likely to be of similar length.

Target refraction

Much attention is paid to accuracy in biometry, and rightly so, but an appropriate choice of target refraction is equally important. It should be noted that the refractive error which appears on the biometry printout is the mean sphere, not the spherical element in the spectacle prescription. The tendency is to choose an IOL power that will give a refractive outcome close to zero, or slightly myopic. However, if the fellow eye has good vision and is significantly hypermetropic, the resultant imbalance may make comfortable spectacle wear impossible.

In leaving a patient deliberately anisometropic, there are two factors to be considered:

1. image size difference (aniseikonia)
2. differential prismatic effect.

All normal spectacle lenses cause some magnification or minification due to the shape and power of the lens, and if the patient is anisometropic, aniseikonia will result. In practical terms, this image size difference does not become a problem until the difference is around 3–4 D. However, differential prismatic effect is likely to become a problem at around 1.50 D.

Prentice's rule tells us that:

$$\text{Prismatic effect (prism dioptres } \Delta) = \text{power (D)} \times \text{distance from optical centre (cm)}$$

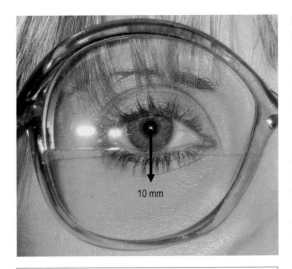

10 mm

Fig. 13.20 Bifocal wearers typically view through a point 10 mm below the distance optical centre when reading.

When using a bifocal lens for close work, the wearer is obliged to use a point approximately 1 cm below the optical centre of the lens, and slightly more for some varifocals (Fig. 13.20).

Each dioptre of vertical power difference thus gives a differential vertical prismatic effect of 1 Δ. Using prismatic lenses from a trial set, readers can readily verify for themselves that the maximum vertical prism that most people can tolerate is 1.5 Δ. Any amount above this produces vertical diplopia.

There are various solutions to this, for example, wearing a contact lens in one eye to balance the prescription; making a special type of bifocal called a slab-off to balance the prismatic effect; or wearing separate pairs of glasses for reading and distance. However, these are all compromises, and it is un-likely that the patient will be happy. In particular, a patient who has comfortably worn varifocals for 20 years will not willingly give them up for a bifocal.

When considering surgery for a first eye, the surgeon must consider:

- the vision in the other eye – is it likely to require surgery also?
- the patient's current glasses prescription and type

For example: a 70-year-old patient who has worn varifocals for 15 years is listed for right cataract surgery. The left shows very early lens opacities, and is thought unlikely to need surgery for several years. His current prescription is:

R +4.00 6/18   L +4.00/–1.00 × 180 6/6   Add 2.50
Mean sphere   L +3.50
Power vertically   L +3.00 which gives 3 Δ base-up
for near at 10 mm below
distance

Note that, when calculating the vertical prism, the effect of the cylinder must be taken into account. A cylinder has maximum effect vertically when its axis is 180, and negligible effect when it is 90. A reasonable estimate may thus be obtained as follows:

To the sphere power, add (for a plus cylinder) or subtract (for a minus cylinder) a proportion of the cylinder power:

For axis 180, all the cylinder power
For axis 45 or 135, half the cylinder power
For axis 90, the cylinder can be ignored

Thus in the example above, the vertical power of the left lens is +4.00 –1.00 = +3.00, giving 3 Δ base-up for near at 10 mm below the optical centre for distance. If we leave this patient emmetropic in his right eye, he will have to overcome 3 Δ of vertical prism for near, which he is unlikely to be able to do. If we leave him +1.50 in the right eye, that differ-ence falls to 1.5 Δ, which he may well cope with. The options of emmetropia and consequent problems, or leaving some hypermetropia, must be discussed with the patient, and recorded in the notes.

Sadly, the 'right' answer may not become apparent until after the surgery. The safest option would be to leave him with the prescription he has now, but provided full discussion has taken place, and recorded in the notes, reducing his hypermetropia is a reasonable choice.

Myopes also require some discussion. The sur-geon should ask myopes of –2.00D or more whether they take their glasses off for close work, even if they have bifocals or separate reading glasses. For example, a –5.00D myope has a near point of 20 cm unaided, compared with 33 cm with a typical reading addition. A patient whose hobby is fine needlework may well not appreciate losing this benefit!

For second-eye surgery, the decision process is similar, but *the prescription for the first eye must be known.*

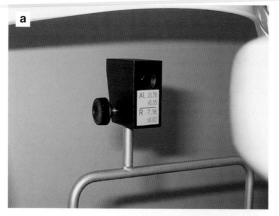

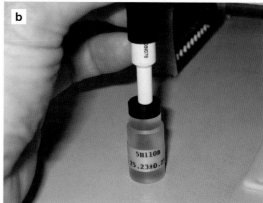

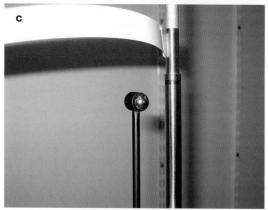

Fig. 13.21 Test pieces for: **(a)** IOL Master; **(b)** ultrasound; and **(c)** keratometer.

Calibration of equipment

It is unusual for biometry equipment to go out of calibration. Rather than giving incorrect readings, the instruments tend not to work at all if they develop a fault. However, it is essential that they are checked for correct function, and that the readings are within the limits stated by the manufacturer.

Most biometry equipment has a test piece supplied (Figure 13.21). Keratometers must also be checked. Commonly, the test piece is a ball bearing of known radius of curvature. True calibration of the machine can only be carried out by a service engineer using a test piece that has itself been calibrated against a gold standard, and at a specified temperature.

The frequency with which function checks are carried out depends on the lead time for surgery. If biometry is done on the same day as surgery, a function check should be carried out daily. If the lead time is 2 weeks, then a weekly function check will allow time for any fault to be discovered in plenty of time.

It is also essential to keep a record that these checks have been done, and of any service visits. Without this evidence, a court may well consider them not to have been carried out.

Summary

Biometry is not an exact science, and it is important to explain this limitation to patients, especially in difficult cases. However, surgeons have a duty to ensure that the biometry they are using is the best that could be obtained. In addition, a careful assessment of patients' requirements is essential to avoid refractive problems postoperatively.

- Biometry is important because the refractive outcome of surgery is one of the key outcomes that will be with the patient permanently
- Biometry is not an exact science. It is based around a normal distribution of measurements about the mean. The practitioner's role is to minimise systematic and measurement error
- It is important to elucidate previous history of laser or other refractive surgery
- Always perform K readings before contact A-scan measurements, as these can disturb the corneal surface

Further reading

Rhonda Waldron has written a comprehensive article on biometry at http://www.emedicine.com/oph/topic486.htm.

See Warren Hill MD's excellent website at www.doctor-hill.com for practical advice on biometry.

Radiological techniques in ophthalmic investigation

GERARDINE QUAGHEBEUR

RADIOLOGY OF THE ORBIT

Introduction

The orbits are bony recesses housing the globes, extraocular muscles, blood vessels, lymphatics, five of the cranial nerves, sympathetic and parasympathetic nerves and most of the lacrimal apparatus.

Each orbit is pyramidal in shape with the apex projected posteromedially and the base or orbital opening projected anterolaterally.

The bony walls separate the orbital cavity from the anterior cranial fossa above; the maxillary antrum/sinus below; the ethmoid and sphenoid sinus and nose medially; and the face and temporal fossa laterally.

Imaging is one cornerstone for diagnosis and should be used in conjunction with clinical signs and symptoms (Boxes 14.1–14.3). The orbit is amenable to radiological investigation by several modalities and it is important to select the appropriate imaging method. Traditionally ophthalmologists have been a low-demand imaging group but advances in imaging

techniques and increasing ability to demonstrate detail will lead to an increase in demand and subsequent reliance on high-quality tailored orbital imaging (Fig. 14.1).

It is important to select the appropriate imaging modality, although this may practically depend on the patient and the availability of the technique. Computed tomography (CT) and magnetic resonance imaging (MRI) are complementary imaging techniques and both may be required for full evaluation of complex lesions. Whichever modality is used, a standardised high-resolution technique is necessary.

Box 14.2

The role of imaging

- To confirm the presence of a lesion
- To define a lesion's anatomical site, thus helping to establish a diagnosis or provide a differential diagnosis
- To define precise anatomical relationships and extent, which allows surgical planning/treatment pathways
- To provide a guide to other imaging techniques

Box 14.1

Common clinical features and presentations

- Trauma
- Pain
- Mass: proptosis, displacement of the globe
- Loss of function: sensory or motor, including diplopia and change in visual acuity

The age of the patient, the chronicity and onset of symptoms and signs are important to the radiologist in interpreting the results

---

Box 14.3

Imaging techniques

- Plain radiographs
- Ultrasound
- Computed tomography (CT)
- Magnetic resonance (MR)
- Contrast studies: angiography, venography/phlebography

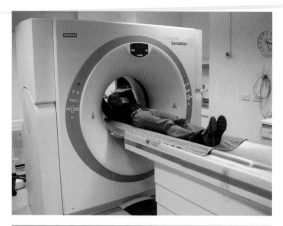

Fig. 14.1 A modern computed tomography scanner.

Good accurate clinical information is essential. At the end of the investigation the following information should be provided:

- Where is the lesion?
- What are its imaging characteristics?
- What is it likely to be?
- Is it confined to the orbit and, if not, what is its extent?

The *anatomical* or *compartment* approach to orbital disease is a useful starting point, but is slightly artificial. Lesions can occur in more than one site and lesions may expand to involve more than one site (Table 14.1).

The classical approach aims to localise a lesion to one of the following regions:

- the globe
- optic nerve or optic nerve sheath complex
- intraconal (within the muscle cone)
- conal (the muscle cone itself)
- extraconal (outside the muscle cone)
- lacrimal gland lesions.

This is a useful starting point but the extent of a lesion must also be described. Bilateral disease may be a pointer to a systemic illness; extension intracranially or elsewhere could be due to direct spread of orbital disease or part of a secondary process.

Plain radiographs

These are less commonly used but retain a role in some cases of trauma, and in evaluation of foreign bodies within the eye. They are not useful in the evaluation of orbital masses or inflammatory conditions. Alterations in size of the orbit can indicate long-standing disease and calcification may sometimes be demonstrated, but these days plain radiographs have been superseded by cross-sectional imaging techniques.

Orbital fractures can be demonstrated on good-quality plain radiographs but the advent of helical CT is leading to a change in practice. Radiation dose to the lens is comparable and the increased resolution on modern sophisticated CT provides far more information. For example, the ability to localise

Table 14.1	Compartments, contents and pathology	
Compartment	**Contents**	**Pathology**
Globe		Retinoblastoma, melanoma, metastases
Intraconal	Optic nerve sheath complex, fat, lymph nodes, vessels, nerves	Optic nerve glioma/meningioma, neurofibroma, lymphoma/angioma, haemangioma, arteriovenous malformation
Conal	Muscles	Thyroid eye disease, pseudotumour, rhabdomyosarcoma
Extraconal	Fat, lacrimal gland, bony orbit	Infection, adenocarcinoma, mucoepidermoid, primary or secondary bone tumours

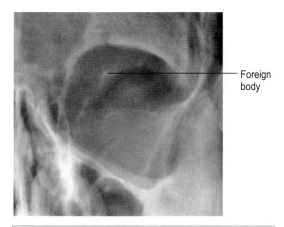

Fig. 14.2 Plain radiograph showing a radiopaque/
metallic foreign body in the left orbit.

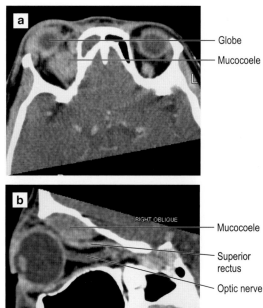

Fig. 14.3 (a) Axial image of computed tomography
data set showing mucocoele in superior right orbit.
(b) Reconstructed image from the axial data set
showing the mucocoele in the sagittal plane.

the extraocular muscles accurately in relation to the
fracture site is not possible on plain X-ray.

Plain films are used to identify radiopaque
(usually metallic) foreign bodies either in addition
to or as an alternative to ultrasound examination. In
many radiology departments plain films are required
prior to any MRI examination if the patient gives
a history of trauma to the eye, or exposure to metal
filings.

A single view can be obtained and reviewed and
a second view (with the eye in a different position)
is only required if doubt exists about the presence of
a suspected foreign body (Fig. 14.2).

ORBITAL COMPUTED TOMOGRAPHY

Introduction to computed tomography scanning

CT scanning was developed in the early 1970s and
is based on ionising radiation. As X-ray beams pass
through tissues they are absorbed or attenuated
(weakened) at different levels depending on the type
of tissue they pass through. CT scanners use multiple
detectors to measure these X-ray attenuation profiles
and produce images. Initially CT scanners could
only produce single slices. Recent developments now
allow continuous rotation of the gantry (the area
of the scanner that detects the information), this is
known as helical or spiral scanning. This means that

entire anatomic regions of the body can be imaged
in a short period of time (for instance, the entire
lungs in 20–30 s). Instead of acquiring a stack of
individual slices these new scanners produce a
volume of data with all the relevant anatomy in one
position. This volume of data can then be reconstructed by computers and sophisticated software
programs to provide images as required. Subsequently pictures can be reconstructed in any plane
or angle. The images can be simple axial, sagittal
or coronal views (Fig. 14.3) or more sophisticated
three-dimensional pictures (Fig. 14.4). This technique is often referred to as multiplanar reformatting
and post-processing. The high acquisition speed
means rapid scanning without motion artefact and
this may allow paediatric scanning without the need
for sedation or anaesthesia. Less patient cooperation
is needed.

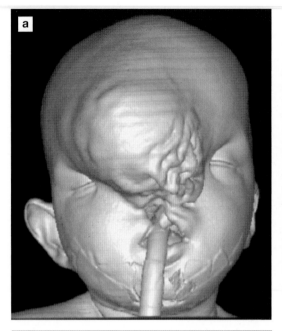

Fig. 14.4 (a) Three-dimensional computed tomography reconstructed image of child with hypertelorism and a facial cleft, showing the 'soft-tissue' window levels. **(b)** Three-dimensional reconstructed image of the same child showing the bony detail.

CT scanning is a readily available technique in most radiology departments and is often the preferred initial imaging method. There are no contra-indications other than pregnancy. All prostheses are safe to scan.

Technique

In most cases a direct axial helical data set will be obtained roughly parallel to the infraorbital–meatal line. This is determined on the lateral scout view and is about –10° to the orbitomeatal base line. The field of view (area to be scanned) should extend inferiorly to include the upper portion of the maxillary sinuses and superiorly to include the pituitary fossa and frontal sinuses. If the patient is asked to elevate the chin as much as possible during the acquisition of the scan, optimal views of the optic nerves and foramina will be obtained. Thin-section axial, sagittal and coronal plane images are produced (1.5–3.0 mm). The information should be displayed on both bone and soft-tissue algorithms.

If helical scanning is not available, then direct axial and coronal contiguous images are acquired with maximum 5 mm slice thickness.

The use of intravenous contrast medium is valuable in most cases where a mass or inflammatory lesion is suspected. The patterns of enhancement of orbital lesions are not that diagnostic but contrast medium provides information about potential vascularity and delineates more precisely the extent of any lesion (Box 14.4). This is particularly relevant where intracranial extension is present.

Contrast is generally not required for scanning in cases of foreign body, trauma and uncomplicated thyroid eye disease or follow-up of known lesions.

If a patient is to undergo combined CT and MRI then non-contrast CT alone is sufficient.

If a tumour is suspected, contrast is essential. If an orbital or ocular tumour is suspected or diagnosed following a scan, additional post-contrast axial scans through the cranial cavity are recommended. Contrast should also be used in cases of orbital infection.

Calcium in
retinoblastoma

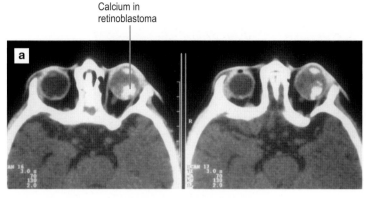

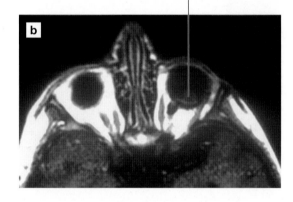

Tumour (retinoblastoma)

Fig. 14.5 (a) Axial computed tomography (CT) scan showing coarse calcification in an enlarged left globe due to retinoblastoma. This is well shown (as opposed to magnetic resonance, in Fig. 14.5b) but CT does not allow an assessment of extension into the optic nerve or through the choroid. Whole-brain imaging is needed to look for metastases and careful evaluation of the opposite eye to looking for bilateral disease is essential. **(b)** Axial T1w magnetic resonance scan of the same child. Calcium is poorly seen but the soft-tissue tumour and its extent are more clearly delineated. Fat suppression technique failed in this small child (see later).

The high intrinsic contrast between bone, muscles, orbital fat and air produces excellent visualisation of orbital structures. CT is excellent for the detection of calcification, which aids in diagnoses such as retinoblastoma (Fig. 14.5) and optic nerve sheath meningioma (Fig. 14.6). CT optimally demonstrates bony structures, including erosion (Figs 14.7 and 14.8), scalloping and bone defects, as in the case of a dermoid cyst (Box 14.5). It is the technique of choice for imaging in preseptal/septal cellulitis.

Box 14.4

Imaging features of an orbital lesion

- Contour and surface: smooth, round, irregular, poorly defined
- Surrounding structures: bony changes, mass effect on globe
- Internal character of lesion: calcium, cystic, vascularity
- Extent of abnormality

Box 14.5

Advantages of computed tomography

- High contrast between bone, muscles and orbital fat produces excellent visualisation of orbital structures
- Quick, readily available
- High spatial resolution: excellent anatomy
- Excellent for bone and calcification
- Less patient cooperation needed
- Multiplanar capability in modern scanners

But:

- Uses ionising radiation

Tramtrack calcification

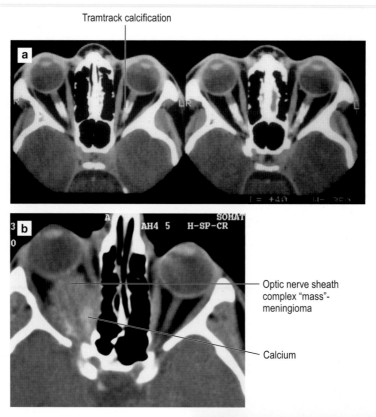

Optic nerve sheath
complex "mass"-
meningioma

Calcium

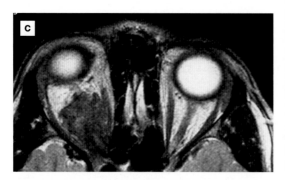

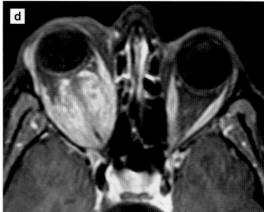

Fig. 14.6 (a) Axial-enhanced computed tomography (CT) scan showing typical tramtrack calcification of the optic nerve sheath complex in a patient with bilateral optic nerve meningioma. **(b)** Axial CT of young female with gradual proptosis showing faintly calcified mass involving optic nerve sheath complex.

A meningioma was diagnosed. **(c)** Axial T2w and **(d)** axial T1w post-contrast magnetic resonance scans of the same patient, delineating the optic nerve sheath meningioma. Calcification is not seen but the extent of the lesion (confined to the extracranial optic nerve) is better demonstrated than on CT.

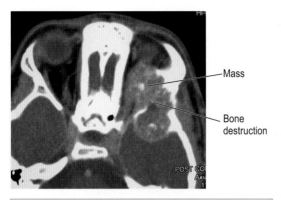

Fig. 14.7 Axial computed tomography image showing an aggressive soft-tissue mass in the left orbit in a young patient with rapidly progressive proptosis. The mass extends through the lateral orbital wall, which is eroded and destroyed, into the infratemporal fossa. Diagnosis: sarcoma.

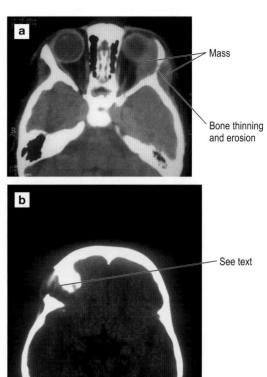

Contrast is essential. Evaluation of the paranasal sinuses to identify the possible source of infection and provide anatomical detail for the ear, nose and throat surgeons if surgery is necessary is possible within the same investigation (Fig. 14.9). It is the investigation of choice for the evaluation of orbital bony trauma (Fig. 14.10) and in the assessment of foreign bodies within the orbit.

Advantages and disadvantages

Irradiation of orbital structures is a potential disadvantage, although the radiation dose to the lens is low. Other limitations are artefact from dental amalgam and relatively low sensitivity for detecting intracranial extension of disease. Detail of the globe and optic nerve may be less good than that provided by MR scanning (Fig. 14.11).

Fig. 14.8 (a) A young child with proptosis. Axial computed tomography image shows a soft-tissue mass in the upper outer quadrant of the left orbit, with thinning and erosion of bone. An aggressive lesion is likely. **(b)** Axial image through brain/skull vault of the same child shows further soft-tissue lesions in the occipital region and right temporal fossa. Multiple lesions are likely in metastases and in histiocytosis, which was the diagnosis here. It is always important to look for other lesions.

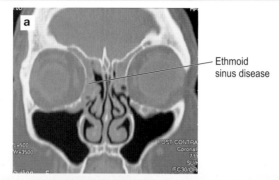

Ethmoid
sinus disease

Preseptal
swelling

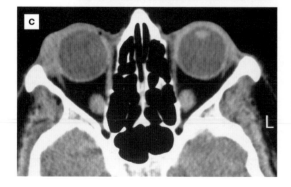

Abscess

Fig. 14.9 (a) Coronal computed tomography (CT) image showing inflammatory disease in ethmoid air cells and demonstrating sinus anatomy prior to ear, nose and throat endoscopic surgery and drainage. **(b)** Extensive orbital infection in an immunocompromised patient with diffuse soft-tissue swelling and disease extending through all spaces, with abscess cavity in the upper outer quadrant. **(c)** Axial CT showing preseptal soft-tissue swelling with no orbital involvement.

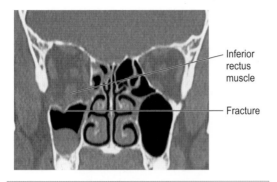

Inferior rectus muscle

Fracture

Fig. 14.10 Coronal computed tomography reformat showing a fracture of the orbital floor with downward displacement of the inferior rectus; fluid in the maxillary antrum.

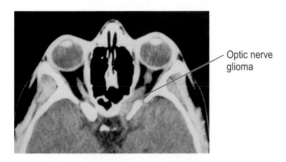

Optic nerve glioma

Fig. 14.11 Computed tomography showing optic nerve glioma extending through a widened optic foramen into the intracranial compartment.

ORBITAL MAGNETIC RESONANCE IMAGING

Introduction to magnetic resonance imaging

In MR scanning the patient is placed within a magnetic field and a radiofrequency coil is used to transmit a radio signal to the body part being imaged. This radiofrequency pulse causes a change in the steady-state proton magnetisation of the tissue and results in a transient small radio signal which is detected by the receiver coil in the magnet. That radio signal undergoes spatial encoding and is subsequently converted into an image by a computer using complex mathematical formulae.

The signal on MR depends on the proton density. Proton density is the concentration of protons in the tissue in the form of water and macromolecules such as fat and protein. The T1 (longitudinal) and T2 (transverse) relaxation times define the way that the excited protons revert to their original state following the radiofrequency pulse.

The most common imaging sequences are T1- and T2-weighted (w) sequences. Signal intensities relate to specific tissue characteristics.

In general, T2w sequences show fluid as a high or hyperintense signal and this will appear bright or 'white' on the images. T2w sequences are sensitive to changes in water content, and thus pathology, but are not very specific. T1w sequences show fluid as a low or hypointense signal, thus it appears dark or black on the images. T1w sequences are excellent at demonstrating anatomical detail and can also be used after administration of intravenous contrast to show enhancement of structures and pathology.

By utilising different radiofrequency pulses it is possible to produce images that are T1- or T2-weighted. Modifications to these pulses can be used to alter the signal return of certain tissues, e.g. fat to change the final image. Fat suppression techniques where the normal bright signal returned from fat is suppressed are useful in orbital imaging to allow improved visualisation of the other orbital structures and disease processes (Fig. 14.12). Fat suppression removes the high signal fat component from the image. This can be achieved in several ways, including short T1 inversion recovery (STIR) and spectral presaturation with inversion recovery (SPIR).

On T2w scans the fluid within the globe (vitreous) is typically high signal or 'white', the lens appears dark, the fat is bright but less so than fluid and the muscles are dark. On T1w scans the vitreous appears dark, the orbital fat is very bright and the muscles are dark (see Fig. 14.21).

Technique

Orbital MR can be obtained on any diagnostic field-strength magnet (0.2–3.0 T) but higher field magnets are preferred as the image acquisition time is shorter and resolution better. The standard head coil (or newer multichannel coils) is used routinely, with surface coils added if needed.

Images should be obtained in axial, coronal and sagittal planes using thin sections (2–4 mm) acquired on a small field of view with a high-resolution matrix.

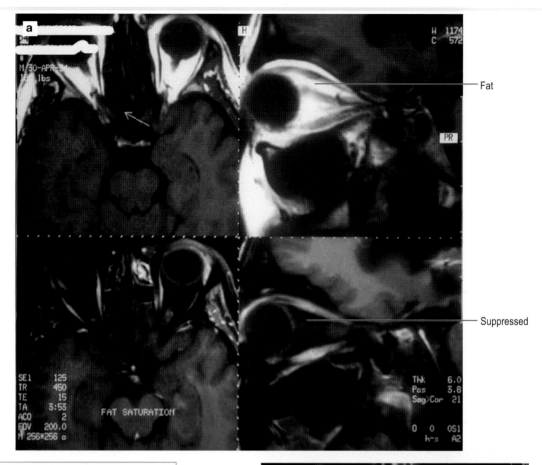

Fat

Suppressed

Fig. 14.12 (a) Demonstration of a fat suppression technique on axial and sagittal magnetic resonance images resulting in better anatomical detail in the lower pictures. (b) The fat suppression technique, now showing the lesion of the right optic nerve with greater clarity in the lower pictures.

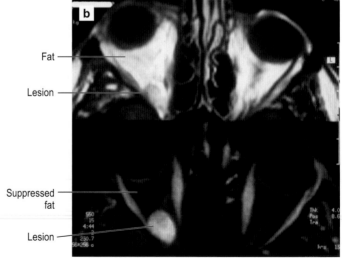

Fat

Lesion

Suppressed fat

Lesion

Axial images should be aligned along the course of the optic nerve, i.e. −10° to the orbitomeatal base line.

Any number of pulse sequences can be used and examinations are often directed by the radiologist's preference and experience. T1w and T2w techniques with and without fat suppression are generally recommended.

The use of fat suppression or STIR techniques may reveal pathology that might be missed if the bright orbital fat signal is not suppressed. Most pathological lesions have a long T1 and T2w relaxation time and thus will appear 'bright or of increased signal intensity' against the dark suppressed orbital fat (Figs 14.12 and 14.13).

Contrast agents are generally used to fully evaluate orbital masses and optic nerve/nerve sheath lesions (Fig. 14.14).

Surface coils can be used to provide higher resolution and detail, particularly of the globe. Images obtained with a surface coil provide better spatial resolution but, because of signal drop-out, apical lesions and intracranial extension may not be as well shown. If surface coils are used the ideal diameter is between 6 and 12 cm to allow both eyes to be imaged; the head should be tilted at 45° to the unaffected eye.

Advantages and disadvantages

The advent of stronger gradients (these determine the magnetic field), faster pulse sequences and surface coils have overcome the earlier limitations of MR in orbital imaging – namely the time taken to obtain the information. MR provides optimal soft-tissue contrast and allows excellent visualisation of the globe, optic nerve and any intracranial extension of disease (Box 14.6). Further advantages include the lack of radiation. There are currently no known biological side-effects to MR. The ease of multiplanar imaging (that is, the ability to view or obtain images in any plane without moving the patient, as in multiplanar CT) and the ability to detect abnormal flow in vessels are additional advantages. The use of specific pulse sequences such as fat suppression and inversion recovery techniques enable abnormalities to be demonstrated with great clarity. The use of a paramagnetic contrast agent may be helpful, particularly in assessing the extension of disease into adjacent structures.

The limitations of MR relate, as with CT, to patient movement and cooperation – most sequences still take several minutes to acquire. This may require the use of anaesthesia in children. Motion artefact significantly degrades image quality. Patients should close their eyes during the examination and keep

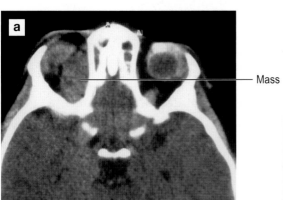

Mass

Fig. 14.13 (a) Computed tomography in a child with proptosis shows an ill-defined homogeneous mass in the upper orbit. The nature of the lesion is unclear. **(b)** Magnetic resonance using T1w fat-suppressed technique shows the mass to be hyperintense or bright – a haemorrhage. There was a history of trauma and the haematoma subsequently resolved.

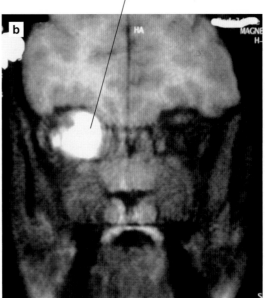

Bright mass due to blood products

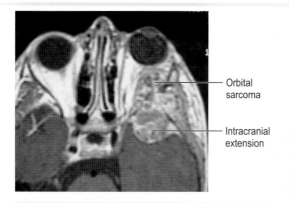

Orbital sarcoma

Intracranial extension

Fig. 14.14 Contrast-enhanced axial T1w magnetic resonance scan in a child with sarcoma, showing extension into the intracranial cavity.

Artefact

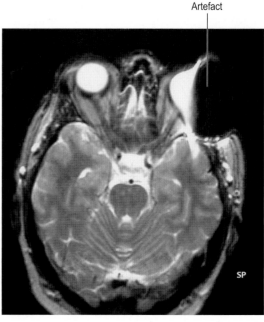

SP

Fig. 14.15 Axial T2w magnetic resonance scan showing susceptibility artefact resulting from a metallic foreign body in the soft tissues over the face. This was not disclosed by the patient.

Box 14.6

Advantages of magnetic resonance

- No radiation
- Multiplanar imaging
- Better ocular and soft-tissue detail; ideal for evaluating optic nerve and extraocular disease, e.g. melanoma extension
- Can see abnormal flow in blood vessels
- Visualisation of anterior optic pathway

But:

- Longer exam times; movement and patient cooperation
- Must be aware of safety issues and contraindications

the eyes still. Eye make-up, including conventional mascara and tattooed eyeliner, can lead to artefacts with distortion of contours. MR is absolutely contra-indicated in patients with possible intraocular foreign body as ferromagnetic foreign bodies are induced to move during the scan and could cause severe injury and death (Fig. 14.15). Additional artefacts may be caused by problems with the scanning process itself, such as inhomogeneous fat suppression. It is important to be aware of the possible appearances caused by such artefacts.

In the axial plane there is often volume averaging of the optic nerve sheath complex and thus correlation with coronal images is essential if lesions are not to be missed.

Contrast studies of the orbit

1. Carotid angiography
2. Orbital phlebography

These have largely been replaced by modern cross-sectional imaging, although carotid angiography is still used in cases of caroticocavernous dural fistula. Intracranial aneurysms may present with orbital pain or proptosis and thus the diagnosis of a carotico-ophthalmic artery aneurysm or cavernous sinus aneurysm may be made by angiography initially, although diagnostic angiography is now often replaced by CT angiography (CTA).

For full evaluation of a dural fistula, selective injection of both internal and external carotid

Superior ophthalmic vein

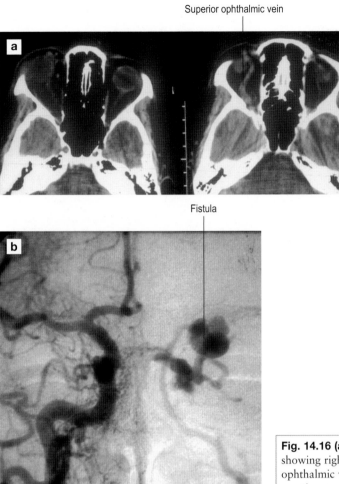

Fistula

Fig. 14.16 (a) Axial computed tomography scan showing right proptosis and an enlarged superior ophthalmic vein, consistent with a caroticocavernous fistula. **(b)** Carotid angiogram confirming the fistula.

arteries and the vertebral arteries may be required (Fig. 14.16).

Interpretation of orbital imaging

Imaging must be supplementary to clinical history and examination. It should not be interpreted in isolation. The best-quality study possible should be obtained. This will be determined by the availability of scanners and the condition of the patient. It is better to obtain a good-quality CT study than a suboptimal MR examination. The techniques are complementary and both may be necessary. MRI potentially has advantages in allowing some physiological assessment to be made, e.g. in thyroid eye disease where 'activity' may be evaluated depending on the signal return from the muscles on T2w and STIR sequences (Figs 14.17 and 14.18).

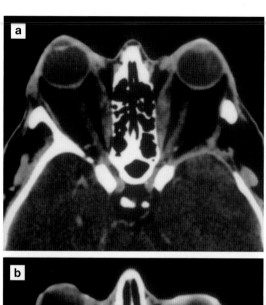

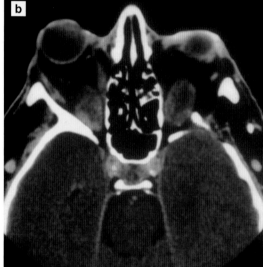

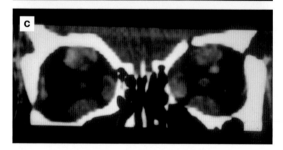

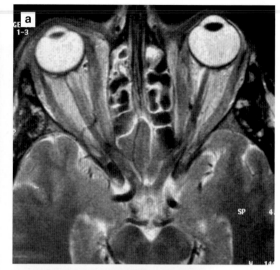

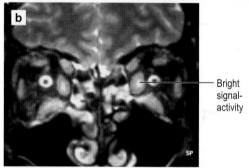

Bright signal-activity

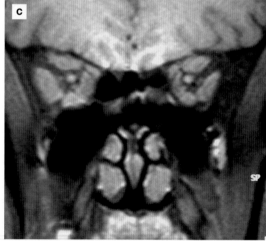

Fig. 14.17 (a) Axial computed tomography showing bilateral proptosis and enlarged extraocular muscles in thyroid eye disease. Note good bony detail at optic foramen. **(b)** From the same patient, showing the inferior recti. **(c)** Coronal reformat showing bilateral muscle enlargement.

Fig. 14.18 (a) Axial T2w; **(b)** coronal T2w; **(c)** T1w fat-suppressed magnetic resonance scans in a patient with acute thyroid eye disease. There is bilateral proptosis, streaky orbital fat and enlarged muscles. The medial recti contain hyperintense (bright) signal suggestive of acute/active disease.

RADIOLOGY OF THE LACRIMAL SYSTEM

Introduction

The lacrimal gland lies in the superior lateral quadrant of the bony orbit within the lacrimal fossa of the zygomatic process of the frontal bone. It comprises two lobes – upper orbital and lower palpebral – connected by an isthmus. The gland secretes lacrimal fluid, which passes over the globe and drains medially. The fluid enters the lacrimal puncta and drains through the inferior and superior canaliculus into the common canaliculus and thus into the lacrimal sac, which lies medially in the orbit. Fluid leaves the sac and drains via the nasolacrimal duct into the nasal cavity, medial to the inferior nasal turbinate (Box 14.7).

Several imaging modalities can be used to supplement clinical evaluation and syringing (see Ch. 8; Boxes 14.8 and 14.9).

Box 14.7

Common clinical features and presentations of lacrimal disease

- Mass lesion of the lacrimal gland or sac
- Pain/inflammatory changes such as dacryocystitis
- Epiphora
- Dry eyes may be associated with systemic conditions such as Sjögren's syndrome and sarcoidosis

---

Box 14.8

The role of imaging

- To confirm the presence of a lesion
- To define a lesion's anatomical site, thus helping to establish the diagnosis or provide a differential diagnosis
- To define precise anatomical relationships, which allows for surgical planning
- May guide to other imaging techniques

Box 14.9

Imaging techniques

- Plain radiographs
- Computed tomography (CT)
- Magnetic resonance (MR)
- Contrast studies: dacryocystography and dacryoscintography

Plain radiographs

Plain radiographs are rarely used these days as cross-sectional imaging is increasingly preferred.

Plain films may reveal evidence of bone changes involving the lacrimal fossa.

Computed tomography

The lacrimal gland can be demonstrated on high-quality orbital CT. It is important to look for associated bony changes in cases of lacrimal gland disease, e.g. sclerosis or destruction of adjacent bone in cases of pseudotumour (Fig. 14.19) or malignant tumour. Lacrimal gland enlargement can be seen on the scan (Fig. 14.20). The normal gland is somewhat almond-shaped in both axial and coronal views, located between the upper outer aspect of the globe

Sclerosis

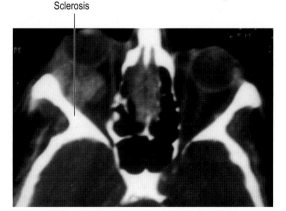

Fig. 14.19 Axial computed tomography demonstrating a pseudotumour. Note the bony sclerosis.

183

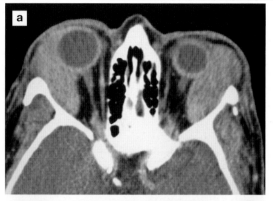

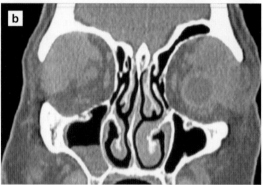

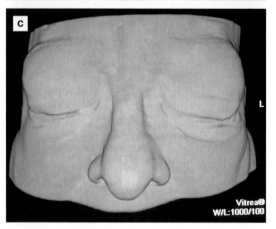

Fig. 14.20 (a) Axial computed tomography showing bilateral symmetrical lacrimal gland enlargement in a patient with sarcoid. **(b)** Coronal reformat of the same patient. **(c)** Three-dimensional soft-tissue display of the patient.

and the lateral orbital wall. It is isodense to extra-ocular muscles. It exhibits contrast enhancement on both CT and MRI. Calcification is well demonstrated on CT and occurs in conditions such as amyloid.

The nasolacrimal ducts are appreciated on inferior sections through the orbit, recognised as rounded structures with cortical margins medial to the anterior orbit. CT also allows evaluation of the adjacent paranasal sinuses and nasal cavity.

Magnetic resonance imaging

The imaging sequences detailed in the previous section apply to lacrimal gland imaging. Surface coils give good detail but may not demonstrate extension of disease. On T1 weighting the gland is of higher signal intensity than the surrounding muscles; on T2 weighting it is barely discernible from fat and muscles. It is better appreciated on fat-suppressed images and best shown in the coronal plane as a low-signal structure lying between the superior and lateral rectus muscle (Fig. 14.21).

The nasolacrimal duct is not well shown on MRI. Bone detail is poor on MRI but images may include detail of other glandular structures such as salivary glands and this may be helpful in evaluating patients with systemic disease such as sarcoid.

Dacryocystography (DCG)

This is used to investigate tear drainage in epiphora. Abnormalities may be functional as a result of poor lacrimal pump function, or anatomical, due to obstruction at any point in the drainage pathway (see Ch. 8).

DCG techniques are largely used to evaluate anatomical disease, although some functional information can be provided, particularly by topical CT DCG.

Contrast dacryocystography

This technique was described by Ewing in 1909 using bismuth subnitrate as a contrast medium (Lloyd, 1984). It has been refined over the past century and remains a useful diagnostic tool today. In essence non-ionic contrast medium is instilled into the inferior canaliculus via a suitable catheter. Contrast is injected gently and a digital subtraction radiographic technique allows the nasolacrimal duct system to be outlined (Fig. 14.22). It is advisable to

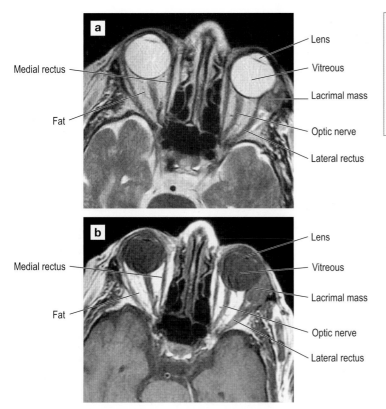

Medial rectus

Fat

Lens

Vitreous

Lacrimal mass

Optic nerve

Lateral rectus

Medial rectus

Fat

Lens

Vitreous

Lacrimal mass

Optic nerve

Lateral rectus

Fig. 14.21 (a) Axial T2w magnetic resonance scan demonstrating a left lacrimal gland lesion, subsequently confirmed as a metastasis. Note also normal anatomy and signal characteristics. **(b)** Axial T1w scan of the same patient.

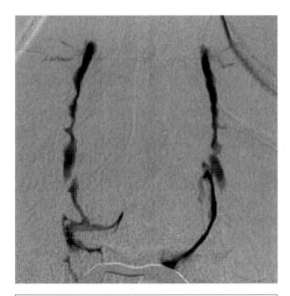

Fig. 14.22 Bilateral dacrycystography demonstrating patency on both sides.

perform bilateral simultaneous DCGs as this allows comparison with the 'normal' side. Topical local anaesthetic drops may be used if the patient cannot tolerate the procedure without. It is advisable to use a standardised imaging technique and include one 'native' or unsubtracted image to demonstrate any relevant bony detail (Fig. 14.23).

Blocks in the inferior and superior canaliculi are recognised when contrast is seen to regurgitate into the conjunctival sac with no filling or outlining of the canaliculus. A common canalicular block is characterised by demonstrating contrast in both inferior and superior canaliculi during injection of dye into the inferior canaliculus. A lacrimal sac blockage is typified by outlining both canaliculi and the common canaliculus with no drainage inferiorly into the nasolacrimal duct. The commonest site of obstruction is at the neck of the lacrimal sac; this may lead to a dilated sac with mucocoele formation. Blocks in the nasolacrimal duct prevent contrast from entering the nasal cavity and may lead to dilation of the portion of duct proximal to the obstruction. The main sites

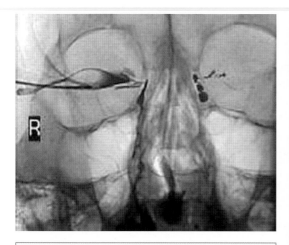

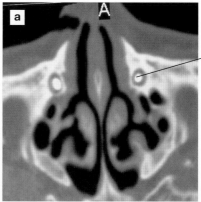

Contrast in nasolacrimal duct

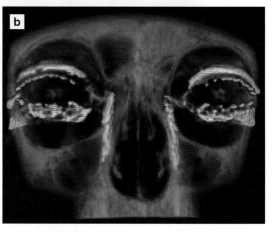

Fig. 14.23 Dacrycystography demonstrating a normal right side but dilated and beaded left lacrimal sac with obstruction. The bone is visible in this 'native' or unsubtracted image.

for blocks or stenosis are at the entrance to the bony canal and at the lower ostium on the nasal wall (Fig. 14.23).

Advantages and disadvantages
The technique requires catheterisation of the canaliculus and is thus invasive.

A dose of ionising radiation is delivered to the lens. The technique provides good anatomical information but limited functional or physiological data.

Computed tomography dacryocystography

CT dacryocystography is a relatively new technique made possible by the advent of multislice helical scanners. Non-ionic contrast medium is dropped on to the conjunctiva and a helical data set is then acquired several minutes later. The axial data allow visualisation of the lacrimal apparatus and give anatomical and functional information. Coronal and sagittal reformats and three-dimensional displays can be provided. The technique is non-invasive and well tolerated by patients. It can be used successfully in the paediatric population without the need for general anaesthesia. The technique does require excellent post-processing software.

Fig. 14.24 (a) Axial data set image of computed tomography dacryocystography showing contrast in both nasolacrimal ducts. **(b)** Post-processed three-dimensional surface shaded display showing patent nasolacrimal duct systems bilaterally.

Advantages and disadvantages
CT dacryocystography requires ionising radiation. Anatomical detail is good but soft-tissue information and functional data less so (Fig. 14.24).

Magnetic resonance dacryocystography

The technique of using either instilled or topically administered MR contrast media into the lacrimal system followed by MRI using fat-suppressed T1-weighted scans has recently been described.

Advantages and disadvantages
The results show good anatomical detail with excellent visualisation of soft tissues. Limited bone

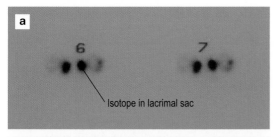

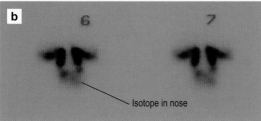

Fig. 14.25 Dacryoscintogram. The early **(a)** and late **(b)** pictures show the flow of isotope through the system. In the late picture isotope is in the nose.

detail is provided but ionising radiation is avoided. It would appear to be a technique that may help with the investigation of patients with epiphora.

Dacryoscintigraphy (DSG)

This is a non-invasive method of assessing patency of the lacrimal system. It provides functional rather than anatomical information.

Images are obtained using a suitable gamma camera. A drop of appropriate isotope solution (99m-technetium pertechnate diluted in sterile saline to a concentration of 10 mCi/ml) is placed in the lateral conjunctival sac using an automatic micropipette. Dynamic acquisition of the images starts immediately; patients are instructed to blink every 5 s. The passage of radioactivity is followed on a video display unit. The isotope enters the canaliculi and progresses along the nasolacrimal drainage system with activity increasing in the lacrimal sac and decreasing in the canaliculi. The examination is terminated when the radiopharmaceutical reaches the nasal cavity. Both eyes tend to be examined together to allow comparison (Fig. 14.25).

Advantages and disadvantages

The technique is non-invasive and sensitive but provides limited anatomical detail. The ease of

performance and relative non-invasive nature encourage routine bilateral studies. Its advantage over dacryocystography is that it produces physiologic information. There is no pressure required to inject the contrast. This may overcome any functional occlusion of the nasolacrimal drainage system in a DCG study. Thus a normal DCG in a patient with epiphora does not provide information related to functional stenosis or obstruction. There is thus an argument for DSG being the first investigation to perform; if it is normal, further investigation with a DCG is unnecessary.

RADIOLOGY OF THE VISUAL PATHWAYS

Introduction

The retrobulbar visual pathway extends from the point where the optic nerve leaves the eye from the posterior surface of the globe to the primary visual cortex which lies within the medial aspects of both occipital lobes. The different parts of this pathway can be affected by a variety of conditions. Depending on their location they tend to give rise to characteristic clusters of clinical symptoms and signs. These should enable the pathologic condition to be localised along the visual pathway with a high degree of certainty. Imaging techniques can thus be tailored appropriately to display the expected condition optimally, provided the referring clinician provides the appropriate information.

CT and MRI have become the mainstays of imaging the visual pathways. CT is excellent in demonstrating the extracranial portion of the optic nerves but MRI is the investigation of choice.

Imaging techniques

The indication and modality for imaging the optic pathways are influenced by clinical findings and symptoms. Visual loss is a characteristic symptom and it is important to indicate the rapidity of onset of visual loss (which suggests the sort of pathology responsible) and the specific visual field deficit (which suggests the location of the process within the visual pathway). For instance, a sudden onset of monocular blindness associated with pain on moving the eyes is suggestive of optic neuritis. A gradually progressive monocular blindness, possibly with proptosis, is more suggestive of a mass lesion within the optic nerve sheath. The identification of papilloedema or optic atrophy may indicate tumour and mass effect or an inflammatory process. If the abnormal findings are unilateral it is likely to be an optic nerve process. If bilateral, then an intracranial cause is more likely.

Bitemporal hemianopia should focus interest on the optic chiasm, and pituitary disease. A homonymous hemianopia suggests disease involving the retrochiasmatic portion of the visual pathway. A sudden onset suggests a vascular cause; a gradual onset is more in keeping with a mass lesion. If the deficit is incomplete and congruent the lesion is more likely to lie in the calcarine cortex. An incomplete and incongruous deficit is likely to involve the optic tracts or lie within the temporal lobe involving Meyer's loop (superior quadrantanopia) or in the parietal lobe, causing an inferior quadrantanopia.

CT and MRI can both be used to evaluate the visual pathways.

Computed tomography

Unenhanced and enhanced studies through the orbits and cranial cavity should be obtained when evaluating a patient with visual pathway symptoms. The unenhanced study is useful to look for a foreign body, haematoma and infarction. Contrast administration is recommended if a mass lesion or abnormal vasculature is identified on the unenhanced scan. If the patient has presented with optic chiasm symptoms and signs, then high-resolution images through this region should be obtained. With the advent of helical CT an examination can be obtained following intravenous contrast administration in the axial plane with subsequent coronal and sagittal reformatting through this area.

In most cases, however, evaluation of the visual pathways will be performed with MRI unless the patient has contraindications to that procedure. CT scans remain useful in that subgroup of the population who present with an acute onset of hemianopia where a vascular cause or stroke is strongly suspected.

Magnetic resonance imaging

This is the modality of choice for visualisation of the visual pathways. Contraindications due to a retained foreign body or ferromagnetic implants must be taken into consideration. In cases of ocular trauma, as discussed in the previous section, MRI is contraindicated.

MRI of the optic pathways will generally include a standard brain examination consisting of images acquired in at least two planes and using at least two different sequences. In many institutions more planes and sequences are used. In addition to the standard brain protocol which will demonstrate most lesions, tailored imaging to the part of the visual pathway that is clinically of interest should be performed.

It is not possible in this chapter to discuss all the imaging modalities and techniques and all the pathologies that can affect the visual pathways. The more common clinical presentations are addressed and illustrated.

Patient presenting with bilateral papilloedema

An intracranial cause giving rise to raised intracranial pressure is most likely. Brain imaging using either CT or MR examination in the first instance is appropriate. Pathologies such as mass lesions, hydrocephalus (Fig. 14.26) or venous sinus thrombosis are the most important conditions to exclude. If the cranial examination reveals no evidence of or cause for raised intracranial pressure then conditions such as benign intracranial hypertension or other causes of swollen discs should be excluded.

Patient presenting with bitemporal hemianopia

This is most likely caused by a disease process involving the optic chiasm. The commonest cause will be a pituitary mass lesion or tumour, although other pathologies do exist in this area. The imaging modality of choice will be MRI. Tailored imaging should include high-resolution sagittal and coronal T1-weighted sequences to demonstrate the optic chiasm and pituitary region. The use of intravenous contrast may be considered if an inflammatory process such as sarcoidosis is suspected. The use of contrast administration is not routine in the evaluation of macroadenomas of the pituitary; in some cases it is useful in the evaluation of microadenomas.

The examination should demonstrate the origin, size and extent of any pituitary-based mass lesion. It should demonstrate the relationship of the lesion to the intracranial portions of the optic nerve, to the optic chiasm and to the cavernous sinus (Figs 14.27 and 14.28).

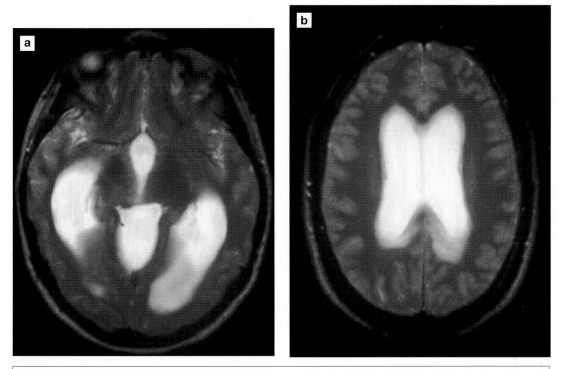

Fig. 14.26 (a) Axial T2w magnetic resonance (MR) scan showing acute hydrocephalus with dilated temporal horns and third ventricle. **(b)** Axial T2w MR scan showing dilated lateral ventricles and high signal in the deep white matter due to fluid transudation in acute hydrocephalus.

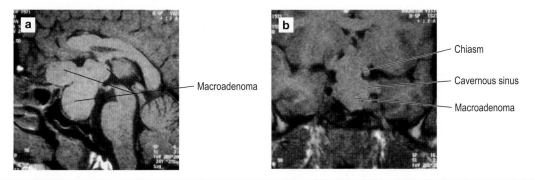

Fig. 14.27 (a) Sagittal T1w magnetic resonance scan demonstrating a pituitary macroadenoma. Note expanded fossa. **(b)** Coronal T1w scan showing a pituitary macroadenoma with distortion and compression of the optic chiasm, and extension into the left side of the cavernous sinus.

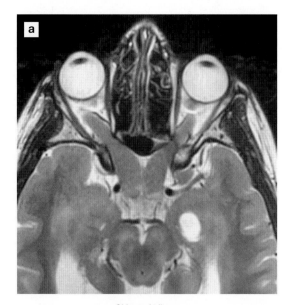

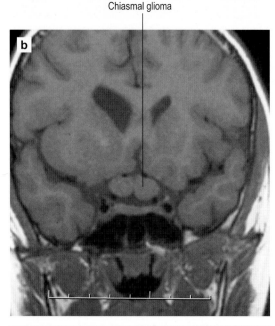

Chiasmal glioma

Fig. 14.28 (a) Axial T2w magnetic resonance (MR) scan showing bilateral optic nerve and optic chiasm glioma in a patient with neurofibromatosis type 1. **(b)** Coronal T1w MR scan showing the optic chiasm glioma.

Patient presenting with homonymous hemianopia

This suggests a disease process involving the retro-chiasmatic portion of the visual pathway. A sudden onset is most likely due to a vascular lesion such as a haemorrhage or stroke. An unenhanced CT brain scan is adequate for diagnosis (Fig. 14.29). A gradual onset is more in keeping with either a mass lesion or underlying vascular malformation and in this case contrast-enhanced CT or MRI is the preferred imaging modality. The precise localisation of the lesion is aided if the radiologist is given all the clinical information. Lesions of the calcarine cortex within the occipital lobe tend to give incomplete congruent deficits. These are best demonstrated on axial and coronal sequences on MR scanning (Fig. 14.30). The use of proton density or fluid attenuated inversion recovery (FLAIR) sequences is

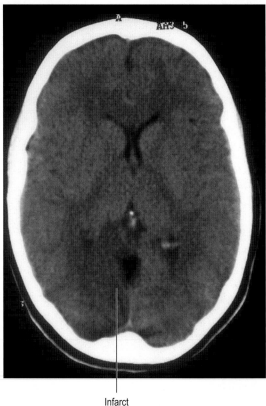

Infarct

Fig. 14.29 Axial computed tomography scan showing an area of infarction in right occipital lobe.

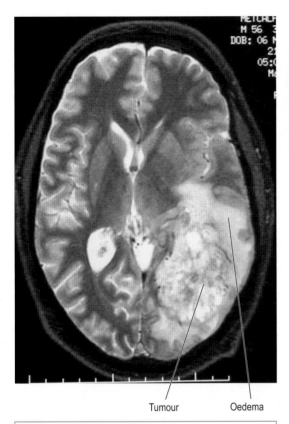

Tumour   Oedema

Fig. 14.30 Axial T2w magnetic resonance scan showing a malignant intrinsic brain tumour in the left occipital and posterior temporal lobes, with associated tumour oedema.

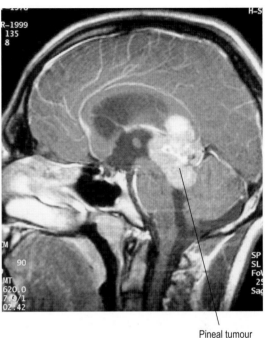

Pineal tumour

Fig. 14.31 Sagittal T1w post-contrast magnetic resonance scan demonstrating enhancing pineal-based tumour (germinoma). The patient presented with Parinaud's syndrome.

helpful as the high signal from an acute infarct is sometimes slightly difficult to appreciate adjacent to the high signal of the overlying cerebrospinal fluid (CSF) within the subarachnoid space (see Fig. 14.35 below). These techniques 'suppress' the bright CSF signal, allowing pathology to be demonstrated more easily. Newer techniques include the use of diffusion-weighted imaging (DWI) which effectively images the movement or diffusion of water molecules in tissues and allows ischaemic changes to be seen within minutes of occurrence.

Patients presenting with eye movement disorders

The final neural pathway for the control of eye movements occurs through cranial nerves 3, 4 and 6.

If a patient presents with an eye movement disorder, imaging should be tailored to demonstrate these structures from their origin in the brainstem nuclei through the intracisternal portions into the cavernous sinus and the orbital apex (Fig. 14.31). Clinical localisation of a nerve palsy is essential and it is also important to inform the radiologist of any accompanying neurological signs. Recognising associated signs and symptoms will aid in a search for the intracranial pathology. For example, a third-nerve palsy with a contralateral hemiparesis would indicate a brainstem lesion. Involvement of multiple cranial nerves would suggest a process in the subarachnoid space and should encourage the radiologist to consider the use of contrast. Ipsilateral third-, fourth- and sixth-nerve palsies will indicate a cavernous sinus process. Associated involvement of the fifth cranial nerve is relevant in localisation of a disease process.

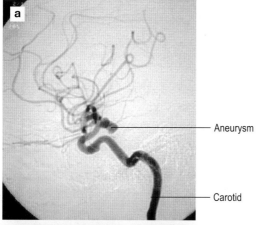

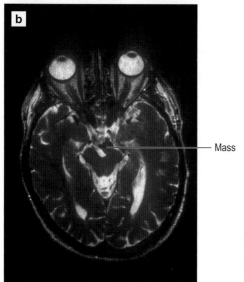

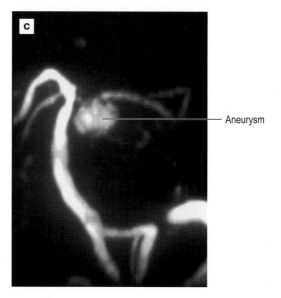

Fig. 14.32 (a) Carotid angiogram demonstrating a posterior communicating artery aneurysm. The patient presented with a painful third-nerve palsy. **(b)** Axial T2w magnetic resonance scan showing 'mass' with flow void in left interpeduncular cistern. **(c)** Magnetic resonance angiography examination confirms an aneurysm of the superior cerebellar artery.

Aneurysm

Carotid

Mass

Aneurysm

In all motility disorders it is important to remember that there are conditions that can mimic lesions of the ocular motor nerves such as thyroid eye disease, myasthenia gravis and drug intoxication.

Third-nerve palsy

The third-nerve nuclear complex is located in the midbrain at the level of the superior colliculus. Fibres from the nucleus coalesce into a fascicle which crosses the red nucleus and the cerebral peduncle before exiting the brainstem. It exits the brainstem between the posterior cerebral and superior cerebellar arteries. It passes through the interpeduncular fossa into the superior portion of the cavernous sinus. It separates into a superior and inferior division in the anterior aspect of the sinus. Radiological evaluation of third-nerve palsy should include tailored imaging of the brainstem, the interpeduncular fossa or cistern and the cavernous sinus.

A pupil involving third nerve palsy may be caused by an aneurysm arising from the posterior communicating artery. Aneurysms may be diagnosed on an MR scan (Fig. 14.32b). Magnetic resonance can also be used to outline blood vessels: the technique is referred to as magnetic resonance angiography (MRA). This can also be used to detect aneurysms (Fig. 14.32c). Conventional angiography using standard radiographic techniques to image

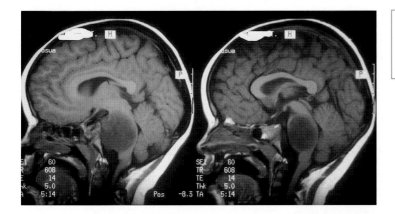

Fig. 14.33 Sagittal T1w magnetic resonance scan showing typical appearance of a brainstem glioma.

blood vessels after the introduction of contrast medium into an artery remains a definitive way to demonstrate an aneurysm, however (Fig. 14.32a).

Microvascular disease is the commonest cause of a pupil-sparing third-nerve palsy and careful evaluation of the brainstem for signal alteration should be considered.

Fourth-nerve palsy

This is the least common of the ocular motor palsies. The fourth-nerve nucleus is located in the midbrain at the level of the inferior colliculus. This cranial nerve exits the brainstem posteriorly and is susceptible to damage in head trauma. It may also be affected in hydrocephalus by dilatation of the aqueduct or compression of the dorsal midbrain.

Sixth-nerve palsy

The sixth-nerve nuclei lie in the dorsomedial aspect of the pons near the pontine reticular formation. Along the floor of the fourth ventricle, the seventh nerve winds around the sixth nerve to form the facial colliculus. The sixth-nerve nucleus also contains interneurones to form the medial longitudinal fasciculus. The nerve passes ventrally from its nucleus to cross the corticospinal tracts and exit the brainstem. From here it passes through the subarachnoid space, bending sharply forward across the apex of the petrous bone lying beneath the petroclinoid ligament with the canal of Dorelo. It enters the cavernous sinus where it lies lateral to the carotid artery.

The cause of sixth-nerve palsy is very age-dependent. In children sixth-nerve palsies may occur after viral infections or as a result of an intracranial

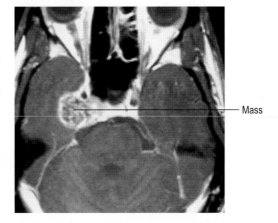

Mass

Fig. 14.34 Axial T1w post-contrast magnetic resonance scan showing enhancing mass related to the right cavernous sinus (chondrosarcoma).

or brainstem tumour (Fig. 14.33). In young adults causes include demyelination, trauma and tumour. In patients over the age of 40 it is usually vascular in origin due to microvascular occlusion and imaging is generally not very helpful.

Isolated sixth-nerve palsies are a difficult problem and imaging must include careful evaluation of the skull base and cavernous sinus region (Fig. 14.34).

Internuclear ophthalmoplegia

The medial longitudinal fasciculus (MLF) connects the nuclei of the third, fourth, sixth and eighth cranial nerves. It lies dorsally near the midline throughout the brainstem. A lesion in the MLF causes an internuclear ophthalmoplegia. In a young

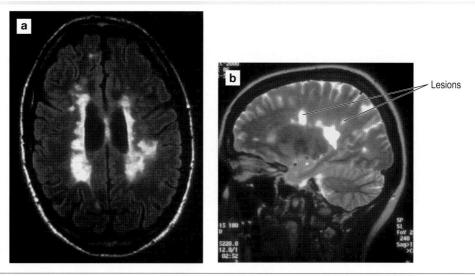

Lesions

Fig. 14.35 (a) Axial FLAIR sequence showing the typical hyperintense lesions of multiple sclerosis. This is a T2w study but the signal from cerebrospinal fluid has been suppressed such that it appears dark. **(b)** Sagittal T2w magnetic resonance scan showing typical lesions of multiple sclerosis in a periventricular location.

Fig. 14.36 Sagittal T1w magnetic resonance scan showing Chiari 1 malformation with the cerebellar tonsils lying through the foramen magnum. Associated hydromyelia (cavity in cord) is present.

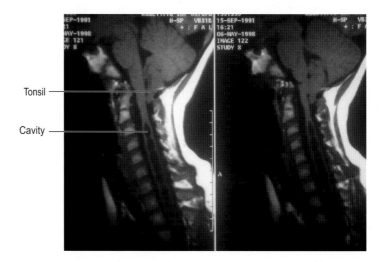

Tonsil

Cavity

person the most likely cause is a demyelinating disorder such as multiple sclerosis. In an elderly patient it is most likely as a result of brainstem infarction. Imaging should include tailored views of the brainstem and midline structures using both sagittal and coronal sequences with T1- and T2-weighted scans (Fig. 14.35).

Nystagmus

Many forms of nystagmus have excellent localising value and as such it is important to indicate to the radiologist as much detail as possible. For example, downbeat nystagmus is associated with lesions of the craniocervical junction. Gaze-evoked nystagmus is associated with vestibular or cerebellar lesions, and rebound nystagmus with lesions of the cerebellum. Imaging can thus be tailored appropriately to demonstrate the relevant areas of interest. In all patients with eye movement disorders it is important to evaluate the craniocervical junction and upper cervical cord carefully, and detailed views of the midbrain and midline structures should be obtained. This is best done by means of high-resolution MRI using sagittal T1- and T2-weighted sequences through the region of interest (Fig. 14.36).

Summary

Modern imaging techniques can provide precise and detailed information for the referring clinician faced with a patient who has symptoms and signs relating to the orbit and visual pathways. The modalities are complementary and in many cases local experience and preference will dictate what imaging technique is used. Close professional relationships between clinicians and radiologists will allow the best outcomes from imaging. A detailed clinical history and examination are vital to the radiologist to ensure that the best technique is used and that the appropriate area of interest is examined.

Further reading

Aviv R, Casselman J. Orbital imaging: part 1. Normal anatomy. Clin Radiol 2005; 60: 854–858.

Aviv R, Miszkiel K. Orbital imaging: part 2. Intraorbital pathology. Clin Radiol. 2005; 60: 288–307.

Forbes G. The orbit. Am Soc Neuroradiol Core Curriculum Course Neuroradiol 1994: 153–161.

Grainger RG, Allison DJ, Dixon AK. Grainger and Allison's diagnostic radiology, 4th edn. Edinburgh: Churchill Livingstone; 2001.

Hosten N, Bornfeld N. Imaging of the globe and orbit: a guide to differential diagnosis. Stuttgart: Thieme; 1998.

Kahaly GJ. Imaging in thyroid associated orbitopathy. Eur J Endocrinol 2001; 145: 107–118.

Lloyd G. The Orbit. In: DuBoulay GH, ed. A Textbook of Radiological Diagnosis. 5th edn. London: HK Lewis & Co; 1984: 288.

Manfre L, de Maria M, Todaro E et al. MR dacryocystography: comparison with DCG and CT DCG. Am J Neuroradiol 2000; 21: 1145–1150.

Mayer EJ, Fox DL, Herdman G et al. Signal intensity, clinical activity and cross sectional area on MRI scan in thyroid eye disease. Eur J Radiol 2005; 56: 20–24.

Osborn A, Hansberger HR (eds). Diagnostic imaging: head and neck. Salt Lake City: Amirsys; 2004.

Som PM, Curtin HD. Head and neck imaging, 4th edn. Philadelphia: Mosby; 2003.

- ■ Imaging is one useful diagnostic approach but must be used in conjunction with the clinical picture and history
- ■ It is important to use appropriate modalities of imaging. Discussion with the radiologist as to the most appropriate test can be helpful
- ■ A combination of computed tomography and magnetic resonance imaging may be necessary to define a pathology fully
- ■ Plain radiographs of the orbit are less commonly used now, except in some aspects of trauma and suspected radiopaque foreign bodies

Clinical visual electrophysiology

RICHARD SMITH and DAVID SCULFOR

Introduction

The first measurement of electrical activity in the visual system is attributed to DuBois-Reymond, who in 1849 discovered that excised fish eyes have a potential difference of about 6 mV between the cornea and posterior scleral surface. In the early years of the twentieth century, it was difficult to measure the small and rapid voltage changes in the eye in response to flashes of light, but even with the relatively crude galvanometers available at the time, Einthoven and Jolly, and later, Granit, described the electroretinogram (ERG) in considerable detail in animal eyes (Einthoven, 1908; Granit, 1947).

By the early 1940s, recording equipment had improved to the point where it was possible to measure the human ERG in the clinical setting. In 1934, Adrian and Matthews had recorded electrical responses from surface electrodes placed over the occipital cortex in a human subject. This and other ground-breaking scientific work formed the basis of a new branch of clinical science, allowing the human visual system to be probed in a way that was not previously possible.

Since the 1940s, technological advances such as solid-state electronics, microprocessors and light-emitting diodes (LEDs) have led to huge improvements in equipment for generating and recording electrophysiological responses, and have contributed to a greatly increased understanding of the workings of the visual system in health and disease.

Visual electrophysiology is now firmly established both as a branch of visual science and as a diagnostic support service to clinical ophthalmology.

Standards in visual electrophysiology

Until the 1980s, clinical visual electrophysiology services often relied on equipment that was 'home-made'. It was difficult to make valid comparisons of data from different laboratories because of wide variations in recording equipment and the way in which tests were performed. In 1989, the International Society for Clinical Electrophysiology of Vision (ISCEV) published the first internationally agreed standard for electroretinography. Standards for other common electrophysiological tests and for calibration of recording equipment have been published more recently.

It is now possible to buy very sophisticated and comprehensive electrophysiology testing systems 'off the peg' from a number of manufacturers, and many of these are designed to comply with ISCEV standards. This has helped to improve the availability of visual electrophysiological tests to ophthalmologists.

It is important to remember, however, that the visual electrophysiologist remains the most important component of the system. No matter how sophisticated the equipment, the process of recording electrophysiological responses requires special training and meticulous attention to detail. Factors such as placement of recording electrodes, ambient lighting levels, pupil size and extraneous electrical interference can have a major influence on responses. Recording equipment must be properly maintained and regularly calibrated. It is still necessary for each laboratory to maintain a database of normal values for each test, which must be updated if the equipment or testing protocols change. The old adage of 'garbage in, garbage out' applies as much to visual electrophysiology as to computing.

The relevance of visual electrophysiology to ophthalmology

When modern cars are serviced, the mechanic interrogates the engine management system by plugging in a diagnostic system connected to a lap-top computer. A variety of faults can be diagnosed and fixed from the data which emerge. There is a common misconception within ophthalmology that visual electrophysiological testing works similarly to a 'black box' into which a general request is made and from which a diagnosis emerges without any further intellectual engagement on the part of the requester.

Unfortunately, the human visual system is much more complex than a car engine and the instruments we use to measure its function are still far from perfect. There are some clinical situations where the results of electrophysiological tests provide the sole and definitive proof of a diagnosis, but they are not common. More usually, the tests provide one piece of a diagnostic jigsaw and the results must be interpreted in the context of the clinical history, examination findings and results of other tests.

The common uses of visual electrophysiology in the clinical setting include the following:

- to provide evidence to confirm or exclude a specific diagnosis
- to monitor the progress of a known condition
- to indicate the level in the visual system at which a problem lies, or the cell populations involved in the disease process
- to provide an approximate objective measurement of visual acuity
- to detect early disease or carrier status in relatives of an affected individual
- to provide an indication of the maturity of the visual system in infants
- to provide an indication of visual potential in an injured or diseased eye.

Before requesting any test, a clinician must be able to make an informed judgement as to whether the test is likely to be capable of answering the question being asked. Electrophysiological tests are non-invasive and very safe, but they tend to be time-consuming to perform and require a reasonable degree of cooperation on the patient's part. There is no point in requesting these tests if the results are unlikely to shed any light on the clinical question being asked, or if the answer can be obtained more easily by other means. It is important to remember, too, that these tests are sometimes used to diagnose, monitor or exclude potentially blinding conditions. From the patient's or parent's perspective, a lot may hang on the results and it is essential that the clinician is able to counsel the patient and family both accurately and sensitively.

The aim of the remainder of this chapter is to help the clinician to obtain the maximum possible benefit from a clinical visual electrophysiology service.

Obtaining informed consent for visual electrophysiological tests

In view of the fact that visual electrophysiological tests are non-invasive, in the UK it is generally regarded as sufficient to obtain verbal consent for testing from the patient (or parent, where the subject is a child under 16) unless general anaesthesia or sedation is being used, in which case formal written consent must be obtained. The person carrying out the test will be able to explain the procedure, but he or she will not necessarily be medically qualified and may not be able to answer detailed questions about the patient's clinical condition.

It is good practice, therefore, when a clinician requests electrophysiological tests, to explain to the patient:

- why the tests are being requested
- what the patient is likely to experience during testing
- how long the tests are likely to take
- that the results have to be analysed before a report can be issued.

The clinician who has observed electrophysiological testing at first hand will be well equipped to provide such an explanation.

Most subjects do not find visual electrophysiological testing distressing, and electrophysiologists are highly skilled at engaging the cooperation of even young children or patients with learning difficulties. The placement of skin electrodes can be mildly uncomfortable at first, though topical anaesthesia is normally used with corneal electrodes (Figs 15.1 and 15.2). Full-field electroretinography and electro-oculography (EOG) require pupil dilatation and a period of dark adaptation. Patients sometimes find bright flashes of light or the process of light adaptation slightly uncomfortable. Although electrophysiological tests avoid epileptogenic flash frequencies, a history of photogenic epilepsy is normally a contraindication to testing. It is safe to test patients with implanted electronic devices such as cardiac pacemakers or cochlear implants, though they are

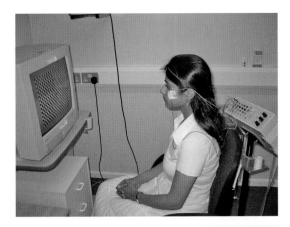

Fig. 15.1 Recording a pattern electroretinogram.

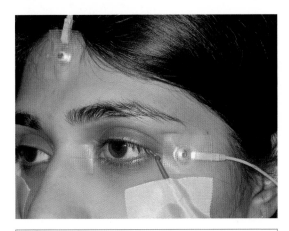

Fig. 15.2 Electroretinogram electrodes showing the reference electrode at the outer canthus, a ground electrode on the forehead, and the active corneal electrodes, in this case, DTL-fibre type.

strong sources of electrical interference which can seriously degrade the recordings. The pattern ERG and pattern cortical evoked potential are easily degraded by defocus, and it is important that the patient wears an appropriate refractive correction for these tests.

Interpretation of electrophysiological recordings

In general, the electrical events that occur in the visual system when a visual stimulus enters the eye

follow an orderly sequence. Hyperpolarisation of the photoreceptors associated with phototransduction starts to occur within the first 12 ms following a flash of light and forms the leading edge of the a-wave of the ERG. The events in the middle and inner layers of the retina which generate the pattern ERG (PERG) occur between 35 and 95 ms following pattern onset or reversal. The cortical visually evoked potential (VEP) to a reversing checkerboard stimulus starts at about 75 ms after the onset of the flash.

There is, of course, much more to the ERG than the transmission of the initial impulse from the photoreceptors to the ganglion cells. There is a complex sequence of electrochemical events in the retina and retinal pigment epithelium which continues for several minutes after a single flash, and the ERG is a composite wave with many components. New features of the ERG are still being discovered. The relative contributions of the various ERG components to the composite wave depend on the recording conditions and it is only possible to interpret an ERG recording in the light of detailed information about the stimulus (e.g. flash intensity, colour, repetition rate and level of background illumination) and the subject (e.g. age, degree of dark or light adaptation, pupil diameter, electrode position). It is possible to select out particular components of the ERG by choosing the stimulus characteristics and recording conditions appropriately, and this sometimes allows information to be gleaned about the function of particular cell types in the retina.

At the level of the occipital cortex, the impulse from a flash or pattern of light projected on to the retina has become considerably modulated, having synapsed in the ganglion cell layer and the lateral geniculate nucleus. The relationship between the type of stimulus and the cortical response is therefore much more complex than in the retina.

Full-field (Ganzfeld) electroretinography

The full-field ERG is a recording of the massed response of the cells of the retina in response to a flash of light. An abnormal ERG implies that the causative disease process is affecting the retina diffusely or extensively. A large macular scar which reduces the visual acuity to hand movements will have little effect on the ERG providing that the function of the peripheral retina is normal. Conversely, a disease process that causes extensive photoreceptor death (such as retinitis pigmentosa) but spares the fovea may almost extinguish the ERG, even though the visual acuity may be 6/5. The ERG is recordable from a healthy retina even in the presence of dense opacities of the ocular media, although the amplitude of the response will be correspondingly reduced.

Ideally, the electrodes used to record the ERG would be placed on the cornea and on the sclera close to the fovea. This is obviously impractical in the clinical situation and instead, one electrode is placed on the cornea and one on the skin at the ipsilateral lateral canthus. Recordings can be made from both eyes simultaneously and a common earth electrode is usually placed in the middle of the forehead. The corneal electrode may be either mounted in a special contact lens, or may consist of a conducting foil or fibre placed at the lid margin in contact with the cornea.

The pupils are maximally dilated and the subject's head is positioned within a bowl with a white, reflective inner surface and a radius that allows the whole retina to be illuminated as evenly as possible by light reflected from the surface. This is known as a Ganzfeld stimulus. The light source for the ISCEV standard ERG is a xenon discharge tube, but arrays of bright LEDs may also be used (Fig. 15.3).

A normal ERG series is shown in Fig. 15.4.

Fig. 15.3 (a, b) Ganzfeld bowl apparatus. (Courtesy of Moorfields Eye Hospital.)

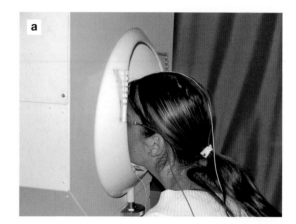

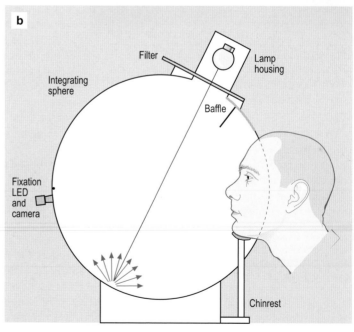

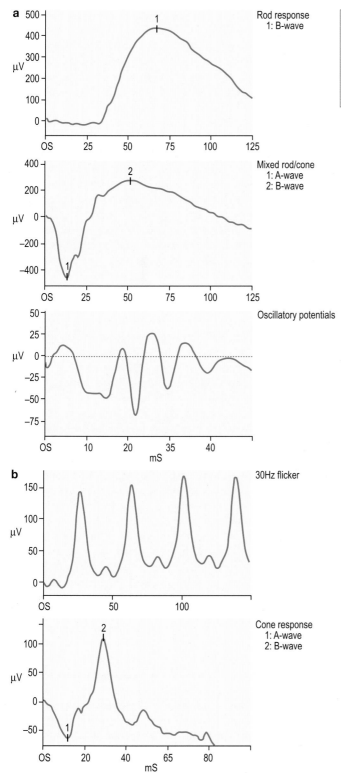

a

Rod response
1: B-wave

Mixed rod/cone
1: A-wave
2: B-wave

Oscillatory potentials

b

30Hz flicker

Cone response
1: A-wave
2: B-wave

Fig. 15.4 Normal electroretinogram series. **(a)** Dark-adapted rod responses to increasing flash intensity and **(b)** light-adapted cone responses. Note the scaling for cone responses compared with rod responses.

Before recording starts, the subject is dark-adapted for 20 min. Recordings are first made of the response to very dim flashes of white or blue light. The only response at this intensity is likely to be the scotopic threshold response (STR), a negative deflection of a few microvolts in amplitude. The response from many flashes must be averaged in order to detect the response above background noise. Further recordings are then made with flashes of progressively higher intensity. The scotopic b-wave appears, increasing in intensity and decreasing in implicit time as the flash intensity increases. At higher intensities, the a-wave appears and also increases in amplitude with increasing flash intensity. Up to this point, the cones have not made a major contribution to the response. Next, a bright white flash (sometimes known as the 'standard flash') is used, which produces a mixed rod and cone response with a large a-wave and b-wave, and wavelets or oscillatory potentials superimposed on the ascending limb of the b-wave. The oscillatory potentials can be recorded separately by repeating the recording with a filter to remove the lower-frequency components of the response. The subject is then light-adapted to suppress rod activity, and a response is recorded to a bright light flickering at 30 Hz. This is a pure cone response. A further recording is made of responses to single flashes of bright light. The cone a-wave and b-wave so generated are of smaller amplitude and are faster than their rod counterparts. There is often a distinct peak (I-wave) on the descending limb of the cone b-wave (Fig. 15.4).

A great deal of research has been conducted into the retinal origins of the components of the scotopic (dark-adapted) and photopic (light-adapted) ERG. Research techniques include the in vitro use of single-cell recordings with microelectrodes and the use of metabolic poisons to block the action of specific cells or receptors. Special test protocols in normal subjects and research on individuals with specific retinal diseases have contributed additional evidence.

The scotopic a-wave is the leading edge of a strong, sustained negative potential. The earliest part of the a-wave originates from the photoreceptors, but the later part (which is normally hidden by the positive deflection of the b-wave) reflects the activity of Müller cells. The scotopic b-wave is probably due to ion fluxes in the middle layers of the retina secondary to the activity of the rod on-bipolar pathway. There is no rod off-bipolar pathway. The cone a-wave also includes a significant contribution from the horizontal cells and cone off-bipolar cells. The cone b-wave is driven largely by the cone on-bipolar cells. The ERG to a 30 Hz flicker contains contributions from both the on- and off-bipolar cells but not from the photoreceptors.

A number of retinal conditions produce specific and predictable abnormalities in the standard ERG. Mutations in rhodopsin found in autosomal dominant retinitis pigmentosa cause progressive death of rods with later secondary damage to cones. The scotopic ERG is severely abnormal or unrecordable from an early stage and the photopic ERG is usually better preserved, but deteriorates as the disease progresses. In contrast, the cone dystrophies reduce or extinguish the photopic ERG while leaving the scotopic ERG relatively well preserved. The rare condition of achromatopsia also results in an absent photopic ERG with a preserved scotopic ERG.

Any process that results in the death of photoreceptors will attenuate the ERG if it is extensive enough. Examples include chorioretinitis, myopic chorioretinal atrophy, extensive laser photocoagulation and autoimmune retinopathies such as carcinoma-associated retinopathy.

Processes that disrupt communication between the photoreceptors and bipolar cells characteristically reduce the amplitude of the b-wave of the standard flash dark-adapted ERG, giving the so-called 'negative ERG' (Fig. 15.5). Conditions which can give rise to this appearance include X-linked retinoschisis, congenital stationary night blindness and retinal vascular occlusions.

The availability of bright LEDs emitting at a variety of wavelengths has made it possible to design special protocols to select out additional features of the cone pathway. These do not currently form part of the standard ISCEV ERG protocol, but are likely to become part of the standard test in the future as their clinical relevance becomes more firmly established.

For instance, a long flash (e.g. 100 ms) under light-adapted conditions produces an onset response (the cone a-wave and b-wave) at the beginning of the stimulus and an offset response (a positive wave, sometimes referred to as the d-wave) as the light switches off. Both the onset and offset components represent an interaction between the on-bipolar and off-bipolar pathways. The complete form of

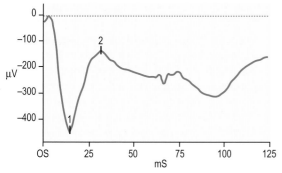

Fig. 15.5 A negative electroretinogram. Note the large a-wave, which is normally attenuated by the rising b-wave.

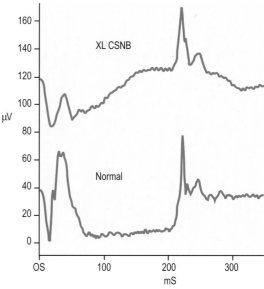

Fig. 15.6 Normal on and off response to a long flash (lower trace) and long flash response in complete congenital stationary night blindness (CSNB: upper trace). (Courtesy of Moorfields Eye Hospital.)

congenital stationary night blindness prevents transmission between rods and cones and on-bipolar cells. As expected, the long flash photopic ERG shows a deep, sustained a-wave with a small or absent b-wave, followed by a large d-wave (Fig. 15.6).

If dim blue flashes are presented against a brighter orange background, an S cone (blue cone) ERG can be recorded because the rods and L and M (red and green) cones are suppressed by the orange background illumination. The S cone ERG is small and its b-wave implicit time is closer to that of the rods than the L and M cones. Like rods, S cones lack an off-bipolar pathway. There is an uncommon form of night blindness known as enhanced S cone syndrome (ESCS) where all the photoreceptors are cones, of which over 90% are S cones. Apart from night blindness, visual function is usually good, although there can be slow deterioration. Predictably, the scotopic ERG is very small as it contains only a cone contribution. The 30 Hz flicker response is reduced and delayed, and the standard cone ERG is also reduced. However, the S cone ERG is abnormally large.

The causative genes for these and many other inherited retinal diseases have been identified in the last decade, and the ERG has provided valuable information on how mutations modify retinal function.

Pattern electroretinogram

The PERG has become established as a standard part of the electrophysiological repertoire since the early 1990s. Placement of electrodes is the same as for a full-field ERG, although foil or fibre corneal electrodes are preferred to contact lens electrodes because a clearly focused retinal image is essential. The stimulus is a pattern of high contrast projected on a monitor. The most commonly used stimulus is a checkerboard pattern where each check alternates between black and white twice every second. For many years, there was controversy as to whether the response recorded to this stimulus was simply a result of interaction between 'mini-ERGs' produced by areas of illuminated retina, but it is now generally accepted that the PERG is a distinct electrophysiological response which contains information about ganglion cell function, although some uncertainty still surrounds its exact origins.

The PERG is a much weaker response than the ERG, rarely exceeding 8–10 µV in amplitude, so an averaged response to a number of pattern reversals is recorded. It is highly susceptible to defocus, so an accurate spectacle correction must be worn for the test where there is any significant refractive error. Unlike the ERG, the PERG is a macula-dominated response.

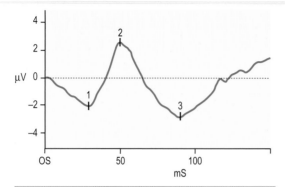

Fig. 15.7 Normal-pattern electroretinogram. The key features are: (1) N35; (2) P50; and (3) N95.

The components of the PERG are conventionally identified by their normal implicit time in milliseconds with a suffix to indicate positive or negative polarity. There is a small negative deflection (N35) followed by a larger, broader positive deflection (P50) and another broad negative deflection (N95) (Fig. 15.7).

The N95 component seems to be closely related to ganglion cell activity and is sensitive to early glaucomatous optic nerve damage. The PERG response is an early casualty of Stargardt's maculopathy and may be profoundly reduced or extinguished before the foveal changes are evident clinically. The PERG can therefore be a useful test in a child who presents with an unexplained reduction in visual acuity.

Multifocal electroretinography

As stated above, the standard flash ERG is a global response from the retina and gives no information about whether some areas of the retina are more involved in a disease process than others. It is not possible to obtain a meaningful focal ERG simply by projecting a beam of light on to a small area of retina, because scattering and reflection of light in the eye result in illumination of a much wider area of retina.

Multifocal electroretinography (mfERG) is an elegant technique by which local ERGs can be extracted simultaneously from a number of areas of the retina. The stimulus consists of an array of scaled hexagons (smaller around the central fixation target, larger in the peripheral field), each element of which flashes in a pseudo-random sequence known as an m-sequence.

Responses are recorded under light-adapted conditions with a similar electrode configuration to the standard ERG. Even with good recording conditions and a high level of patient cooperation, it is necessary to record for several minutes to obtain stable recordings. The raw mfERG response is undecipherable to casual analysis, but because each hexagon follows an m-sequence, a computer can be used to extract an ERG trace from each hexagon by a mathematical process known as kernel analysis. Each focal ERG obtained in this way is a composite wave which contains responses to single flashes (first-order responses), on top of which is superimposed the effects of earlier flashes in the sequence (second- and higher-order responses, i.e. adaptation effects; Fig. 15.8).

Superficially, the first-order kernel of the mfERG resembles a conventional photopic ERG with a negative deflection followed by a positive deflection. Clinical evidence suggests that these components are equivalent to the a-wave and b-wave of the full-field ERG, but it must be remembered that mfERG traces are mathematically derived responses rather than directly recorded ERGs. The amplitude of the mfERG response is also very small – a few hundred nanovolts at best – and great care has to be taken to achieve a good signal-to-noise ratio.

Although used extensively as a research tool, the mfERG is generally less useful than the full-field ERG in routine clinical practice. It distinguishes between healthy and poorly functioning areas of retina quite well, but gives little information about the function of different retinal cell types. It is degraded by defocus, media opacity and patient movement.

Electro-oculography

When the retina is illuminated by a sustained light source following a period of dark adaptation, the ERG a-wave and b-wave are followed by three distinct slower potentials known as the c-wave, fast oscillation and slow oscillation (or light rise). The c-wave is a cornea-positive potential which peaks at about 2 s from the light onset and represents the sum of a retinal component and a retinal pigment epithelial component. The fast oscillation is a cornea-negative potential which reaches a trough at about 1 min from light onset and the light rise is a

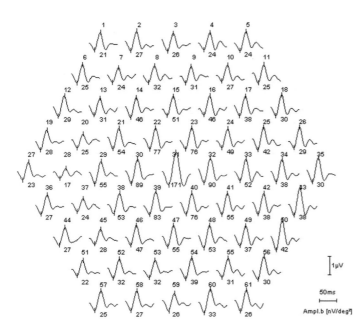

Fig. 15.8 Normal multifocal ERG trace array. (Courtesy of Moorfields Eye Hospital.)

1µV

50ms

Ampl.b [nV/deg²]

cornea-positive potential which peaks at 10–15 min from light onset. The fast oscillation and light rise are both due to changes in ion concentrations across the retinal pigment epithelium cell membrane.

The c-wave and fast oscillation are technically difficult to record in conscious subjects and are of limited clinical usefulness. However, the light rise can be measured more easily by an indirect technique known as electro-oculography (EOG), developed by Arden (Arden, 1962).

If electrodes placed at the lateral canthus and medial canthus are connected to a galvanometer, adduction of the eye will cause a deflection of the galvanometer in one direction while abduction of the eye will result in a deflection in the opposite direction. This is because, even in the dark, the living eye has a potential difference of about 6 mV between the cornea and the retina (DuBois-Reymond, 1849). The light rise is superimposed on this standing potential, and, for the same degree of adduction or abduction of the eye, will result in an increased deflection of the galvanometer.

In the clinical EOG protocol, the subject is seated in front of a diffuser, behind which is a bank of fluorescent light tubes (Fig. 15.9). In the centre of the diffuser, there is an LED to act as a fixation target. Another pair of LEDs either side of the central fixation target can be illuminated alternately to help the

subject make excursions of the eyes to left and right of a constant amplitude. For most of the time during the test, the subject looks at the central LED, but every minute, the left and right LEDs illuminate alternately to prompt the subject to make a series of excursions of the eyes to left and right. The potential difference between the lateral and medial canthal electrodes is measured on a slow time base and the periods of eye movement appear as deflections above and below the baseline. During dark adaptation, the amplitude of the deflections on the trace gradually diminish to a constant level, referred to as the dark trough. The lights are then turned on and the amplitude of the deflections on the trace start to increase, reaching a maximum after about 10 min of light adaptation. The ratio of the maximum amplitude in the light to the minimum amplitude in the dark is an indirect measurement of the retinal pigment epithelium light rise and is commonly known as the Arden index (Fig. 15.10).

The lower limit of the Arden index in normal subjects is about 1.7, but it can be as high as 4.0, and may vary in the same individual between tests performed on different occasions. Any condition resulting in a substantial reduction in the ERG will also reduce the EOG light rise. The EOG is influenced by a number of pharmacological agents, notably acetazolamide and ethanol. The variability

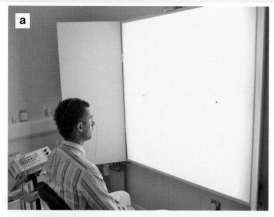

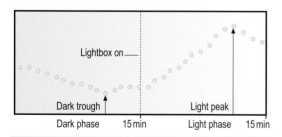

Fig. 15.9 (a) Electro-oculogram recording and **(b)** electrode positions. The two red fixation light-emitting diodes can just be seen on the light box.

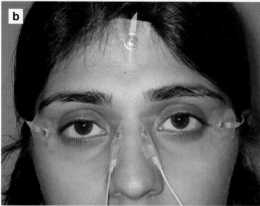

Fig. 15.10 Normal electro-oculogram response.

of the EOG and the fact that it is a tedious test to perform limits its clinical utility, but it has proved useful in Best's vitelliform dystrophy, where the EOG light rise is consistently subnormal, while the ERG is usually unaffected. VMD2 (bestrophin), the product

of the gene commonly implicated in Best's vitelliform dystrophy, is a chloride channel protein found in the basal cell membrane of the RPE. Mutations in this gene result in reduced conductivity and hence an impaired EOG light rise.

The visually evoked cortical potential (VECP or VEP)

It is possible to record electrical responses from the primary and secondary visual cortex in response to visual stimuli of various types. This is facilitated by the fact that several areas responsible for the processing of visual information, notably the primary cortex serving the macula, lie on the outer surface of the brain close to the skull. The brain is, of course, an electrically busy organ and the VEP has to be extracted from a cacophony of electrical noise, particularly the alpha rhythm of the electro-encephalogram (EEG).

To record the VEP, a midline occipital skin electrode is placed and is referenced to a mid frontal electrode. Additional electrodes may also be placed over the occipital and parietal areas of both hemispheres. Recordings are time-locked to a repetitive stimulus which allows alpha rhythm and other unwanted noise to be averaged out, leaving a response that is attributable to the visual stimulus. The primary visual cortex gives particularly strong and repeatable responses to a reversing checkerboard pattern, as described for the PERG. Another commonly used stimulus is referred to as 'pattern onset', where a checkerboard pattern alternates with a uniform grey screen of the same mean luminance.

VEPs originating from the secondary visual areas have been recorded to many other types of stimulus including motion, stereopsis and colour. It is also possible to record multifocal VEPs with a similar apparatus to that used for the multifocal ERG. These specialised VEPs are used in research studies but have not yet found their place in routine clinical practice.

The waveform of the VEP depends on the type of visual stimulus, the position of the electrodes used to record it, the maturity of the visual cortex and the level of alertness of the subject. Even where the stimulus characteristics and placement of recording electrodes are carefully standardised, considerable interindividual variability in the waveform is common because the calcarine cortex is highly and variably convoluted, and because the relationship between anatomical landmarks on the skull and surface features of the brain is imprecise. It is not possible to assign functional significance to particular components of the VEP waveform; instead, the VEP can be analysed in terms of implicit time of components, vector (direction of spread of components through the brain, where multiple electrodes are used) and tuning characteristics (optimum stimulus conditions for producing the strongest possible response).

A typical adult pattern reversal VEP trace has three main components, which are named according to their polarity and implicit time as N75, P100 and N135 (Fig. 15.11). Of these, the P100 component is usually the largest and most reproducible response when recorded with a midline occipital electrode. Because the macula projects to the most posterior part of the occipital cortex, the P100 is a macula-dominated response. Both retinas project to both hemispheres, so one eye must be tested at a time in order to compare responses between the two eyes .

The pattern reversal VEP can be used as an approximate objective measure of visual acuity. When the size of the checks is reduced to the point where the contrast borders can no longer be resolved, the cortical response disappears. At a check size which subtends a visual angle of 15 min arc, a visual acuity of approximately 6/18–6/24 is required for a clear cortical response. At a check size of 60 min arc, a visual acuity of 3/60–6/60 is required for a clear cortical response.

Demyelinating optic neuritis impairs conduction in the optic nerve. In the acute phase, where visual acuity is significantly reduced, the VEP is often undetectable. When the visual acuity has returned to normal, the VEP from the affected eye usually recovers, but remains permanently delayed, typically by 30 ms or more (Fig. 15.12).

Ocular albinism is associated with a variable degree of misrouting of optic nerve fibres. Fibres from the temporal retina which would normally project to the ipsilateral hemisphere instead decussate in the chiasm and project to the contralateral hemisphere. There is not a close relationship between the extent of misrouting and the visual acuity or amplitude of nystagmus, but misrouting can often be detected using the pattern VEP. As well as a midline occipital electrode, electrodes are placed over the left and right occipital lobes and the responses resulting from stimulation of either eye are compared at each electrode position. In the most obvious examples of misrouting, stimulation of the right eye will result in a response predominantly over the left occipital lobe and vice versa. Sometimes the misrouting is more subtle and is only evident on careful measurement of the traces (Fig. 15.13).

Abnormalities in the visual pathway at or posterior to the chiasm can be detected with the pattern VEP using hemifield stimulation. The patient views a fixation target in the centre of the screen and the checkerboard stimulus occupies either the left or right half of the screen. Hemifield responses must be recorded with an array of electrodes (normally five) over the occipital lobes.

The pattern VEP can be used to monitor the maturation of the visual system in infants. Its development fairly closely parallels the development of visual acuity recorded by other tests, such as preferential looking.

The pattern VEP is degraded by uncorrected refractive error, unsteady fixation and drowsiness. It is possible to record a VEP to simple flashes of light. This is useful where the visual acuity is too poor to perceive even large checks or where fixation or concentration is poor. The flash VEP is much less

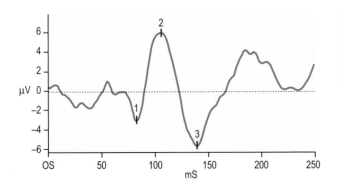

Fig. 15.11 Normal pattern visually evoked potential to 60 min arc reversing checkerboard stimulus. The key features are: (1) N75; (2) P100; and (3) N135.

Fig. 15.12 Pattern visually evoked potential in right optic neuritis. Note the delayed P100 in the right eye compared to the normal trace in the left.

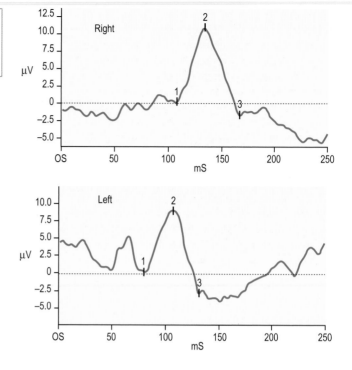

Fig. 15.13 Visually evoked potential responses showing misrouting of the visual pathway. **(a)** The result of subtracting the response from the right hemisphere from that of the left, with the right eye being stimulated. **(b)** The lower trace is similarly obtained while stimulating the left eye. The asymmetry is obvious.

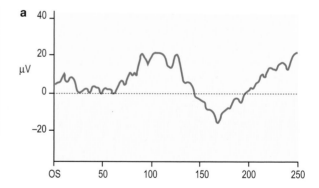

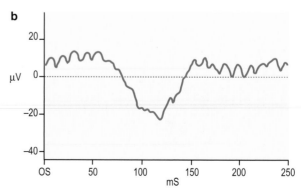

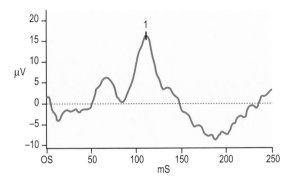

Fig. 15.14 Normal flash visually evoked potential. The key feature is: (1) P2.

macula-dominated than the pattern VEP and can be recorded through cataracts or corneal scars. Unfortunately, it is much more variable in appearance than the pattern VEP and, in general, it is used as a basic indication of the integrity of the visual pathway from the eye to the occipital cortex. The most consistent feature is a positive component, designated P2, which usually occurs at around 125 ms after the flash, but identification of even this component is not always easy (Fig. 15.14).

With the exception of demyelination, the VEP gives little help in differentiating the type of lesion affecting the optic nerves or other parts of the visual pathway. It will not, for instance, distinguish between an ischaemic lesion and a compressive lesion. It can be useful, however, for monitoring the progress of a known condition affecting the visual pathways.

Dark adaptometry

Dark adaptometry is a psychophysical measurement rather than an electrophysiological test, but it is usually performed in electrophysiology departments. The human eye has a remarkable ability to detect small increments and decrements in brightness or contrast across a range of about 6 log units (1 million times) of light intensity. This is achieved to a small extent by altering pupil diameter and to a larger extent by bringing rods or cones into or out of play, but the most important mechanism for adjusting the gain of the visual system is the balance between bleach and regeneration of visual pigment.

Dark adaptation is measured by bleaching the retina with an intense light, turning out the light, then periodically recording the brightness at which a test light projected a few degrees away from fixation can just be perceived, until the eye is fully dark-adapted. A typical dark adaptation threshold curve is shown in Chapter 1. The curve is biphasic, with the first part due to the cones and the second part to the rods. The step between the cone and rod parts of the curve is referred to as the 'rod–cone break'.

In achromatopsia, the cone component of the dark adaptation curve is absent and recovery from bleach occurs rapidly. In rod–cone dystrophies, such as autosomal dominant retinitis pigmentosa, and in the various types of congenital stationary night blindness, the rod part of the dark adaptation curve is absent, resulting in an elevated dark adaptation threshold even after prolonged dark adaptation.

Oguchi's disease is a rare form of night blindness due to mutations in the genes which encode either arrestin or rhodopsin kinase. It is characterised by a metallic sheen of the retina on fundoscopy which disappears on prolonged dark adaptation (Mizuo's phenomenon). The dark adaptation curve is greatly prolonged, but eventually reaches a normal threshold level after several hours of dark adaptation.

Summary and suggestions for further reading

This chapter has given an overview of visual electrophysiological investigations and their application in a clinical setting, with a number of specific examples of diseases of the visual system which show characteristic electrophysiological features. Visual electrophysiology is a rapidly developing field of visual science and the scientific literature can be daunting for the trainee ophthalmologist. The ISCEV website (www.iscev.org) gives details of the electrophysiological standards referred to in this text and contains other educational resources. There is a superb online textbook on the organisation of the human retina by Helga Kolb et al. at http://webvision.med.utah.edu. For up-to-date references on specific inherited ocular diseases, consult the Online Mendelian Inheritance in Man (OMIM) website at www.ncbi.nlm.nih.gov.

- Despite the sophistication of the recording equipment available, a critical aspect of the process of electrophysiology is the training and experience of the electrophysiologist. Meticulous attention to detail is required for repeatable and reliable results
- Electrophysiology is a part of the diagnostic process. It does not, often, provide the diagnosis per se and clinical guidance as to the tests required is critical
- The International Society for Clinical Electrophysiology of Vision (ISCEV) website (www.iscev.org) provides standards as referred to in this chapter and other useful information and resources for the trainee

References

Arden GB, Barrada A, Kelsey JH. New clinical test of retinal function based upon the standing potential of the eye. Br J Ophthalmol 1962; 46: 449–467.

DuBois-Reymond E. Untersuchungen uber die thierische Elektrizitat, Vol. 2. Berlin: Reimer; 1849: 256–257.

Einthoven W, Jolly W. The form and magnitude of the electrical response of the eye to stimulation at various intensities. Q J Exp Physiol 1908; 1: 337–416.

Granit R. Sensory mechanisms of the retina with an appendix on electroretinography. London: Oxford University Press; 1947.

16

Fluorescein angiography

LARRY BENJAMIN

Introduction

Fluorescein angiography is used to examine vascular structures in the eye such as the iris, retina and choroid. Injected fluorescein dye remains within normal blood vessels, thus leakage into surrounding tissue indicates vascular pathology. The time taken for the dye to pass from the arterial to the venous circulation (and, indeed, the time taken just to reach the eye) may also provide some functional information about the circulatory system. It is most commonly used to investigate retinal diseases such as diabetic retinopathy.

Principles

The principles of this technique were first described by MacLean and Maumenee and later developed by Novotny and Alvis. Fluorescein has the property of absorbing light in the blue wavelength and emitting it in the green wavelength (fluorescing). Fluorescein is a vital dye: its characteristics are shown in Box 16.1.

Dye injected into a peripheral vein passes into and through the choroidal and retinal circulation. A blue light projected into the eye causes the fluorescein to emit a green light. This is photographed through a yellow barrier filter. This removes any reflected blue light but allows the fluorescent green wavelength through. The picture is captured on to black and white film or the charge-coupled device (CCD) of a digital camera. Fluoroscopy is the direct viewing of the fluorescence without recording it. This can be done with an indirect ophthalmoscope fitted with a blue filter. The principles of fluorescein angiography are shown in Figure 16.1.

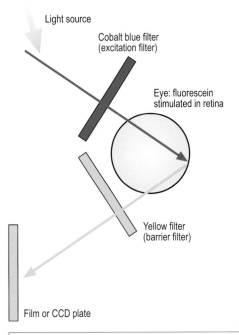

Fig. 16.1 The principles of fluorescein angiography. CCD, charge-coupled device.

Box 16.1

Properties of sodium fluorescein

Nature
Crystalline hydrocarbon dye
Colour
Orange/red
Molecular weight
376 kDa
Wavelength of excitation
465–470 nm
Emission wavelength
520–530 nm

Table 16.1	Side-effects and risk factors of fluorescein injection
Side-effects of fluorescein injection	**Risk factors**
Vasovagal attack Nausea Anaphylaxis Wheezing Itching	Allergy to shellfish Previous reaction

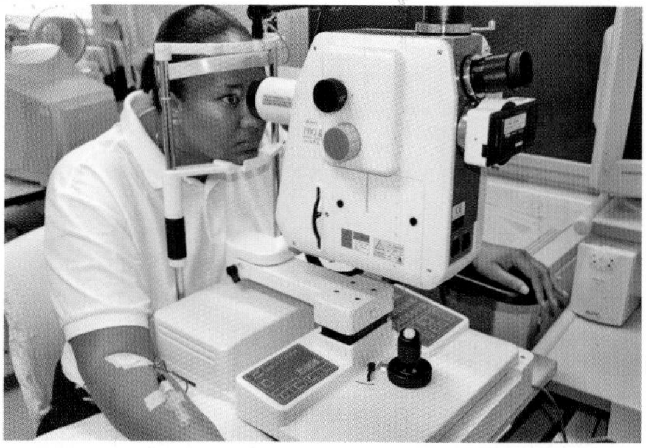

Fig. 16.2 The patient seated comfortably at the fundus camera.

The technique

There is both a morbidity (Table 16.1) and a mortality (1 in 200 000) associated with this technique. Its use should be limited to diagnosis in patients whose management may be altered by the results or subjects included in an ethically approved research study. Some of the indications are shown in Box 16.2. Full resuscitation facilities must be available close at hand.

The patient is comfortably seated at the retinal camera (Fig. 16.2). The blue exciter filter and the yellow barrier filter are appropriately positioned in the camera. Injection of dye (5 ml of 10% fluorescein) is best given in the antecubital fossa, ensuring that the patient feels no discomfort as this may signify extravasation of dye into the tissues, which can be very painful. A test injection of 1–2 ml of normal saline is useful to confirm correct placement of the cannula before fluorescein is given.

The dye can cause nausea as it reaches the cerebral circulation and patients should be warned of this. In addition it colours the skin yellow for 12–24 h and is excreted in the urine, turning it a bright yellow colour. Sublingual administration of Stemetil 3–5 mg 1 h before the administration of dye may abolish the nausea.

The sequence of the angiogram

The sequence shown in Figure 16.3 demonstrates the different phases of an angiogram. Abnormalities may occur at different stages, and the stage at which an abnormality appears may be important diagnostically.

The protocol starts with a normal colour image (Fig. 16.3a) and a red-free picture, taken with only the green filter in place to give a black-and-white image of the fundus prior to fluorescein injection (Fig. 16.3b). The dye is then injected. Image capture begins again at the time it is anticipated that the dye will reach the eye. This will vary in patients according to their age and the state of their cardiovascular system; it is typically 8–12 s.

The earliest fluorescence is seen in the choroidal circulation and vessels arising from it, for example, a cilioretinal artery or a subretinal neovascular membrane. Choroidal fluorescence may be patchy initially but in health should be uniform at the start of the venous phase. The xanthophil pigment of the

---

Box 16.2

Common indications for fluorescein angiography

- To diagnose and demarcate choroidal neovascular membranes
- To differentiate between collateral vessels (non-leaky) and new vessels (leaky) in the retina
- To diagnose subclinical cystoid macula oedema
- To define the extent of macular leakage after branch retinal vein occlusion
- To define the site of subretinal leakage in central serous retinopathy before laser treatment
- To identify ischaemia in diabetic maculopathy

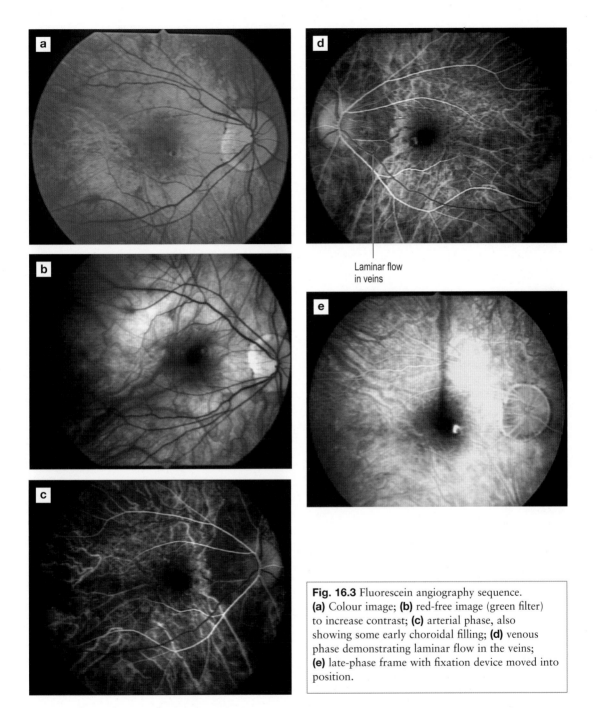

Laminar flow
in veins

Fig. 16.3 Fluorescein angiography sequence.
(a) Colour image; **(b)** red-free image (green filter)
to increase contrast; **(c)** arterial phase, also
showing some early choroidal filling; **(d)** venous
phase demonstrating laminar flow in the veins;
(e) late-phase frame with fixation device moved into
position.

central macular region masks the fluorescence from
the choroid; this region therefore remains dark.

The arterial phase of the retinal circulation is
seen next (Fig. 16.3c), followed by the arteriovenous
or capillary phase and subsequently the venous

phase which initially demonstrates laminar flow
(Fig. 16.3d). Late-phase pictures (after 5 min) are
also taken (Fig. 16.3e). In this particular sequence
a subfoveal neovascular membrane lights up early
in the sequence and remains brightly fluorescent into

the late phase. In the late-phase picture a fixation device has been placed in the camera for the patient to fix on. This enables the spatial relationship to be established between fixation and the pathological lesion being examined.

Stereo pairs may help visualise pathology that causes an elevation of retinal or choroidal structures. These are constructed by taking two successive pictures, altering the horizontal angle of the camera between the two. This can be done either with an Allen separator, a piece of optical-quality glass which electrically flips between two pre-set positions moving the fundus image 30° between positions, or by physically moving the fundus camera between exposures by the full sideways travel of the joystick.

Interpretation of the angiogram

Images captured on black-and-white film are seen as negatives when the film is developed. Consequently, fluorescein, which has been stimulated and effectively glows (fluoresces), is dark on the negative. The negatives can be reversed or printed to show fluorescein as white. Examples of this can be seen in Figure 16.4. Digital systems are usually set up to produce positive images (Fig. 16.3) but can be manipulated to produce negatives.

It is important to have a system for analysing angiograms. The 'what, where and when' approach is recommended. This involves looking at:

- the phase of the angiogram (the *when*)
  - choroidal
  - arterial
  - arteriovenous or capillary
  - venous
  - late
- the site of the lesion (the *where*)
  - nasal/temporal
  - superior/inferior
  - the level in the retina/choroid/pigment epithelium
- the nature of the lesion (the *what*)
  - normal vessel
  - abnormal (leaking) vessel
  - window defect
  - blocking defect.

Hypofluorescence (Figs 16.5 and 16.6)

The retinal pigment epithelium (RPE) allows a limited amount of fluorescence through from the choroid. This is blocked in RPE hypertrophy. In the same way retinal haemorrhages, exudates and media opacities block fluorescence (Fig. 16.5b). Large drusen may initially block choroidal fluorescence

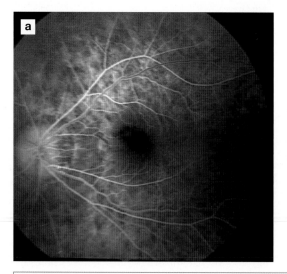
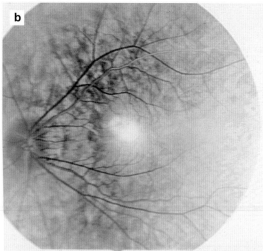

Fig. 16.4 (a) A positive frame from an angiogram (the usual image type in digital systems). **(b)** The same frame but as a negative (fluorescein is dark). This is how angiography looks on negative film.

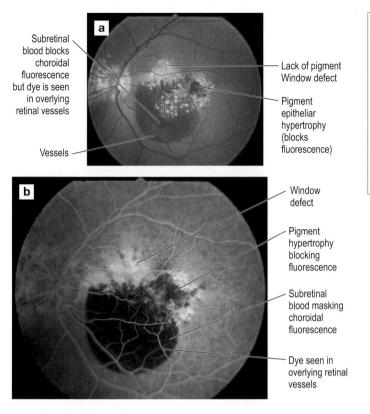

Subretinal blood blocks choroidal fluorescence but dye is seen in overlying retinal vessels

Vessels

Lack of pigment Window defect

Pigment epitheliar hypertrophy (blocks fluorescence)

Window defect

Pigment hypertrophy blocking fluorescence

Subretinal blood masking choroidal fluorescence

Dye seen in overlying retinal vessels

Fig. 16.5 (a) A colour fundus picture showing an acute bleed from a disciform lesion. **(b)** The fluorescein angiogram. Note the presence of haemorrhage and hypertrophied pigment epithelium, both of which block fluorescence on the angiogram. Note too how the retinal vessels are seen coursing over the blood, indicating its subretinal location and how the drusen stain with fluorescein.

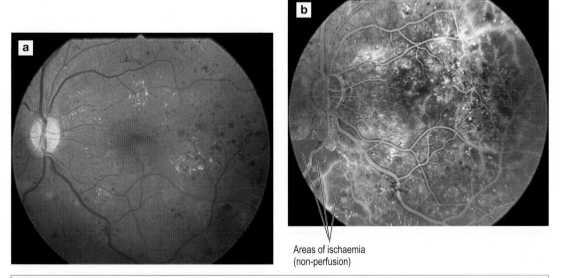

Areas of ischaemia (non-perfusion)

Fig. 16.6 (a) Ischaemia in a diabetic patient: the colour fundus photograph of the left eye. **(b)** A later frame from the angiogram of the same eye, showing areas with no retinal fluorescence. Complete capillary shutdown has occurred in these areas.

but in later phases of the angiogram they stain and hyperfluoresce (Fig. 16.5b). Choroidal infarcts will produce sectors of hypofluorescence early on in the angiogram.

In the capillary bed of the retina, ischaemia and capillary shutdown, found in central retinal vein occlusion or diabetic retinopathy, hypofluoresce (Fig. 16.6b).

Hyperfluorescence (Figs 16.5 and 16.6)

The absence of pigment (pigment epithelial drop-out) is seen as a brightly fluorescent patch as the choroidal vasculature is seen through the 'window defect' of the missing pigment (Fig. 16.5b). Abnormal new blood vessels or inflamed vessels may also hyperfluoresce.

A subretinal neovascular membrane growing through the RPE from the choroid fluoresces early in the sequence as the vessels arise from the choroid (Fig. 16.3). Disc and retinal new vessels will fluoresce later in the sequence (Fig. 16.7).

Fluorescein leakage may result in pooling of the dye if a fluid-filled space exists. The margins around the leaking dye are sharp. This is seen in a pigment epithelial detachment (Fig. 16.8), retinal detachment (for example, central serous retinopathy: Fig. 16.9) and cystoid macular oedema (Fig. 16.10).

Leakage of fluorescein into tissue causes staining; here the borders are ill defined, for example staining of retinal drusen or non-cystoid retinal oedema.

Sometimes abnormalities may demonstrate auto-fluorescence (fluorescence without injection of fluorescein dye). Optic nerve head drusen are an example of this phenomenon (Fig. 16.11).

The causes of hypo- and hyperfluorescence are summarised in Figure 16.12.

Iris angiography

The same set-up used for posterior-segment work can be used. Most fundus cameras have a supplementary lens incorporated into the optical pathway for viewing and photographing the anterior segment.

Iris vessels can be imaged and abnormal leakage (for example, from rubeotic vessels) can be photographed. It is important not to dilate the pupil before iris angiography and thus it must be carried out on a separate occasion to fundus angiography. Alternatively a dedicated anterior-segment camera is used with the appropriate filters built into the system. Figure 16.13 shows an iris tumour and a frame from its angiogram with some leakage from the tumour circulation.

Indocyanine green angiography

Indocyanine green is a tricarbocyanine dye which is useful for examining the choroidal circulation. It

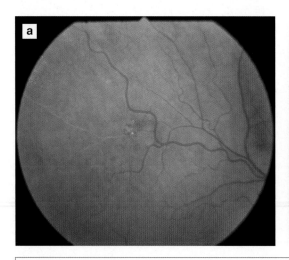
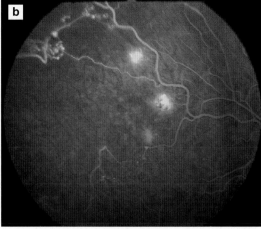

Fig. 16.7 (a) A colour photograph showing an ischaemic vessel and new vessels growing from the retina. **(b)** Leakage from the new vessels on angiography.

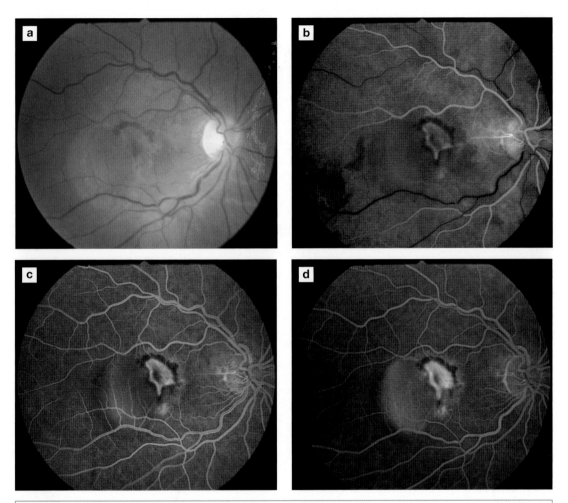

Fig. 16.8 (a) A colour fundus photograph of a pigment epithelial detachment (PED). The well-demarcated border of the PED is clearly seen. **(b)** The arterial phase of the angiogram demonstrates a vascular net or choroidal neovascular membrane. It first appears with the initial choroidal flush as fluorescein enters the eye. The edge of the PED is better demarcated. **(c)** The late venous phase of the angiogram shows fluorescein gradually filling the PED, persistent, bright fluorescence of the membrane and blockage of fluorescence by the rim of blood at the superior edge of the membrane. **(d)** Late-phase frame showing filling of the PED with fluorescein.

uses the same fundus camera set-up but the camera is also sensitive to the infrared wavelengths and requires different filters. It can also be used in conjunction with the scanning laser ophthalmoscope to produce videoangiography. The technique is not widely used clinically. It is particularly useful in assessing choroidal disease.

Pitfalls and complications

Mistiming the run

A common pitfall is mistiming the run. As the view through the camera is effectively blank when the injection is given, anticipating the timing of the first photograph can be difficult, especially if the patient loses fixation and the camera is not lined up at the

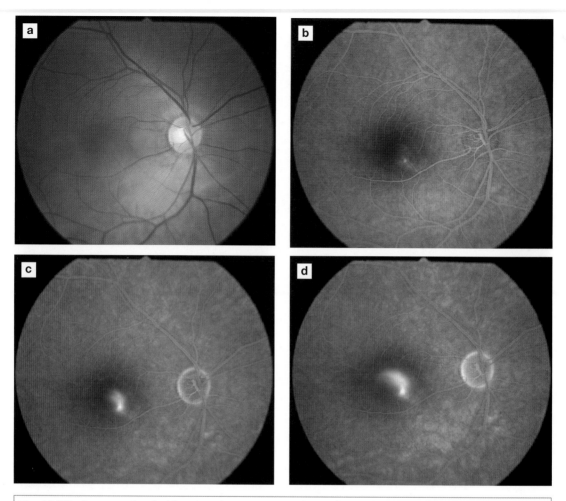

Fig. 16.9 Leakage associated with a central serous retinopathy. **(a)** Colour fundus photograph. **(b–d)** Progressive leakage from the defect in the retinal pigment epithelium has caused a detachment of the neurosensory retina; note how fluorescein leaks into the space, causing a smokestack appearance. Eventually the entire space would fill.

time when fluorescein first appears in the retinal circulation.

To avoid this, it is important to:

- ask the patient to keep fixing on either the internal fixation device or an external fixation light
- keep the barrier filter out until a few seconds after the injection to allow the fundus to be visualised (some cameras do this automatically, only placing the barrier filter as the frame is exposed)

- commence taking pictures before the appearance of the dye
- take pictures every second or so, warning the patient of the frequency and ensuring refixation after blinks.

Extravasation of dye

This may be very painful, and any discomfort experienced by the patient at the beginning of the injection should alert the person injecting to this possibility. Remember that, if there is any doubt about the placement of the needle, it is useful to

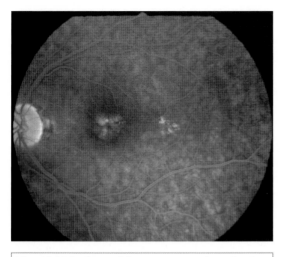

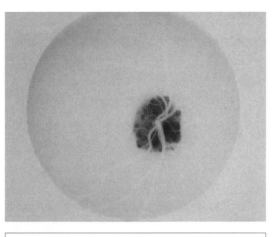

Fig. 16.11 Autofluorescence from an optic nerve head drusen.

Fig. 16.10 Leakage of fluorescein into the retina in cystoid macular oedema.

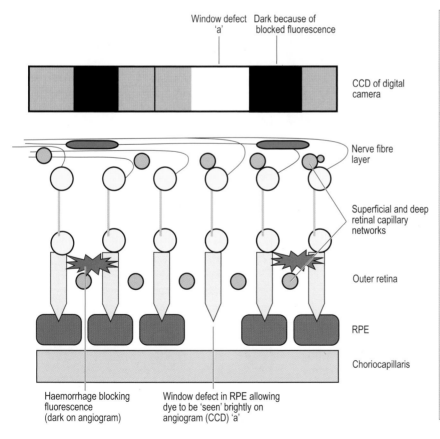

Fig. 16.12 A section of the retina showing potential sources of fluorescence (the choroid and retinal vessels in yellow) and origins of hypo- and hyper-fluorescence. The effect of this on film with fluorescence shown as bright (positive) is indicated. A window defect can be seen at position 'a' with a resultant bright spot on the angiogram as dye is seen through the window. Haemorrhage and pigment hypertrophy will block fluorescence. CCD, charge-coupled device; RPE, retinal pigment epithelium.

219

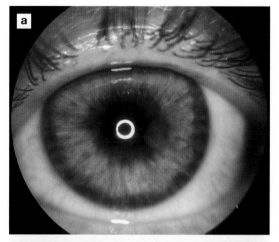

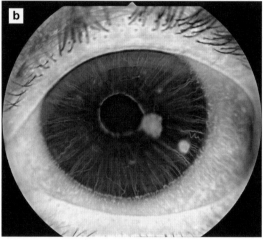

Fig. 16.13 (a) Colour photograph of an iris tumour. **(b)** Iris angiogram showing some leakage from the tumour vasculature.

test for correct siting by administration of 1–2 mls of normal saline before the fluorescein.

Intra-arterial injection

The dye appears in the retinal circulation very quickly and the patient will often complain of a hot flush in the affected limb which will turn a bright-orange colour. Intra-arterial siting of the cannula is also suggested by a rapid and extensive flush-back of blood into the tubing, even after removal of the tourniquet.

Nausea

This is very common, occurring as the dye reaches the cerebral circulation. It is unusual for patients actually to vomit. The nausea passes off after around 30 s and may be lessened or abolished if Stemetil is administered pre-angiography.

Anaphylaxis

Two people should always be involved in the performance of angiography in case of anaphylaxis or a vasovagal response. The patient should be warned of the possibility of nausea before the injection is given and the photographer should be prepared to stop if it occurs.

A standard drug stock should include adrenaline (epinephrine), Piriton, hydrocortisone and access to suction and a fully stocked and maintained cardiac arrest trolley.

Summary

Fundus fluorescein angiography is a very useful investigation in helping to delineate vascular abnormalities of the retina and choroid. It requires specialised equipment, access to resuscitation facilities and trained staff to carry it out. Analysis of the angiograms requires experience but is easily learned through a logical approach to a description of the site, size and phase of the lesion in terms of dye circulation. With stereo-angiograms the site of lesions can be further delineated in terms of depth

- A useful adjunctive investigation to clinical examination but as it carries some morbidity and a small mortality rate it should only be used where management may be altered or as part of an ethically approved study
- A systematic approach to interpretation of the angiogram is essential
- Clinical data supplied on the request form are helpful to the technician performing the angiogram. It is especially important to outline the site of the pathology and on which eye should be the main angiographic run
- Cooperation from the patient is helped by a careful and thorough explanation of what is to be expected during the angiogram

of the pathology within the layers of the vascular and pigmented coats of the eye.

Stereo-angiograms are useful to characterise further elevated lesions of the retina and choroid.

References and further reading

Cohen SY, Quentel G. Angiographic diagnosis of retinal disease. Paris: Elsevier; 1998.

Maclean AL, Maumenee AE. Hemangioma of the choroids. Trans Am Ophthalmol Soc 1959; 57: 171–194.

Maumenee AE. Doyne memorial lecture. Fluorescein angiography in the diagnosis and treatment of lesions of the ocular fundus. Trans Ophthalmol Soc UK 1969; 88: 529–536.

Novotny HR, Alvis DL. A method of photographing fluorescence circulating blood in the human retina. Circulation 1961; 24: 82–86.

Richard G. Fluorescein and ICG angiography. New York: Thieme; 1998.

Schatz H, Burton C, Yannuzzi LA et al. Interpretation of fundus fluorescein angiography. St Louis: Mosby; 1978.

17

New imaging techniques

ANDREW MCNAUGHT

Introduction

Over recent years there have been significant developments in the techniques that are available to image the eye. In this chapter digital photographic imaging, particularly as it is applied to screening for eye disease, is described. The application of confocal microscopy techniques has allowed the optic nerve and macula to be analysed three-dimensionally with the retinal tomograph. Optical coherence tomography (OCT) provides a different means of three-dimensional analysis of the optic nerve, retina and, more recently, the anterior segment. The structure of the nerve fibre layer can also be analysed by observing its effect on polarised light, the principle underlying the nerve fibre analyser. These new techniques are beginning to play a role in clinical practice.

Digital fundus photography

Fundus photography is an indispensable component of modern ophthalmological practice worldwide. The capability to document and monitor the appearance of the retina and optic nerve head (ONH) allows the detection and recording of retinal features associated with diseases causing visual loss, e.g. diabetic retinopathy, age-related macular degeneration and glaucoma. It also allows the structural changes in response to treatment to be objectively recorded. Modifications to the basic fundus camera apparatus have also allowed developments, including fluorescein angiography and stereo-imaging.

The recent development of digital fundus cameras offers clear advantages in some applications over traditional 35 mm film photography. These advantages are evident in screening for diabetic retinopathy.

Screening for diabetic retinopathy using digital fundus photography

Diabetes affects approximately 3.5% of the UK population. Diabetic retinopathy is the leading cause of blindness in the working age group (Evans, 1990–1991). Screening for diabetic retinopathy has been shown to be effective in preventing visual impairment (Rohan et al., 1989; Singer et al., 1992; Ferris, 1993). If a photographic approach to screening is adopted, there are advantages in adopting digital fundus photography (Fig. 17.1):

- Digital images have been compared favourably to Polaroid photography (Ryder et al., 1989)

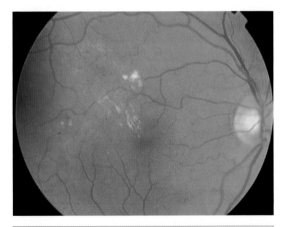

Fig. 17.1 Fundus image of a diabetic patient from Gloucestershire showing exudates close to the fovea. This patient was detected using portable digital fundus photography by a technician using a non-mydriatic camera undertaken at the patient's general practice premises. The patient was referred to the Cheltenham General Hospital where argon laser photocoagulation was undertaken. (Courtesy of Peter Scanlon, Director of the UK Diabetic Screening working party.)

- Instant image availability ensures that optimal images are captured at the time of the patient's visit. This also permits the patient to see the picture, helping with education, which may eventually encourage improved diabetic control
- The digital technique facilitates efficient storage and retrieval of images: this benefits all professionals involved in the patient's care – the ophthalmologist, diabetologist and ultimately, as images become available online, the patient's general practitioner.

There are practical advantages in the use of cameras designed for non-mydriatic photography for diabetic screening: the cameras allow useful images to be obtained in patients whose pupils are not able to be fully dilated (common in diabetics). They are also more portable than conventional cameras, which are optimised for fully dilated pupils (Scanlon, 2000).

Principle

All digital cameras utilise conventional fundus camera optics to capture an image of the retina on to a charge-coupled device (CCD) camera. The resolution, and hence the smallest feature that can be distinguished by any digital camera is determined by the number and size of the pixels in the CCD chip. There is debate as to whether the resolution of the captured image of presently available digital cameras is adequate to capture retinal features important in diabetic retinopathy, e.g. exudates, microaneurysms and neovascularisation.

The smallest features composing a retinal image may be assumed to be the individual photoreceptors – approximately 2 μm. Imaging through the ocular media limits the optical resolution of a healthy eye to 10 μm.

A 45° field covers approximately 15 mm diameter of retina, therefore a minimum of 1500 × 1500 pixels would be required to achieve the maximum resolution. Because the retinal image occupies just 75% of the horizontal resolution of the CCD, this suggests that an array of around 2000 × 2000 pixels would be required. This would result in an unacceptably large uncompressed file size of around 15 MB per image. Storing and transferring large numbers of such large files would be prohibitively expensive today.

Currently, compromise between resolution and image file size is required. UK guidelines (UK National Screening Committee) for diabetic screening digital fundus photography suggest a minimum resolution of 20 pixels per degree of retinal image. The recommended field of view is 45° horizontally, and 40° vertically. This translates to a field of approximately 900 pixels along its longest, horizontal, axis. In view of the circular images produced, a slightly larger imaging chip is required to accommodate the image: the existing 1360 × 1024 sensor does accommodate the image. This is the smallest imaging chip that satisfies the current standard (Scanlon, 2000).

The current UK guidelines do allow some image compression to ensure a manageable final image file size. Compression using the jpeg standard of up to 20-fold has been shown not to reduce the image quality for diabetic screening purposes. The final file size is between 1 and 2 MB. However, future technological developments in CCD size, cost, compression software and ease of storage and transport of larger files may allow practical use of higher-resolution imagers.

Other applications of digital fundus photography

The digital fundus camera is increasingly used for all of the applications previously undertaken using conventional 35 mm fundus photography. Imaging systems that allow digital fluorescein angiography with powerful image manipulation software are now commonly found in UK ophthalmology departments (e.g. Imagnet) (see Ch. 16). The decisive advantage is instant image review by the operator, ensuring a good-quality image at the initial visit. Patient education is also enhanced, as patients can view the image during the consultation.

Other applications include:

- Red-free fundus photography to enhance visualisation of the retinal nerve fibre layer (RNFL). This imaging technique, using 35 mm film, previously required specialist, time-consuming acquisition and printing techniques: the same, or superior results can now be achieved using image-processing techniques on a digital image (Fig. 17.2).
- Optic disc photography in glaucoma patients. The image is captured using the higher magnification afforded by the 20° field, and allows documentation and follow-up of

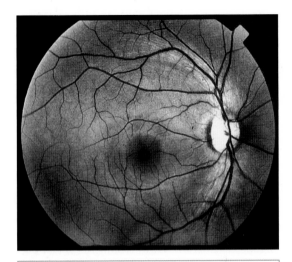

Fig. 17.2 Red-free image of a normal fundus showing the radiating fibres of the retinal nerve fibre layer. These axon bundles are thickest at the upper and lower poles of the optic nerve head. Wedge-shaped defects are highly suggestive of glaucoma; although when more diffuse loss occurs, it is more difficult to detect. The utility of red-free photography in individual glaucoma suspects is severely limited by the quality of the ocular media, whether the image is captured on to 35 mm film or a charge-coupled device.

glaucoma patients and suspects. There is undoubtedly an advantage to be had if a stereo-image of the ONH is captured (see below), but even monoscopic images are much more useful than drawings.

Stereo-imaging

Stereoscopic imaging is of particular importance in the diagnosis and monitoring of glaucomatous changes at the ONH. Use of stereoscopic ONH images in glaucoma is an accepted component of best clinical practice in guidelines produced by both the European Glaucoma Society and the American Academy of Ophthalmology (Abrams et al., 1994). Stereoscopic assessment of ONH changes is also a key clinical endpoint in a number of important glaucoma treatment trials, e.g. the Ocular Hypertension Treatment Study (OHTS).

Stereoscopic images of the ONH can be obtained using conventional 35 mm fundus photography by the sequential capture of two images taken at different angles (spatial shift) to generate stereopsis, and hence depth information. Alternatively, and optimally, the two images of the ONH can be captured simultaneously using a specialised fundus camera equipped with an Allen separator. This is a prism mounted on a motor-driven actuator which moves the image a fixed number of degrees between frames. Two separate images taken at different angles are captured sequentially. This produces the required spatial shift, though it reduces the field of view by positioning the two images in a single 35 mm frame. Subsequent analysis of the images, especially if digitised post hoc (even if not originally captured using a digital fundus camera), can be performed using increasingly sophisticated computer software. Images can even be displayed using modified visual display unit screens to allow simultaneous viewing by a panel of clinicians (Sheen et al., 2004).

Quantitative analysis of stereo-images of the ONH involves *planimetry*. Prior to digital image capture, or digitisation of 35 mm slides, planimetry involved the use of paired viewers/projectors and an operator who outlined the disc and cup margin manually. Planimetry of digital stereo-images now requires less cumbersome equipment as the whole process can be accomplished using the appropriate computer software. The operator still needs to outline the edge of the disc and the optic disc cup, and does need good stereo-acuity to exploit the images fully (Coleman et al., 1996).

Most currently available 35 mm (and digital) fundus cameras will allow sequential stereo-imaging of the ONH. Manually moving the camera head between the two component exposures means the stereo-base distance may not be constant: this limits the reproducibility of sequential stereo-pairs for quantitative measurements of depth. There is a simultaneous 35 mm stereo-camera made by Nidek (Fig. 17.3 was obtained with a Nidek camera). There is currently no digital simultaneous stereoscopic fundus available, but there is a sequential digital stereoscopic fundus camera, with custom software to allow quantitative analysis of the stereo-images (Discam, Marcher Enterprise, UK).

Documentation and monitoring of qualitative glaucomatous ONH changes, e.g. presence and progression of neuroretinal rim notching, haemorrhages and estimates of the cup-to-disc ratio can be made with conventional (and digital) mono fundus

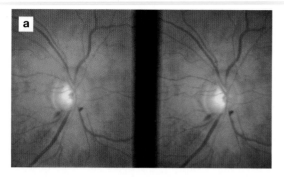

Fig. 17.3 (a) Stereoscopic image of glaucomatous optic nerve head obtained with a Nidek simultaneous stereoscopic fundus camera. Images was digitised post hoc using a slide-scanner. Note the haemorrhage at the inferior disc margin, notching of the neuroretinal rim at upper and lower poles, and a wedge-shaped retinal nerve fibre layer defect extending inferiorly from the site of the haemorrhage. (Courtesy of Prof. David Mackey, Glaucoma Inheritance Study in Tasmania.)

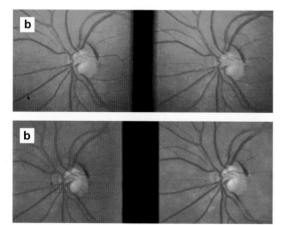

Fig. 17.3 (b) Stereoscopic images of the same optic nerve head (ONH) with an interval of 18 months between the upper and lower pairs (Nidek camera). Note the deepening and inferior extension of the notch at the lower pole of the ONH. These images demonstrate optic disc progression, and these changes were associated with progression of the associated superior arcuate visual field defect. The patient had previously declined a trabeculectomy for this eye. (Courtesy of Prof. David Mackey, Glaucoma Inheritance Study in Tasmania.)

cameras, and this approach is clearly superior to simple sketching of the ONH features in the patient's notes. However, the lack of stereopsis excludes any quantitative analysis of changes in depth, and so precludes planimetry.

Scanning laser ophthalmoscope

The scanning laser ophthalmoscope (SLO) is a confocal optical system designed to obtain three-dimensional images of the posterior segment of the eye. A laser beam is scanned across the fundus, and the reflected light at each point is quantified. The reflected light has to pass through a narrow aperture (the confocal pinhole) before reaching the CCD detector. The optical system is designed so that only light from a thin 'slice' of the total retinal thickness is allowed to reach the detector at any time: light from the 'slices' just in front and behind the target area is excluded. This technique ensures clear resolution of structures at a particular depth within the retina – in effect, an 'optical section' through the retina, analogous to the X-ray section through a body organ created during a computed tomography or magnetic resonance imaging scan.

The device allows continuous alteration of the scanning depth so that eventually a three-dimensional layered representation of the scanned retinal tissue is reconstructed. At each topographic location in the scan the reflected light intensity varies: it is assumed that the intensity variation is maximal at the structure surface. The completed scan is then subject to topographic analysis (Fig. 17.4).

The most widely available scanning laser tomograph (SLT) is the Heidelberg retinal tomograph II (HRTII, Fig. 17.5). This device has been developed for the diagnosis and monitoring of glaucomatous optic neuropathy, and retinal imaging, specifically macular disease. The following discussion relates to the HRTII unless stated.

Principle

The HRTII performs up to 64 separate optical sections at an interval of 1/16 mm. The spatial resolution of each optical slice is 384×384 pixels and the maximal image field width is $15 \times 15°$. The topography is inferred by measurement of the intensity of reflected light at each pixel in the image resulting from each optical slice. When imaging the ONH, three separate complete scans are performed

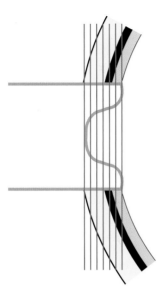

Fig. 17.4 The confocal principle. The microscope takes a picture at different planes; tissue above and below that plane is not imaged. Combining these planes allows a three-dimensional image of the structure to be constructed.

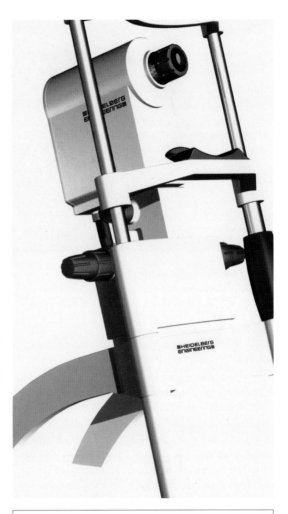

Fig. 17.5 Heidelberg retinal tomograph II. (Courtesy of Heidelberg Engineering.)

automatically. These three separate scans are used to determine the repeatability of the overall acquisition process, and to help determine the statistical significance of any changes in topography detected on follow-up examinations. The HRTII has been shown to produce highly reproducible measurements in human subjects (Sihota et al., 2002), and the topographic measurements of the ONH correlate with histological measurements in primate eyes (Yucel et al., 1998).

Importantly, the scanning method of image acquisition allows capture of adequate ONH topography through an undilated pupil (Fig. 17.6). Unlike conventional ONH fundus photography, the scanning method allows usable images to be obtained with the HRTII in the presence of moderate cataract. Furthermore, unlike conventional fundus photography, there is no bright 'flash': this is popular with patients as it allows for more comfortable imaging. Careful positioning of the patient's head, as well as relaxed accommodation, is important as these variables can affect the quality and reproducibility of the acquired images.

Interpretation

The HRTII incorporates software which analyses the result of the optical scans produced by confocal imaging. There is a significant research base underpinning the software.

To allow interpretation of the three-dimensional data obtained by the HRTII, the operator must first manually outline the outside edge of the optic disc. The optimal surface marking for this line is the scleral rim. This structure is, however, not always easily discerned. This somewhat subjective task

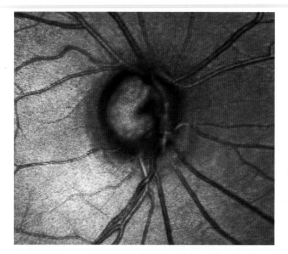

Fig. 17.6 Single optical 'slice' from Heidelberg retinal tomograph II topographic analysis. This image is at the level of the retinal nerve fibre layer and the typical striations representing axonal bundles are well seen.

may eventually be performed automatically by the software itself (Swindale et al., 2000).

A defined 'reference plane' in three-dimensional space within the ONH boundary (as drawn by the operator) must also be constructed. Structures anterior to this are defined 'neuroretinal rim' and posterior to this plane as 'cup' (Fig. 17.7).

There is ongoing research into the optimal software technique to provide a reference plane which maximises reproducibility, and is the most valid plane to document ONH progression accurately over time. The options currently within the HRTII software are as follows.

The 'standard' (default) reference plane

This imaginary plane is located 50 μm below the ONH boundary line, at the temporal disc edge, on the horizontal midline. This location corresponds to the centre of the papillomacular bundle of the RNFL. The rationale behind the selection of this site is that visual acuity is preserved until late in glaucoma, and therefore the papillomacular bundle, which serves the fovea, would be expected to have a stable height over time. Unfortunately, more recent research has shown thinning of the papillomacular bundle in progressive glaucoma in spite of preserved visual acuity (Chen et al., 2001). This reference plane may not therefore be ideal for quantifying glaucoma progression; the plane will decrease in height in line with the rest of the neuroretinal rim, and thus underestimate the true rate of neural loss.

Alternative reference plane: 320 μm reference plane

This plane is 320 μm posterior to a fixed ring centred on the ONH. This plane is at a greater eccentricity and is thus proportionately less affected by the loss of RNFL height with glaucoma progression. It is also associated with higher between-image reproducibility. Unfortunately, oblique insertion of the ONH as seen with tilted discs may produce artefactual underestimation of the cup size, and overestimation of the neuroretinal rim volume.

The HRTII software uses the chosen reference plane and operator-drawn ONH margin to allow automatic delineation of the optic cup margin, and then calculates a large number of ONH parameters. These include cup area, shape, volume and neuroretinal rim area and volume. The calculations are made for the whole disc and allow more detailed

Fig. 17.7 The colour map on the left produced by the Heidelberg retinal tomograph II shows the neuroretinal rim as blue and green and the cup as red. The operator has outlined the margin of the disc, shown on the right-hand picture by the green line.

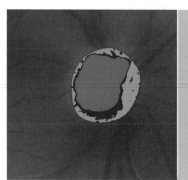
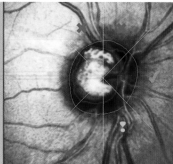

examination. The disc is also divided into six sectors and the parameters calculated for each sector.

The HRTII as a diagnostic tool

The accurate separation of a normal ONH from a glaucomatous one remains the holy grail of glaucoma imaging. Undertaking studies to examine the ability of a technique to do this requires the investigator to define, in advance, using clinical measures *other* than HRTII parameters, a group of 'glaucomatous' subjects, and a group of 'normals'. This itself poses problems. If a glaucomatous visual field defect is required to classify the subject as 'glaucoma' then, inevitably, the ONHs of these subjects will demonstrate more damage, and will require less exacting analysis to separate them from the 'normal' subjects. If, however, criteria such as the presence of a RNFL defect, or 'expert' panel assessment of ONH abnormality are used in the presence of an undamaged visual field, then separation of the 'glaucoma' group from the 'normal' group will be a greater challenge for the HRTII analysis.

The currently available diagnostic software supplied with the HRTII offers alternative parameters which are based on clinical research using different group definitions of 'glaucoma', as described below.

Discriminant function analysis

This is a statistical technique that attempts to predict membership of a glaucomatous, or normal, group by adopting one (or more) of the parameters provided by the HRTII, and combining these measures to optimise discrimination between groups. Several formulae combining neuroretinal rim volume (for the whole disc, or sectors of the rim), cup shape measure and cup area have been described. Perhaps the most successful was the formula devised by Lester et al. (2002), which principally uses sectorial differences in neuroretinal rim volume.

Moorfields regression analysis

This analysis uses a database of HRTII results from 112 normal subjects only. All subjects in the database are Caucasian and have refractive errors of < 6 D. The neuroretinal rim area was calculated for each normal eye, and then underwent a logarithmic transformation to normalise the distribution. The limits of normality from the distribution are derived from the prediction intervals of a regression analysis of log neuroretinal rim area against ONH area, and age. Prediction intervals representing 95%, 99% and 99.9% likelihood of normality are generated for the neuroretinal rim area as a whole, and for each of six pre-defined sectors around the ONH circumference.

Using this analysis, an ONH is classified as 'within normal limits' if the total and segmental area analysis are all in excess of the 95% prediction interval. ONHs with neuroretinal rim values globally, or at any sector, between the 95% and 99% intervals, are classified as 'borderline'. ONHs with neuroretinal rim values less than the 99.9% interval are labelled 'outside normal limits' (Woolstein et al., 1998). The HRTII software provides a graphical representation of the patient's sectorial and global neuroretinal rim results with the three prediction intervals shown on the chart (Fig. 17.8).

The Moorfields regression analysis has been evaluated in an independent group of 48 normal and 104 eyes with early glaucoma. In all, 81% of the normal eyes were classified as 'within normal limits' but 19% were designated 'borderline' or 'outside normal limits'. In the glaucoma group, 78% were classified as either 'outside normal limits' or 'borderline', but 22% were described as normal by the software (Ford et al., 2003).

Whilst the Moorfields regression analysis is the most widely used analysis within the HRTII software, and the classification is clinically very useful, there are glaucomatous discs that are misclassified as 'normal' and normal discs wrongly designated as glaucomatous. The software does often misclassify either very large and/or tilted ONHs (Fig. 17.9), and this may reflect the relatively small database, with correspondingly small numbers of anomalous but otherwise non-glaucomatous discs.

Indications

1. Documentation of the ONH in glaucoma: the HRTII is an ideal means of documenting the ONH in new glaucoma patients, and providing a baseline for subsequent detection of ONH progression. However, because of the current relative shortcomings of the current HRTII analysis software, the gold standard *diagnostic* test for signs of glaucomatous optic neuropathy remains biomicrosopy performed by the experienced clinician

2. Detection of glaucoma progression: recent research has demonstrated the ability of

Fig. 17.8 Moorfields regression analysis of glaucomatous optic disc with inferior neuroretinal rim thinning. The segmental analysis has highlighted the thinned sectors accurately (red crosses) and indicated those healthier superior sectors (green ticks). The graphical representation shows the prediction intervals for normality as well as the subject's measurements for both disc and rim area.

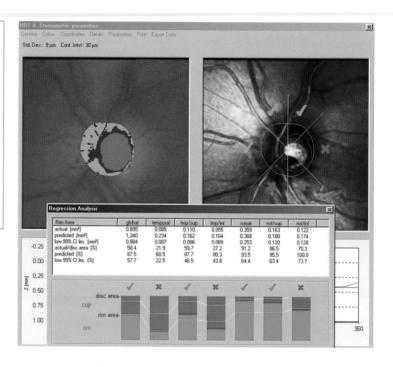

Fig. 17.9 Tilted and glaucomatous disc classified as 'within normal limits' by the Moorfields regression analysis.

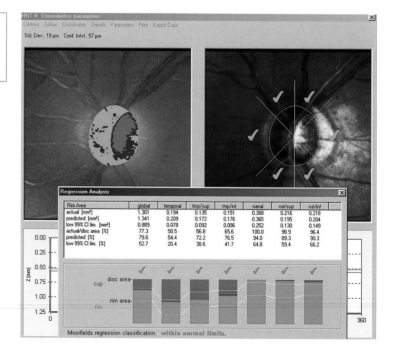

sequential HRTII images to detect and quantify glaucomatous optic disc changes. There is evidence that the HRTII may detect progressive disease at an earlier stage than visual field analysis. Kamal et al. (2000) quantified the inter-test variability inherent in sequential measurement of normal eyes and derived

parameters for significant deterioration above the 'background' variability. Other approaches have been described, and the later versions of the HRTII software do allow for analysis of sequential images (Fig. 17.10). The criterion for clinically significant change is the subject of further research

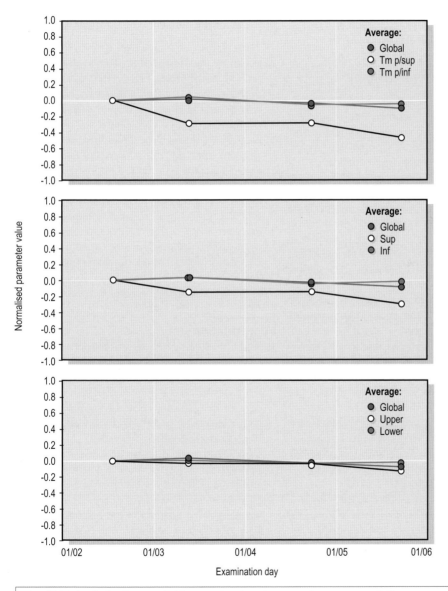

Fig. 17.10 Analysis of sequential images showing change and an average of all parameters with time. The global rim area is represented by the red line. Different sectors of the optic nerve head can also be displayed and are represented by the other lines.

3. A more recent application of the essentially unmodified HRTII is in the imaging of the macula. The HRT II 'macula module' software is designed to detect elevations, and increases in retinal thickness secondary to conditions including macular oedema, macular holes and age-related macular degeneration. This application of the HRTII is currently undergoing evaluation as a possible modality for secondary screening of diabetic patients for sight-threatening diabetic macular oedema.

Optical coherence tomography

Principles

OCT is a means of obtaining high-resolution cross-sectional images through the thickness of the retina. The image is produced through the use of a low-coherence light source and application of interferometry to the reflected light from the retina (see Ch. 13).

Essentially the imaging beam is split in two. One beam is projected on to the retina, the other to a reference mirror that moves back and forth. It is the interference between the two reflected light beams, one from the retinal tissue under scrutiny, the other from the reference mirror, which has made excursions of known magnitude. If the light pulses from the retina and reference mirror reach the interferometer simultaneously, a signal is detected due to constructive interference. These signals, corresponding with optical interfaces within the retina, are reconstructed into the A-scan, corresponding with a scan of the retina at one point (analogous to A-scan ultrasound). As the process is repeated at neighbouring points, a B-scan is constructed as the scanning process continues along a short line across the retinal surface. Recent development of a 'white' laser of very low coherence has allowed 'ultra-high'-resolution OCT (Drexler, 2001).

The signal intensity depends on the optical characteristics of tissues scanned: these differences often correspond to different histological layers within the retina. The final OCT image is generated by a logarithmic plot of the signal intensities and is presented as a colour-coded scale (Fig. 17.11).

Performance

The depth resolution of the most widely available commercial OCT (Stratus, Carl Zeiss Meditec, Dublin, CA, USA) is quoted at < 10 µm. The A-scans are acquired at a rate of 400 per second. Various options for the resolution of the B-scans are available in the software: 128, 256 and 512 A-scans to each B-scan. There is clearly a trade-off in terms of resolution if the faster B-scan acquisitions are chosen. The highest lateral resolution is approximately 20 µm.

Various patterns of B-scan are available in the software for the different retinal regions of interest:

1. A circular scan for the ONH RNFL: 'RNFL thickness' and 'fast RNFL' (diameter 3.4 mm, centred on the ONH). This generates a plot of the peripapillary RNFL thickness, which is important in glaucoma diagnosis and monitoring (Fig. 17.12; Leung et al., 2004)
2. Radial lines through the ONH 'optic disc' and 'fast optic disc': this consists of 6–24 slices through a common central point on the ONH. The 'fast' option scans only six lines at the lowest lateral resolution (Fig. 17.13)
3. Macular 'radial lines' are used to measure macular thickness (Fig. 17.11). Options include 6–24 scans of adjustable length at adjustable lateral resolution through the central macula. The 'fast macular thickness map' comprises six 6 mm radial line scans, and is completed within 2 s.

Interpretation

1. RNFL thickness: these measurements around the ONH are compared with an age-matched database of normal eyes (Fig. 17.12). Early research work has suggested discrimination between normal subjects and glaucoma patients with a sensitivity of 89% and specificity of 92% (Budenz et al., 2005)
2. OCT ONH 'optic disc' has also been shown to demonstrate useful discrimination between normal and glaucomatous eyes (Schuman et al., 2003)
3. Qualitative examination of images from the macular 'radial lines' scans has demonstrated clear visualisation of macular holes, macular oedema and lesions associated with age-related macular degeneration (Fig. 17.14). These retinal images provide clinical information which is not obtainable from alternative methods of retinal imaging; therefore the OCT does seem destined to become increasingly important in the management of retinal disease (Box 17.1).

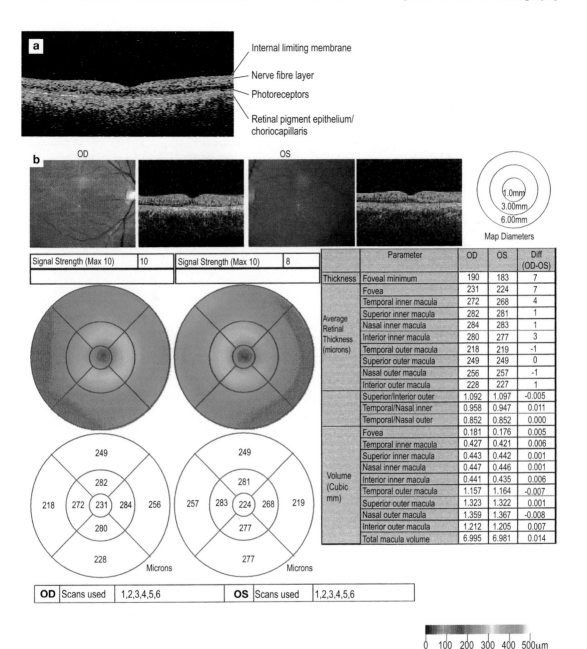

Internal limiting membrane

Nerve fibre layer

Photoreceptors

Retinal pigment epithelium/
choriocapillaris

Parameter		OD	OS	Diff (OD-OS)
Thickness	Foveal minimum	190	183	7
Average Retinal Thickness (microns)	Fovea	231	224	7
	Temporal inner macula	272	268	4
	Superior inner macula	282	281	1
	Nasal inner macula	284	283	1
	Interior inner macula	280	277	3
	Temporal outer macula	218	219	-1
	Superior outer macula	249	249	0
	Nasal outer macula	256	257	-1
	Interior outer macula	228	227	1
	Superior/Interior outer	1.092	1.097	-0.005
	Temporal/Nasal inner	0.958	0.947	0.011
	Temporal/Nasal outer	0.852	0.852	0.000
Volume (Cubic mm)	Fovea	0.181	0.176	0.005
	Temporal inner macula	0.427	0.421	0.006
	Superior inner macula	0.443	0.442	0.001
	Nasal inner macula	0.447	0.446	0.001
	Interior inner macula	0.441	0.435	0.006
	Temporal outer macula	1.157	1.164	-0.007
	Superior outer macula	1.323	1.322	0.001
	Nasal outer macula	1.359	1.367	-0.008
	Interior outer macula	1.212	1.205	0.007
	Total macula volume	6.995	6.981	0.014

Signal Strength (Max 10) 10   Signal Strength (Max 10) 8

OD   Scans used   1,2,3,4,5,6   OS   Scans used   1,2,3,4,5,6

0 100 200 300 400 500μm

Fig. 17.11 (a) An optical coherence tomography (OCT) scan through the macula. This has been annotated to show the different layers of the retina, represented by different colours on the scan. **(b)** A typical retinal thickness report. A picture of the area scanned and an OCT image are shown above. The circular plots below show the thickness contour maps centred on the fovea.

a

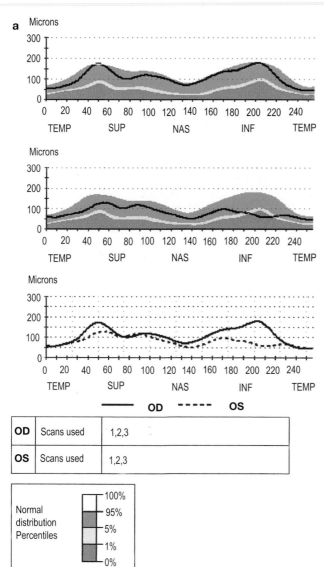

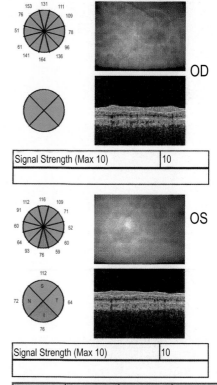

	OD (N=3)	OS (N=3)	OD-OS
Imax/Smax	1.04	0.76	0.27
Smax/Imax	0.96	1.31	-0.35
Smax/Tavg	2.75	2.11	0.64
Imax/Tavg	2.86	1.61	1.24
Smax/Navg	1.82	1.79	0.03
Max-Min	134.00	83.00	51.00
Smax	172.00	128.00	44.00
Imax	179.00	98.00	81.00
Savg	132.00	112.00	20.00
Iavg	147.00	76.00	71.00
Avg. Thick	108.84	80.29	28.56

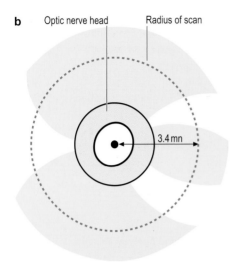

b

Optic nerve head   Radius of scan

3.4 mn

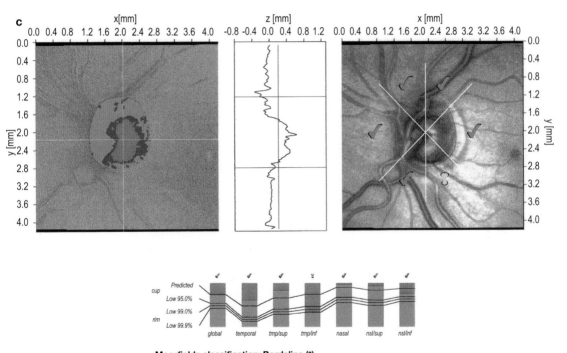

c

x[mm]
0.0 0.4 0.8 1.2 1.6 2.0 2.4 2.8 3.2 3.6 4.0

z [mm]
-0.8 -0.4 0.0 0.4 0.8 1.2

x [mm]
0.0 0.4 0.8 1.2 1.6 2.0 2.4 2.8 3.2 3.2 3.6 4.0

y [mm]
0.0
0.4
0.8
1.2
1.6
2.0
2.4
2.8
3.2
3.6
4.0

y [mm]
0.0
0.4
0.8
1.2
1.6
2.0
2.4
2.8
3.2
3.6
4.0

cup
rim

Predicted
Low 95.0%
Low 99.0%
Low 99.9%

global temporal tmp/sup tmp/inf nasal nsl/sup nsl/inf

Moorfields classification: Bordeline (*)

(*) Moorfields regression classification (Opthalmology 1998;105:1557-1563). Classification
based on statistics. Diagnosis is physician's reponsibility.

Fig. 17.12 (a) The optic nerve head retinal nerve fibre layer (RNFL) thickness scan. **(b)** The scan is produced
by scanning a circle around the optic nerve. This is then 'unwound' to produce the linear picture shown in
Figure 17.12a. The RNFL thickness is compared to a normative database and the statistical chance of the
nerve fibre thickness being normal is displayed graphically, on the left-hand side. In this case the RNFL is
abnormally thin inferiorly in the left eye. The black line on the graph indicates the patient's RNFL thickness.
Inferiorly in the left eye it dips into the red band. Fewer than 1% of normal subjects would have an RNFL
thickness as thin as this. **(c)** Note that the RNFL thickness scan corresponds with the Heidelberg retinal
tomograph II image, showing a reduced neuroretinal rim area inferiorly in the left eye.

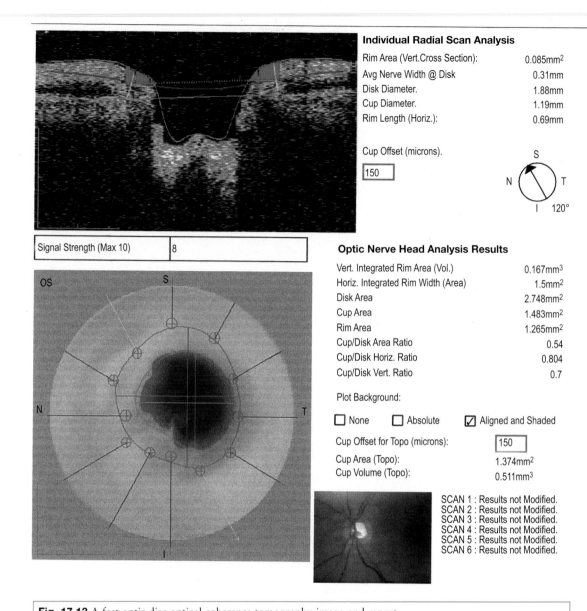

Individual Radial Scan Analysis

Rim Area (Vert.Cross Section):	0.085mm^2
Avg Nerve Width @ Disk	0.31mm
Disk Diameter.	1.88mm
Cup Diameter.	1.19mm
Rim Length (Horiz.):	0.69mm
Cup Offset (microns).	

150

Signal Strength (Max 10) | 8

OS   S   N   T   I

Optic Nerve Head Analysis Results

Vert. Integrated Rim Area (Vol.)	0.167mm^3
Horiz. Integrated Rim Width (Area)	1.5mm^2
Disk Area	2.748mm^2
Cup Area	1.483mm^2
Rim Area	1.265mm^2
Cup/Disk Area Ratio	0.54
Cup/Disk Horiz. Ratio	0.804
Cup/Disk Vert. Ratio	0.7

Plot Background:

☐ None   ☐ Absolute   ☑ Aligned and Shaded

Cup Offset for Topo (microns):   150

Cup Area (Topo):	1.374mm^2
Cup Volume (Topo):	0.511mm^3

SCAN 1 : Results not Modified.
SCAN 2 : Results not Modified.
SCAN 3 : Results not Modified.
SCAN 4 : Results not Modified.
SCAN 5 : Results not Modified.
SCAN 6 : Results not Modified.

Fig. 17.13 A fast optic disc optical coherence tomography image and report.

In common with all imaging modalities, the quality of OCT images is dependent on the clarity of the ocular media. Current technology allows lateral scanning (with a trade-off between speed and resolution) through the retinal thickness, but clearly there are situations where a larger area of retina could usefully be imaged. En-face OCT techniques are under development, which, combined with lateral scans, will allow three-dimensional reconstructions of large 'blocks' of retinal thickness. This development will allow more clinically interpretable representations of the retina in depth.

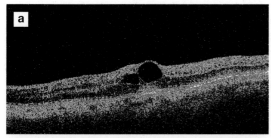

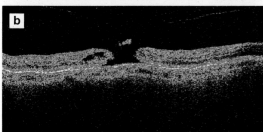

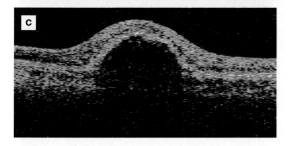

Fig. 17.14 (a) The appearance of macular oedema on an optical coherence tomography (OCT) scan. **(b)** An OCT scan of a macular hole. **(c)** The OCT appearance of a pigment epithelial detachment.

Nerve fibre analyser

(GDx and GDx VCC, Carl Zeiss Meditec, Dublin, CA, USA)

The RNFL is thought to exhibit birefringence because of parallel cylindrical structures within the axons (Weinreb et al., 1990). This property forms the basis of the measurement of RNFL thickness by the GDx, and the recently modified version, the GDx VCC.

The essential imaging device is a scanning laser polarimeter using a near-infrared laser (780 nm). The scan raster covers an image field of 40° horizontally and 20° vertically. This field encompasses the ONH, peripapillary RNFL and the macula. The retina is illuminated with linearly polarised light that undergoes birefringence as it passes through the cornea, lens and, importantly, the nerve fibre layer. Reflected rays, polarised so that they are travelling perpendicular to the ONH fibres, travel at a different speed from those that are parallel to the fibres. The degree of polarisation in the reflected light is quantified using two analysers to measure light polarised parallel and perpendicular to the illuminating laser. The difference in velocity between these two differently polarised beams is termed retardation. It provides a measure of RNFL thickness: the greater the retardation, the thicker the nerve fibre layer.

Principle

The retardation image (Fig. 17.15), which allows estimation of the RNFL thickness, is produced by calculations involving the relative signal detected by the two analysers. A confounding factor is anterior-segment birefringence, mainly produced by the cornea, which will obviously confuse the results. In the first machines this was compensated for in a uniform fashion but this did not work for all patients. The GDx VCC employs a variable corneal compensator to neutralise this birefringence. Essen-

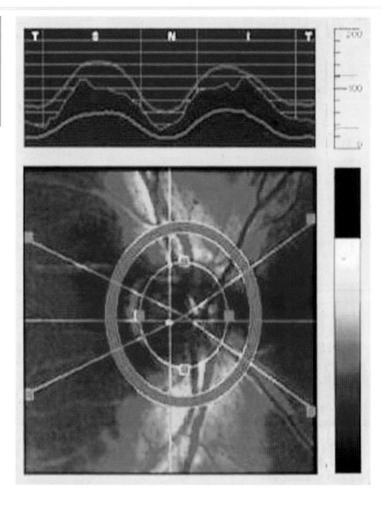

Fig. 17.15 GDx image from a normal eye with a normal retinal nerve fibre layer (RNFL) thickness map. The image shows a healthy 'double hump' of thickest RNFL at the upper and lower peripapillary regions.

tially it measures the change in polarisation from the macular region, where there are no nerve fibres, to calculate the birefringence of the cornea. During imaging the compensator is adjusted to abolish the bright 'bowtie' macular reflectance, which is characteristic of anterior-segment artefact.

Interpretation

The GDx and the GDx VCC express the overall result of the retinal scan using the nerve fibre index (NFI). This is a single statistic, which is the output of the 'support vector machine' which uses data from hundreds of scans of normal and glaucomatous eyes. Values range from 0 (unequivocally normal) to 100 (advanced glaucoma). NFI has been shown

to be the best single parameter for distinguishing between normal and glaucomatous eyes. Research has shown that glaucoma-affected eyes rarely have an NFI of < 35, and normal eyes rarely have an NFI of > 44. Clearly, there will be a group of eyes with intermediate values between 35 and 44 which are not classified by the device. The likelihood of glaucoma in these eyes may be indicated by analysis of other output parameters, though undoubtedly, the original GDx failed to discriminate normals from glaucoma eyes in a significant proportion of cases. The more recently described GDx VCC is subject to investigation. Early indications suggest a more clinically useful imaging device (Reus and Lemij, 2004).

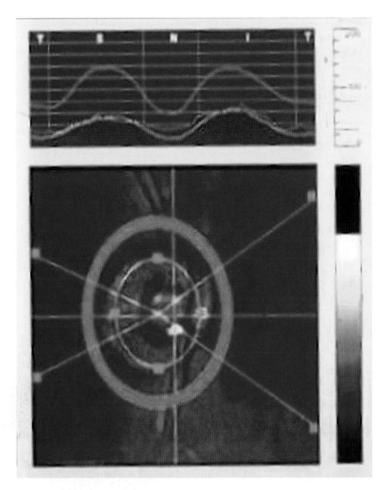

Fig. 17.16 GDx image from a glaucomatous eye showing global reduction in peripapillary retinal nerve fibre layer (RNFL) thickness. There is relative loss of the characteristic RNFL thickness relationships at the upper and lower poles of the optic nerve head.

The original GDx device was sensitive to artefactual birefringence produced by anterior-segment structures, especially the cornea. Severely affected GDx scans did not allow accurate discrimination between healthy and glaucomatous eyes. The GDx VCC may have overcome this difficulty, but further research is required. As with the HRT, software to look for progressive change in the RNFL is incorporated into the technology.

Indications

The original GDx is not recommended as a reliable discriminator in the early diagnosis of glaucoma. The GDx VCC may be more accurate, and may eventually have an important role in the early diagnosis of glaucoma eyes prior to the development of gross ONH damage and/or visual field defects (Fig. 17.16).

- Advantages of digital fundus photography include:
  - Instant image review, ensuring good-quality images at the initial visit
  - Better patient education, as patients can view the images as well
  - Instant recall of images from databases in different locations
- The Heidelberg retinal tomograph scanner is not only useful for optic disc analysis but also has new applications in analysing macular pathology
- The optical coherence tomography scanner can be used to monitor:
  - Postoperative cystoid macular oedema
  - Macular holes pre- and postoperatively
  - Optic disc anatomy
  - Retinal nerve fibre layer changes in glaucoma

References

Abrams L, Scott I, Spaeth G et al. Agreement among optometrists, ophthalmologists and residents in evaluating the optic disc for glaucoma. Ophthalmology 1994; 101: 1662–1667.

Budenz D, Michael A, Chang R et al. Sensitivity and specificity of the STRATUSoct for perimetric glaucoma. Ophthalmology 2005; 112: 3–9.

Chen E, Gedda U, Landau I. Thinning of the papillomaular bundle in the glaucomatous eye and its influence on the reference plane of Heidelberg retinal tomography. J Glaucoma 2001; 10: 386–389.

Coleman A, Sommer A, Enger C et al. Interobserver and intraobserver variability in the detection of glaucomatous progression of the optic disc. J Glaucoma 1996; 5; 384–389.

Drexler W, Morgner U, Ghanta R et al. Ultra-high resolution ophthalmologic optical coherence tomography. Nature Med 2001; 7: 502–507.

Evans J. Causes of blindness and partial sight in England and Wales. London: HMSO; 1990–1991.

Ferris L. How effective are treatments for diabetic retinopathy? JAMA 1993; 269: 1290–1291.

Ford B, Artes P, McCormick T et al. Comparison of data analysis tools for detection of glaucoma with the Heidelberg retina tomograph. Ophthalmology 2003; 110: 1145–1150.

Kamal D, Garway-Heath D, Hitchings R. Use of sequential Heidelberg retina tomograph images to identify changes at the optic disc in ocular hypertensive patients at risk of developing glaucoma. Br J Ophthalmol 2000; 84: 993–998.

Lester M, Mardin C, Budde W et al. Discriminant analysis formulas of optic nerve head parameters measured by confocal scanning laser tomography. J Glaucoma 2002; 11: 97–104.

Leung C, Yung W, Ng A et al. Evaluation of scanning resolution on retinal nerve fibre layer measurement using optical coherence tomography in normal and glaucomatous eyes. J Glaucoma 2004; 112: 3–9.

Reus N, Lemij H. Diagnostic accuracy of the GDx VCC for glaucoma. Ophthalmology 2004; 111: 1860–1865.

Rohan TE, Frost CD, Wald NJ. Prevention of blindness by screening for diabetic retinopathy: a quantitative assessment. BMJ 1989; 299: 1198–1201.

Ryder R, Kong N, Bates A et al. Instant electronic imaging systems are superior to Polaroid at detecting sight threatening diabetic retinopathy. Diabetic Med 1996; 15: 254–258.

Scanlon P. Screening for diabetic retinopathy by digital imaging photography and technician ophthalmoscopy. Diabetes Technol Ther 2000; 2: 283–287.

Schuman J, Wollstein G, Farra T et al. Comparison of optic nerve head measurements obtained by optical coherence tomography and confocal scanning ophthalmoscopy. Am J Ophthalmol 2003; 135: 504–512.

Sheen NJL, Morgan JE, Poulsen J et al. Digital stereoscopic analysis of the optic disc: evaluation of a teaching module. Ophthalmology 2004; 111: 1873–1879.

Sihota R, Gulati V, Agarwal H et al. Variables affecting test–retest variability of Heidelberg retina tomograph II stereometric parameters. J Glaucoma 2002; 11: 321–328.

Singer DE, Nathan DM, Fogael HA, Schachat AP. Screening for diabetic retinopathy. Ann Intern Med 1992; 124: 164–169.

Swindale N, Sjepanovic G, Chin A et al. Automated analysis of normal and glaucomatous optic nerve head topography images. Invest Ophthalmol Vis Sci 2000; 41: 1730–1742.

Tan J, Hitchings R. Approach for identifying glaucomatous optic nerve progression by scanning laser tomography. Invest Ophthalmol Vis Sci 2003; 44: 2621–2626.

Weinreb R, Dreher A, Coleman A et al. Histopathologic validation of Fourier-ellipsometry measurements of retinal nerve fibre layer thickness. Arch Ophthalmol 1990; 108: 557–560.

Woolstein G, Garway-Heath D, Hitchings R. Identification of early glaucoma cases with the scanning laser ophthalmoloscope. Ophthalmology 1998; 105: 1557–1563.

Yucel Y, Gupta N, Kalichman M et al. Relationship of optic disc topography to optic nerve fiber number in glaucoma. Arch Ophthalmol 1998; 116: 493–497.

Index